W9-DFE-176

Endovascular Skills

Endovascular Skills

Guidewire and Catheter Skills for Endovascular Surgery

Third Edition

PETER A. SCHNEIDER

Division of Vascular Therapy
Kaiser Foundation Hospital
Honolulu, Hawaii, USA

informa
healthcare

New York London

Informa Healthcare USA, Inc.
52 Vanderbilt Avenue
New York, NY 10017

© 2009 by Informa Healthcare USA, Inc.
Informa Healthcare is an Informa business

International Standard Book Number-10: 1-4200-6937-3 (Hardcover)
International Standard Book Number-13: 978-1-4200-6937-2 (Hardcover)

Library of Congress Cataloging-in-Publication Data

Schneider, Peter A.
Endovascular skills : guidewire and catheter skills for endovascular surgery / by Peter Schneider. – 3rd ed.
    p. ; cm.
  Includes bibliographical references and index.
  ISBN-13: 978-1-4200-6937-2 (hb : alk. paper)
  ISBN-10: 1-4200-6937-3 (hb : alk. paper)
  1. Blood-vessels–Endoscopic surgery. 2. Blood-vessels–Interventional radiology.
  3. Peripheral vascular diseases–Endoscopic surgery. I. Title.
  [DNLM: 1. Vascular Surgical Procedures–methods. 2. Angiography–methods.
  3. Catheterization–methods. 4. Endoscopy–methods. 5. Stents. WG 170 S359e
  2008]

RD598.5.S36 2008
617.4′130597 – dc22
                                       2008042737

For Corporate Sales and Reprint Permission call 212-520-2700 or write to: Sales Department, 52 Vanderbilt Avenue, 7th floor, New York, Ny 1017.

Visit the Informa Web site at
www.informa.com

and the Informa Healthcare Web site at
www.informahealthcare.com

Foreword

This third edition of Dr. Schneider's text does an excellent job of providing a comprehensive and carefully updated book addressing the goals expressed in the title, *Endovascular Skills: Guidewire and Catheter Skills for Endovascular Surgery*. It is straightforward and easy to read and takes a step-by-step approach. The book not only provides a review of basic catheter and guidewire skills for those entering the endovascular arena, it thoroughly updates new endovascular techniques and devices for those experienced in endovascular therapy.

In this third edition, Dr. Schneider captures the progress that has been made in recent years and incorporates the expanding knowledge base in a detailed discussion of instruments, technical capabilities, and a developing range of therapeutic applications. There are new chapters that provide a thorough discussion of .014 wire and monorail technologies for treating tibial, visceral, renal and carotid lesions. There is also extensive discussions of techniques for treating occlusive lesions in the iliac, SFA, and subclavian arteries. There is also a comprehensive section on evolving technologies including lasers, cryotherapy, reentry devices, etc. that may offer advances following further investigation.

In the chapters relating to stent and endovascular device applications to vascular beds where the technologies are not FDA approved for these applications, Dr. Schneider appropriately comments on the current status of techniques while recognizing that these remain "off-label" applications for individual use in patients for whom no alternative treatment is available. As is needed in discussing an evolving technology, there is a careful balance between describing the state of the art and evolution while providing disclaimers regarding currently approved utilization. Throughout the text, Dr. Schneider does an excellent job of addressing these issues while describing the fundamental knowledge required to adopt the methods.

As a single-author text written by a vascular surgeon experienced in endovascular methods, there is a continuity of thought and conceptual approach to patients with vascular disease that emphasizes the selection of the best method of treatment for an individual patient. From this perspective Dr. Schneider provides a practical approach to individual lesions, with the option for treatment ultimately being determined by the potential success of the endovascular procedure contrasted with that of a conventional open repair.

The text is well illustrated. It addresses issues regarding the performance of endovascular procedures in an operating room versus an interventional suite, a topic of particular interest to physicians and centers initiating endovascular programs. It also contains a section that provides additional information regarding manufacturers of instrumentation and imaging modalities. The book focuses on techniques, basic instrumentation, balloons, and stents rather than on the use and indications for endovascular prostheses or similar endovascular technologies. From this perspective, it is a valuable source of information for any interventionalist or vascular specialist who is training for or has a practice focused on the use of endovascular techniques.

I strongly recommend this book for individuals and institutions providing endovascular care and congratulate Dr. Schneider for producing a high-quality text that addresses the fundamental issues important to training and continued evolution in endovascular therapy.

Rodney A. White, M.D.
Chief of Vascular Surgery
Harbor-UCLA Medical Center
Torrance, California, U.S.A.

Preface to the Third Edition

Endovascular Skills is meant to provide a "step-by-step" approach to techniques and procedures that comprise one of the most exciting and rapidly developing specialties in medicine today: minimally invasive management of vascular disease. Endovascular technique has gone from a novelty to a mainstay of vascular care and the Third Edition of *Endovascular Skills* has been revised and expanded to reflect these changes. This book serves as a "how-to" guide for endovascular intervention and aims to assist clinicians in the development and refinement of skills that are now essential to modern vascular practice.

Since *Endovascular Skills* was first compiled in the mid-1990's, endovascular intervention has gone through a tremendous phase of development. Significant advances have been made in re-opening and re-lining vessels in every vascular bed. More extensive patterns of vascular disease are being treated, many of which would have required open surgery in the past. The endovascular approach has become more broadly accepted by patients, medical professionals, scientists, engineers, and the public at large. The technical skills and the device innovations that make endovascular practice possible have advanced and developed over the past few years, providing new treatment options that are safer and better tolerated. These skills and devices will likely continue development for the foreseeable future. Simultaneous growth in the public health challenge of an enlarging patient population at risk for vascular disease will likely prompt wider adoption and new applications.

The skills to perform endovascular techniques are based on several principles that are outlined in *Endovascular Skills*. The book begins with strategy, vascular access, guidewire–catheter handling, and arteriography in a multitude of vascular beds (Part I). The knowledge base builds as the text progresses in much the same manner that the skill of the professional builds as experience is gained by performing more complex cases and managing complicated patterns of disease. Part II of the book is devoted to endovascular therapy, including; sheath access, balloon angioplasty, stents, and other treatment modalities. These sections are the same as previous editions in concept but they have been thoroughly revised to incorporate the most contemporary practices. In the same manner that endovascular has matured as a field, an entirely new major section has been added to the Third Edition which covers Advanced Endovascular Skills. Part III focuses on more recently developed imaging and endovascular treatment techniques, including; use of 0.014 guidewires and monorail platforms for noncoronary arteries, cryoplasty, atherectomy, stent-grafting, subintimal angioplasty, carotid bifurcation stenting, and many others.

The possession of endovascular skills by clinicians dedicated to the management of vascular disease is one of the keys to advancing patient care in this area. The Third Edition of *Endovascular Skills* is meant to assist in that challenging and rewarding endeavor.

New illustrations and updated drawings by Meadow Green.

Contents

19.   The Infrarenal Aorta, Aortic Bifurcation, and Iliac Arteries: Advice About Balloon Angioplasty and Stent Placement   317

20.   The Infrainguinal Arteries: Advice About Balloon Angioplasty and Stent Placement   341

21.   Advice About Endovascular Salvage of Previous Reconstructions   351

Part I

Basic Endovascular Skills

1

Endovascular Concepts

Endovascular Skills in Practice

Endovascular skills are an integral part of vascular patient care and will continue to be for the foreseeable future. As the scope of catheter-based treatment broadens, the ability to manage more complex lesions with these techniques will continue to increase, and hopefully drive better overall results of care. The development of guidewire–catheter skills is not an easily definable goal, but is a dynamic process. As the array of possibilities in the endovascular field has blossomed, the necessary skills included under the heading of *guidewire–catheter skills* have likewise increased substantially. On the basic level, guidewires and catheters are the universal instruments of success in endovascular work. A more advanced approach includes an amazing and expanding myriad of devices passed over the guidewire to help manage vascular disease.

Knowledge and facility must be achieved in several areas that are not necessarily intuitive, including coordinating *fluoroscopic–eye–hand movements*, predicting guidewire–lesion interactions, understanding the behavior of various guidewire and catheter combinations, and learning the limits of each technique (knowing when to quit). These are the basic *endovascular skills*. Part I of this book provides an overview of basic endovascular skills. Part II presents techniques in endovascular therapy that build upon the basic skills, such as guiding sheath access, balloon angioplasty, stenting, and how to use these techniques in various vascular beds. Part III covers advanced endovascular techniques and devices in an effort to assist the reader in becoming familiar with more recently available, and rapidly evolving, technology.

Reinvention of Vascular Care

Endovascular concepts are reshaping treatment. The potential for simple, low-morbidity solutions to complex clinical problems is a common goal among vascular specialists. Near-term progress in reconstructive capability is likely to result from advances in endoluminal technique. Guidewires and catheters form the technical and conceptual basis of endovascular intervention and technology, while device and skill development are taking the field to the next level. Endovascular procedures have dramatically changed the spectrum of vascular practice. Iliac angioplasty and stenting have almost completely replaced aortofemoral bypass. Stent–graft repair of abdominal aortic aneurysms have dramatically altered the management paradigm for aneurysm disease. It is not yet clear what the role of carotid stenting will be, but this will play an important role in treating carotid occlusive disease, both how it is assessed and how it is managed. Although some endovascular procedures are not currently durable enough to offer long-term solutions, such as many of the infrainguinal treatment options, they may still be adequate for patients with multiple comorbidities or limited life expectancy. These techniques also hold hope for becoming more clinically useful as they are refined.

Endovascular techniques were initially complementary to open vascular surgical techniques in terms of the spectrum of disease that could be treated. Endovascular options were available for those with less severe vascular pathology. In addition, there were many patients treated who had severe medical comorbid conditions and otherwise would not have been possible to treat. Now endovascular intervention appears to be a reasonable alternative to open surgery in most patients with open operations reserved for endovascular failures and complications.

Our focus is on making vascular treatment safer and more durable, whether it involves medical, endovascular procedures, open surgical procedures, or a combination of these. Lack of familiarity with a variety of approaches encourages advocates of a specific technique to crusade for the exclusive application of that technique, regardless of whether it includes medical, endoluminal, or operative technology. Our focus is on reducing disability, disease, and death by providing full spectrum vascular care and doing so without bias.

Qualifications

How many times do you need to do a procedure before you know how to do it? Should that number differ for someone who already spent years learning every other aspect of a disease process and its management? How many Whipple procedures or esophagectomies or pelvic exenterations does the average surgeon perform prior to performing the first one in practice? How about something really complicated and challenging like open suprarenal aneurysms? Reason suggests that the more procedures have been performed in training, the better the results ought to be. How do we balance the need to provide safe patient care (by having well-trained specialists) with the need to have reasonable requirements for workforce training (so that a decent size workforce is available)? The answers to these questions are being developed by diverse institutions with differing points of view. Not everyone is going to be happy with the answers and they will be somewhat arbitrary. The issue becomes more complicated by two factors. The technology and techniques are evolving and becoming more sophisticated, and therefore require more time and effort to learn to the level of state-of-the-art. The other factor is that many of the specialists practicing vascular interventions are also practicing cardiology or radiology or other things that are unrelated or distantly related to vascular. How do you get good results as a part-timer? How will certification be maintained? How will the field advance? Clearly, we still have work to do in each area.

Table 1 Case Requirements to Perform Endovascular Interventions

	SIR	SCAI	ACC	AHA	SVS
Angiograms	200	100/50[a]	100	100	100/50[a]
Interventions	25	50/25[a]	50/25[a]	50/25[a]	50/25[a]

[a] As primary interventionist.
Abbreviations: SIR, Society of Interventional Radiology; SCAI, Society for Cardiac Angiography and Interventions; ACC, American College of Cardiology; AHA, American Heart Association; SVS, Society for Vascular Surgery.

Each society has its own recommendations for how many endovascular cases it takes to become qualified to perform endovascular procedures (Table 1).

Carotid stents have been separated from the listed requirements. There are varying recommendations from different societies on how many carotid arteriograms and how many carotid stents must be performed to claim proficiency. The number accepted by the Society for Vascular Surgery and the American heart Association is 30 carotid arteriograms and 25 carotid stents, approximately half as first operator. Likewise with thoracic stent–grafts, specific numbers of procedures will likely be required.

When a new technique or treatment modality becomes available, the specialists in that field make arrangements for incorporating the new technique into practice. When coronary stents initially became available, the cardiologists who placed them and trained others in how they should be placed had no residency training in these areas. They learned through courses and on-the-job training. The key is that most of these physicians had a foundation in endovascular skills to build upon.

Ultimately, it will be those who have strong interest in this field and are passionate about vascular care who advance it to its fullest potential.

Selected Readings

Bates ER, Babb JD, Casey DE Jr, et al. American College of Cardiology Foundation Task Force; American Society of Interventional & Therapeutic Neuroradiology; Society for Cardiovascular Angiography and Interventions; Society for Vascular Medicine and Biology; Society for Interventional Radiology. ACCF/SCAI/SVMB/SIR/ASITN 2007 Clinical Expert Consensus Document on carotid stenting. Vasc Med 2007; 12(1):35–83.

Calligaro KD, Toursarkissian B, Clagett GP, et al. Clinical Practice Council, Society for Vascular Surgery. Guidelines for hospital privileges in vascular and endovascular surgery: Recommendations of the Society for Vascular Surgery. J Vasc Surg 2008; 47(1):1–5.

Hobson RW II, Howard VJ, Roubin GS, et al. CREST. Credentialing of surgeons as interventionalists for carotid artery stenting: Experience from the lead-in phase of CREST. J Vasc Surg 2004; 40(5):952–957.

Lewis CA, Sacks D, Cardella JF, et al. Position statement: Documenting physician experience for credentials for peripheral arterial procedures—what you need to know. A consensus statement developed by the Standards Division of the Society of Cardiovascular and Interventional Radiology. J Vasc Interv Radiol 2002; 13:453–454.

Rosenfield KM; SCAI/SVMB/SVS Writing Committee. Clinical competence statement on carotid stenting: Training and credentialing for carotid stenting–Multispecialty consensus recommendations. J Vasc Surg 2005; 41(1):160–168.

White RA, Hodgson KJ, Ahn SS, et al. Endovascular interventions training and credentialing for vascular surgeons. J Vasc Surg 1999; 29:177–186.

2

Case Preparation and Room Setup

Set Yourself Up for Success

The success of the case depends in part on a few things that happen before you get to the procedure. The evaluation of the patient and the preprocedure analysis makes a difference. Decisions about access and strategy, how compelling the indications are for treatment, and the expectations of the patient and family all play important roles. Throughout this book, there is advice about these issues. Chapter 3 details access choices and how to use them. Chapter 12 covers issues of treatment strategy. Chapter 13 is about where we work and related issues. This chapter deals with some of the logistical issues that everyone faces in performing endovascular surgery.

Sizing Up the Case

Issues to address with regard to medical management of the patient may be numerous. The ones that occur most frequently are management of diabetes, renal insufficiency (contrast tolerance), and anticoagulation or antiplatelet agents. Each of these must be appropriately balanced based on your estimation of what needs to be done, how long it will take, how extensive it will be, and whether or not it will solve the patient's problem. In the midst of all this, the patient must be prepared by the physician and staff for the shortest possible hospital stay, maybe only a few hours. Logistical issues around transportation, mobility, and accompaniment home by a family member must be addressed. In preparing for the technical part of the case, check old angiograms and procedure notes. Examine the patient and perform a complete vascular examination. Palpate the arteries and assess perfusion to limbs intended for treatment and those that will be distal to likely puncture sites. Obtain and analyze some type of preprocedure noninvasive study to assist with planning.

Prior to the Puncture

Informed consent is best obtained in the office when the patient is afforded time to consider issues and to consult with family. Patients on Coumadin™ or antiplatelet agents should be considered on a case-by-case basis. It is usually safe to perform either arteriography or endovascular intervention in patients on antiplatelet therapy, as long as there are no other factors that are likely to promote hemorrhage, such as dialysis dependency. If the antiplatelet agent must be stopped, it should be 10 days or more prior to the procedure. If endovascular intervention is required, Coumadin should be stopped approximately five days prior to the procedure. Patients who require anticoagulation to be continued except for a "window" when it is stopped may often be treated with outpatient Lovenox to shorten the hospital stay. At the operator's discretion is whether a protime should be obtained on the day of the procedure. Patients with renal insufficiency are managed with preoperative hydration with normal saline and mucomyst. Methods of preprocedural evaluation are available that help to limit the contrast required for the study. These are discussed in chapter 10. A contrast agent that is less toxic to the kidneys, CO_2, should also be considered. Patients with a history of contrast allergy should be treated before the procedure with prednisone and Benadryl™. This protocol is detailed in chapter 15.

Percutaneous or Open?

Whether access should be gained through percutaneous needle puncture or open exposure was an unrewarding preoccupation that was based upon an arbitrary division of labor. This dilemma was prompted by the fact that most vascular workshops were prepared to carry out percutaneous exposure or open exposure, but not both. Vascular specialists are now facile with both methods of access, and the vascular workshop should be set up to handle the full range of approaches. More about the vascular workshop is presented in chapter 13.

The goal of arterial access is the smallest incision that provides safe and effective entry. Access site complications occur when the operator is committed to one approach, and the intended procedure is forced to conform. There is some increase in the risk of puncture site complications with progressively larger arteriotomies. Arterial access sheaths up to 10 Fr can usually be placed safely using a percutaneous approach. For access devices larger than 10 Fr (greater than 3.3 mm), open access is advisable. Recently developed arterial closure devices may permit safe percutaneous access for larger devices.

Working Environment

Surgeons understand that top performance is something that does not just happen. It develops only with preparation. Judgment and technical skills take time, effort, and enthusiasm to develop. The staff that assists you, the equipment available, and the facility where you use those skills can either promote or detract from your ability to get sick patients through difficult situations. These preparations help to limit the variables and facilitate excellent results. Endovascular work is no different. There is a substantial learning curve associated with each procedure. Creating that working environment where high quality endovascular practice can be carried out is essential.

It is necessary to assure the presence of the proper interventional equipment when performing endovascular interventions. The necessary catheters, guidewires, guiding catheters and sheaths, balloons, and stents must be available. The room must be equipped to adequately monitor the patient. Medications must be available, including anticoagulants, antiplatelet agents, hemodynamic medications as needed, and sedation as required. The staff must be knowledgeable in the inventory of the supplies, devices, and equipment used during interventional procedures. The surgeon must be comfortable with the ability of the staff to assist in performing these procedures. Educating the staff beforehand on the nature of the procedure to be performed, the important points of the case and the specific assistance that will be necessary are critical to assuring smooth progression through the case. Adequate monitoring of the patient allows rapid assessment of the patient's status, thereby allowing intervention for hemodynamic problems early, and limiting their impact upon the outcome. Some surgeons find themselves more comfortable performing these procedures for this reason in an operating room setting with the assistance of an anesthesiologist or nurse anesthetist. It is important that the person performing the intervention be confident that the people assisting can quickly deal with hemodynamic or other problems. Fixed imaging equipment is not mandatory but is best and facilitates performance of endovascular procedures. A room stocked with adequate disposable inventory is desirable. It is helpful to develop a method of arranging the room for different procedures, depending on the proposed access site and the area of intended imaging.

Equipment

The patient must adequately be monitored before, during, and after the procedure. Otherwise, the attractive advantages of a less morbid and less invasive procedure may be readily negated by some unfortunate complicating event. It is imperative to have monitoring equipment in both the procedure room and the recovery room. Monitoring necessitates the presence of someone in the room whose primary responsibility is assessing and managing the patient. This person has a significant role in assuring that the subject is stable and that the monitoring equipment is functioning properly. Resuscitation equipment must be available should it become necessary. This includes a functioning suction device, oxygen, and intravenous solutions along with a cart equipped with standard emergency resuscitation material. One should have standard oxygen saturation monitoring equipment. This probe is placed away from the extremity in which arterial access is obtained to assure that distal vessel spasm or disease, if present, does not impair the readings of this monitor. It is necessary to have continuous monitoring of the electrocardiographic tracing. In some cases, it may also be mandatory to have the ability to continuously monitor the arterial pressure. This may be obtained with a separate arterial line, and this may be useful in performing carotid stents or major aortic cases. This arterial pressure system is also part of the manifold system used to connect to the arterial sheath. It is helpful to have this additional port off the manifold that allows pressure monitoring.The pressure system can, however, be added to the sidearm of the sheath attaching the side port of the sheath to a separate pressure monitoring system. In addition to this invasive arterial pressure monitor, it is necessary to have a noninvasive method of monitoring the pressure in case the invasive system is not functioning or is impaired for a period of time during the procedure.

Imaging equipment is described in chapters 8 and 13. The table should be a floating-point table that is carbon fiber and allows imaging in all rotations. Performing these procedures without a carbon fiber table adds to the complexity of the case and will limit the angles in which images can be obtained. Floating-point tables allow rapid surgeon positioning of the table and decreases the time necessary for performing the procedure. If using a mobile system, a floating-point, carbon fiber table will be helpful.

It is also helpful to have a sterile tabletop upon which to work. In order to move expeditiously through the performance of these procedures, arranging two tables behind the team is helpful. The space offered by an additional "back table" provides an area upon which the items to be used are prepared and placed, available in the order of use. The time saved not searching for an item on a crowded surface will easily offset the small space loss incurred by the additional table.

Facilities and Room Setup

Prior to the procedure, inventory items should be assembled. The procedure is previewed in a step-by-step manner. It is important to have the facility and room arranged so that the surgeon is comfortable performing the procedure and has all equipment necessary for the procedure is readily available. The room should be large enough to allow movement around the patient and sterile field. The patient should be comfortably positioned. Safety straps and side restraints help maintain patient position and safety. The interventionalist is positioned tableside with easy access to the equipment tables. It is essential to have adequate assistance during these procedures and to assure that the assistant is well versed in the technique. The assistant should be positioned to the side of the interventionalist and should also have easy access to equipment. The image system is best positioned opposite the side of the table where the surgeon is located and the monitor bank for images positioned at eye level opposite the surgeon. The monitor bank should include three monitors. The first should contain the working images. The second monitor is a reference monitor to allow posting of reference images that can be used to assist with positioning catheters and guidewires. The final monitor should be a physiologic monitor, which contains the output of any hemodynamic measurements, oxygen saturation, electrocardiographic tracing, and pressure measurements. Maximize the potential for success in each case. Preprocedure analysis makes a difference. Practice settings that have some particular disadvantage with respect to setup or equipment can still be made to work, but planning around those issues is essential.

Selected Readings

Bonatti J, Vassiliades T, Nifong W, et al. How to build a cath-lab operating room. Heart Surg Forum 2007; 10(4):E344–E348.

Dietrich EB. Endovascular suite design. In: White RA, Fogarty TJ, eds. Peripheral Endovascular Interventions. St. Louis, MO: Mosby, 1996:129–139.

Mansour MA. The new operating room environment. Surg Clin North Am 1999; 79:477–487.

Sikkink CJ, Reijnen MM, Zeebregts CJ. The creation of the optimal dedicated endovascular suite. Eur J Vasc Endovasc Surg 2008; 35(2):198–204.

3

Getting In:
Percutaneous Vascular Access

Get on the Vascular Superhighway

Use of the vascular system itself to assist the therapist in arriving at the site of the lesion for treatment has tremendous appeal. It is simple, direct, less morbid, and leaves little external evidence of what has taken place. Much resources and development has been brought to bear in order to make standard open surgery a thing of the past and this effort has been relatively successful. As devices are miniaturized, access becomes simpler. A well-placed access site sets the operator up for success. A poorly chosen or conducted access can make a simple case complicated and possibly make a complicated case impossible. Access site issues must be considered for every case. Access-related complications are still the most common complications of endovascular intervention. An access mistake is nearly a guarantee of a complication. Consider the need for access a breach of the vascular system, a necessary evil, that ought to be minimized to the extent possible. Although a percutaneous access site is much less than a standard surgical incision, it is still what the patient notices most during the recovery process.

ANGIO CONSULT: WHAT ARE THE PRINCIPLES OF PERCUTANEOUS ACCESS?

1. Choose the puncture site with the individual patient's needs in mind.
2. Determine the likelihood of performing an endovascular intervention during the angiogram procedure and take that into account when choosing a puncture site.
3. Pick the access site that is far enough from the lesion so that a sheath may be placed without encountering the lesion itself.
4. Feel the artery intended for puncture so you know what to expect. Is it soft or hard and what is the quality of the pulse?
5. Palpate the anatomic landmarks. For example, with every femoral puncture, the anterosuperior iliac spine and the pubic tubercle and the inguinal ligament should be defined by physical examination and palpation.
6. Visualize the artery and its relationship to anatomic landmarks before skin puncture.
7. Standardize your technique.
8. Use fluoroscopy for guidance.
9. Do not be afraid to abandon the access and puncture elsewhere if the risk is too high.
10. No one gets in every single time.
11. If there is a problem, hold pressure for a few minutes and start again.
12. It is rare to have any significant damage to the access artery from the needle alone. Larger problems occur when a poor puncture placement is not recognized and larger devices are placed through that site.

Table 1 Percutaneous Puncture Site Choices

Puncture site	Approach	Provides access to...	Comments
Femoral	Retrograde	Aorta and its branches	When either femoral artery can be used, most right-handed operators will stand on the patient's right side and puncture the right common femoral artery.
Femoral	Antegrade	Ipsilateral infrainguinal	Contraindicated when there is inflow disease or a high profunda origin or when the patient is obese.
Brachial	Retrograde	Aorta and its branches	Prefer the left side. Access site for sheath larger than 7 Fr should be closed through open exposure. Risk higher than with femoral puncture.
Subclavian	Retrograde	Aorta and its branches	Risk higher than with femoral puncture. Alternative to brachial or axillary artery puncture.
Retrogeniculate popliteal	Retrograde	Ipsilateral SFA	Patient in prone position.
Common carotid	Retrograde	Aorta and its branches	Increased risk of stroke and bleeding.
	Antegrade	Carotid bifurcation	Minimal working room to bifurcation.
Translumbar		Aorta and its branches	Prone position, limited to arteriography, increased risk of bleeding.

Choosing Your Approach

The most important maneuver for successful vascular access occurs prior to the procedure: that is, choosing the puncture site. The optimal puncture site choice should provide a low risk of complications and reasonable proximity to the site of intended intervention. Table 1 provides a list of puncture site choices. The retrograde femoral puncture is the most commonly used since it is safest and offers the highest degree of versatility. Brachial artery punctures are usually the second choice, with preference for the left brachial artery since the pathway from the right brachial artery crosses the origin of the right common carotid artery and the innominate artery.Many procedures are also being performed using the radial artery, especially diagnostic cardiac catheterization. When upper extremity access is required for a large sheath, it may be obtained using open exposure of the brachial artery. Other puncture sites that have been used less commonly include the retrogeniculate popliteal artery and the common carotid artery. Even less commonly, the tibial or pedal arteries have been used for retrograde access to the lower extremity and the axillary artery or subclavian artery has been used for upper extremity access. Translumbar access is only rarely performed

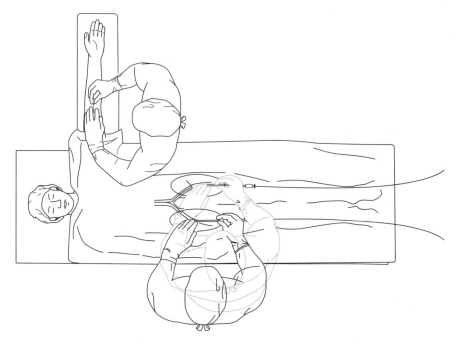

Fig. 1 Working forehand. The operator works forehand whenever possible. In this example, the right-handed surgeon stands on the patient's right side to puncture either femoral artery. Brachial puncture is also performed forehand.

for diagnostic procedures but has recently been performed for commonly to gain access to a patent aneurysm sac in a patient with an endoleak after stent–graft exclusion of an abdominal aortic aneurysm. Chapter 10 includes a detailed discussion of puncture site evaluation prior to arteriography. Once the puncture site has been chosen, the operator should set up the case so that the work may be performed forehand if at all possible. This usually helps to avoid needless struggle. Figure 1 demonstrates options for a forehand approach.

Femoral Anatomy for Arterial Access

The most common complications following arteriography or endovascular intervention occur at the puncture site. An understanding of anatomy helps avoid complications. The goal is a single perfect pass of the entry needle on every case. The operator should visualize the femoral artery passing from beneath the inguinal ligament. The inguinal ligament extends from the anterosuperior iliac spine to the pubic tubercle. This landmark is usually possible to define and is essential in helping to determine how far superior or inferior the puncture should be. The desired needle entry location in the common femoral artery is 1 or 2 cm distal to the level where the inguinal ligament crosses the common femoral artery. Once the location of the inguinal ligament has been defined, the landing of the needle on the artery depends upon the angle at which the entry needle passes from the skin to the artery.

The quality of the artery may be understood prior to the procedure by palpating it. The artery may be rolled under the fingers. The thicker-walled or calcified artery will present a firm structure that can be rolled a little back and forth, which has more body than just the palpation of a pulse. If the patient has a poor femoral pulse and has stronger pulses more distally, at the popliteal or pedal levels, the common femoral artery may be calcified. If the patient has a femoral bruit and yet the femoral pulse is stronger than expected, it may be the waterhammer effect cause by a lesion in the distal common femoral artery, just distal to the point of palpation. If the artery is not easy to locate because of a diminished pulse, there are several steps that may be taken. These are outlined in the later section "Puncture of the Pulseless Femoral Artery" of this chapter.

Fluoroscopy may also be used prior to puncture to locate the head of the femur and to identify the artery. Puncture of the artery proximal to the femoral head is likely to be too far proximal and to enter the external iliac artery. The artery usually passes over the medial side of the femoral head. The temptation is to use the groin crease to determine the location of the puncture. Obese patients often have a groin crease that is significantly distal to the location of the inguinal ligament, and this may lead to a puncture that is too low (Fig. 2). The fossa ovalis may also be palpated as a discontinuity in the fascia of the leg at the location where the saphenous vein dives toward the deeper common femoral vein. Since this is directly over the lower aspect of the common femoral vein, it may also be used as an anatomic marker, with the femoral artery just lateral (usually the proximal superficial femoral artery is present at this level). Occasionally, it is helpful to use a skin marker to define the inguinal ligament and location of the common femoral artery.

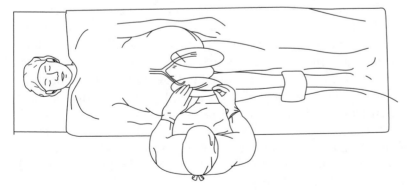

Fig. 2 Identify the anatomic landmarks before arterial puncture. Identification of landmarks for arterial puncture may be challenging in the obese patient. The groin crease is usually substantially distal to the actual inguinal ligament and this must be taken into account when planning femoral access.

Percutaneous Retrograde Puncture of Femoral Artery

Both groins are prepared and draped. A towel holding each of the items immediately required for puncture and guidewire placement (a syringe for local anesthetic, a scalpel, a mosquito clamp, a puncture needle, and a guidewire) is placed on the patient's lap. Intravenous antibiotics are administered if the patient has a prosthetic graft or heart valve in place or if an endovascular device implantation is anticipated. The right-handed operator stands on the patient's right side for the puncture of either groin so that the forehand approach can be used (Fig. 3). The femoral artery of choice is palpated and the inguinal ligament is traced from the anterosuperior iliac spine to the pubic tubercle. The goal is to puncture the proximal to middle common femoral artery. In most patients this represents a segment 4 to 8 cm in length. The operator must anticipate the trajectory of the needle with an angle of approach of 45 degrees or steeper. The more calcified or scarred the artery, the more a steep trajectory of the needle approach is required to spear the artery and so the needle does not simply bounce off it. Fluoroscopy also helps in this situation, because as the needle pushes the hardened artery, the whole structure can be seen moving.

The operator uses the nondominant hand to trap the common femoral artery. The right-handed surgeon uses the left hand to trap the common femoral artery between the forefinger and the third finger. The third, fourth, and fifth fingers fan out on one side of the artery and the thumb and forefinger on the other side of the artery to hold back the surrounding tissue. The hand is adjusted until the impression of the pulse is equal on the tips of the second and third fingers. Once the left hand (or nondominant hand) is correctly placed, it is not moved again until pulsatile backbleeding is coming from the needle. Plain lidocaine (1%) is injected into the skin and subcutaneous tissues in the area for the prospective puncture between the forefinger and the third finger of the operator's left hand. Infiltration with local anesthetic causes induration and this increases the transmission of femoral artery pulsation to the surrounding soft tissue, which can be appreciated if the fingers are in the correct location. A No. 18 straight angiographic entry needle is then used to approach the artery at a 45-degree angle. Either a single-wall or a double-wall puncture needle may be used (Fig. 4). The vessel is usually 2 to 5 cm beneath the skin entry site. The anterior wall of the common femoral artery can usually be palpated with the tip of the needle and identified by the pulsation of the artery against the needle. The needle tip is advanced through the anterior wall of the artery.

Because the anterior wall is usually softer and the posterior wall more firm, the needle may immediately abut the posterior wall of the common femoral artery. Occasionally, the needle must be withdrawn just slightly to allow guidewire passage (Fig. 5).

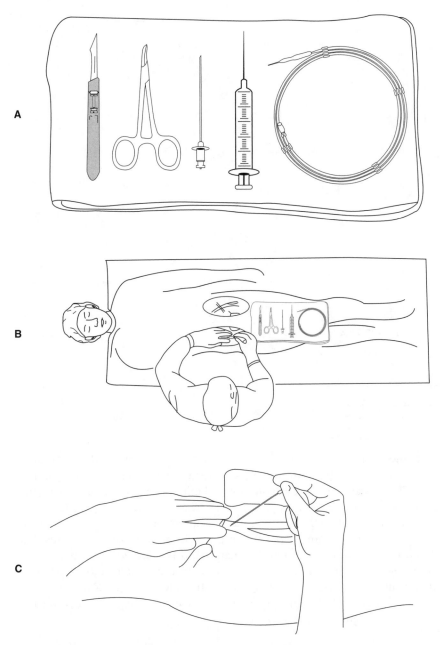

Fig. 3 Percutaneous retrograde puncture of femoral artery. (**A**) A sterile towel is placed on the patient's lap with the tools immediately required for percutaneous arterial entry *(from left to right):* a scalpel, a hemostat, a percutaneous entry needle, a syringe with local anesthetic, and a guidewire. (**B**) The right-handed operator stands on the patient's right side for puncture of either femoral artery to permit a forehand approach. If the left femoral artery requires puncture, the operator leans over the patient. (**C**) The prospective location of the middle to proximal common femoral artery puncture is evaluated by tracing the inguinal ligament from the anterosuperior iliac spine to the pubic tubercle. The artery is trapped between the forefinger and

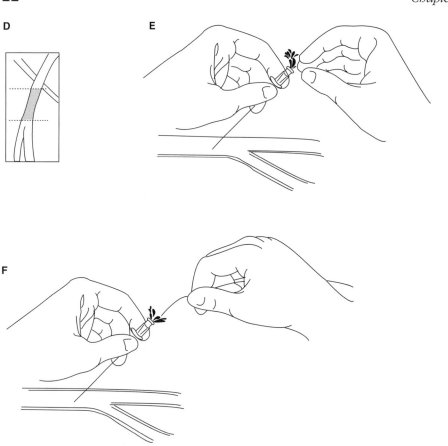

Fig. 3 Continued   third finger of the operator's nondominant hand. The thumb and forefinger hold back the surrounding soft tissue, as do the third, fourth, and fifth fingers. When local anesthetic is administered into the subcutaneous tissue, the femoral pulse usually becomes more pronounced. The entry needle approaches the artery at a 45-degree angle. (**D**) The femoral arteriotomy is safest in the proximal to middle common femoral artery. (**E**) When pulsatile backbleeding indicates that the needle tip is in the artery, the nondominant hand is released from its position trapping the artery. The nondominant hand accepts the needle and steadies it. (**F**) The dominant hand retrieves the guidewire, straightens the guidewire tip, and inserts it into the needle hub. The guidewire tip may be straightened using the maneuver shown in Figure 4 of this chapter.

When pulsatile backbleeding is achieved, the operator's nondominant hand is released from its location over the common femoral artery. The nondominant hand is then used to hold the needle until the guidewire can be passed through the needle. At this point, the needle must be held by the nondominant hand since the needle is in an unstable position in the artery and must be secured. The contralateral hand will be busy grabbing, inserting, and advancing the guidewire. The several-centimeter floppy-tip portion of

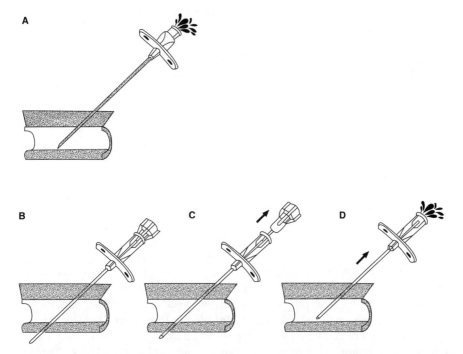

Fig. 4 Single-wall or double-wall puncture technique. (**A**) The single-wall puncture needle has a beveled tip that is placed into the anterior wall of the artery. (**B**) The double-wall puncture needle has a trochar with a sharp beveled tip that is inserted through the artery. (**C**) The needle is removed. (**D**) The blunt tip outer casing is then gradually withdrawn until its tip is in the arterial lumen and pulsatile backbleeding is evident.

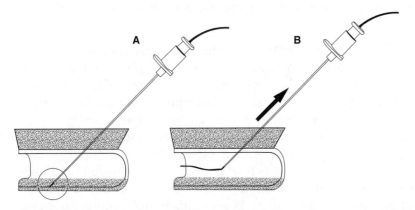

Fig. 5 Guidewire hits posterior wall. The tip of the needle often pushes the softer anterior wall of the common femoral artery against the thicker posterior wall before it enters the lumen. (**A**) When the guidewire is advanced through the needle, it hits the posterior wall of the artery and is unable to pass. (**B**) The needle is withdrawn 1 to 2 mm and the guidewire is passed again.

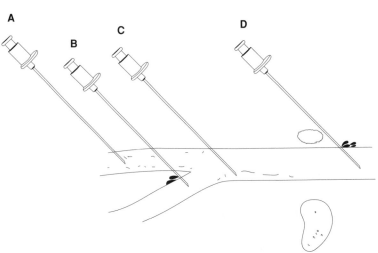

Fig. 6 Incorrect femoral artery punctures. Entry site complications result from poorly placed femoral artery punctures. (**A**) Proximal superficial femoral artery puncture is too low and may cause puncture site thrombosis. The proximal superficial femoral artery is frequently the site of significant plaque formation. (**B**) A proximal deep femoral artery entry is difficult to compress and may result in hemorrhage. (**C**) The needle tip may disrupt posterior wall common femoral artery plaque. This is more likely in proximity to the bifurcation. (**D**) Puncture of the distal external iliac artery is contiguous with the retroperitoneal space and is prone to hemorrhage.

the guidewire is advanced through the needle until the stiffer portion of the guidewire is traversing the arterial entry site. If the lesion is near the puncture site (e.g., distal external iliac artery lesion), fluoroscopy is initiated immediately.

Most puncture site complications are related to arteriotomies that are too high, too low, or forced into an area too hostile for simple puncture (Fig. 6). The anterior wall of the common femoral artery often has a soft spot, even when the femoral artery and its bifurcation are heavily diseased. Puncture of the external iliac artery is difficult to compress and it is surrounded by the potential space of the retroperitoneum (Fig. 7). Hemorrhage from a high puncture may require a stent–graft or surgical control. Unfortunately, an external iliac artery puncture is often not recognized until after the access is removed and the patient develops pain or vital sign instability. The proximal profunda femoral artery is also difficult to compress because of its deep course. The proximal superficial femoral artery is usually calcified and often a site of substantial plaque formation. Puncture site compression at the superficial femoral artery origin may cause thrombosis. Since common femoral artery plaque forms preferentially along the posterior wall, double-wall puncture confers no advantages and may add some risk. Double-wall puncture should also be avoided if thrombolytic therapy is a possibility.

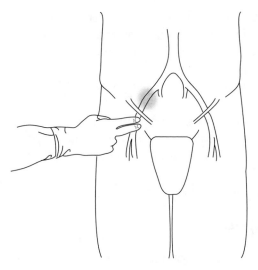

Fig. 7 Retroperitoneal hemorrhage from a proximal groin puncture. A groin puncture that is too far proximal may enter the external iliac artery and cause hemorrhage into the retroperitoneal space. If it is unrecognized, pressure at the skin puncture site, which is somewhat distal to the arterial puncture site, may exacerbate hemorrhage by creating additional outflow resistance downstream from the bleeding arteriotomy, as in the example shown. If the abdominal wall is relaxed, manual pressure can often be held satisfactorily over a distal external iliac artery puncture site with a little extra effort.

PLAN OF ATTACK: GUIDEWIRE WILL NOT PASS THROUGH THE NEEDLE

1. If the tip of the entry needle is against the posterior wall of the artery, withdraw the needle 1 to 2 mm very slowly while gently attempting to pass the guidewire (Fig. 5). As the needle pulls back far enough, the guidewire will pass easily.
2. If the guidewire encounters a common femoral artery lesion, irregular posterior wall plaque may be disrupted, form a dissection plane, or embolize. Do not force the guidewire.
3. Withdraw the guidewire to ensure that the needle tip is still intra-arterial and that backbleeding is pulsatile.
4. Establish that arterial return is consistent with the clinical impression of inflow to that level (e.g., dampened arterial inflow should be expected if the patient has aortoiliac disease on physical examination).
5. Reinsert the guidewire and use fluoroscopy to see where the guidewire hangs up. Sometimes the guidewire goes just beyond the needle tip and into a medial or lateral collateral. If the guidewire tip forms a loop or appears to go on a circuitous course just after it exits the needle, do not force it. The guidewire is probably subintimal and you will probably have to pull it out.

6. If there is appropriate blood return from the needle, put an extension tube on the hub of the needle and puff contrast while under fluoroscopy or use road mapping. Visualize the puncture site and the cause of the obstruction.

7. Consider a new puncture at the same location or a different approach altogether.

8. The needle may be too low and hitting femoral bifurcation plaque. Pull the needle and hold pressure at the arterial puncture site. Repeat the puncture 1 to 2 cm more proximally along the common femoral artery.

Micropuncture Technique

A coaxial micropuncture set (Cook, Inc., Bloomington, Indiana, U.S.A.) includes a 21-gauge needle to enter the artery, a 0.018-in. guidewire with a floppy tip, and a 4 Fr short catheter with an inner smaller diameter dilator that passes over the 0.018-in. guidewire (Fig. 8).

The 21-gauge needle is placed in the artery. When backbleeding occurs, the soft tipped, steerable 0.018 in. guidewire is advanced through the needle under fluoroscopic guidance. Arterial backbleeding through a 21-gauge needle is usually much less pulsatile than through the larger 18-gauge needle. The needle is removed and the 4-Fr short catheter with the 3-Fr inner dilator is passed over the guidewire. After the catheter is in place, the dilator and guidewire are removed. The short 4-Fr access catheter is flushed with heparinized saline and a longer, appropriately sized guidewire (usually 0.035-in. diameter) is passed. The short 4-Fr catheter is removed and the desired access is placed. Puncture sites beyond the femoral artery, including the brachial or radial artery, bypass grafts, and alternative access sites, are preferentially approached using the micropuncture technique.

When should micropuncture technique be used? Some operators use it for every case and some use it selectively. It is particularly useful for brachial or radial access, for pulseless arteries, scarred groins, and calcified arteries, or for antegrade access to the lower extremity.Advantages of micropuncture technique include a smaller initial arterial hole, use of a steerable wire, and graduated enlargement between the inner stiff trochar and the 4- or 5-Fr dilator. There are disadvantages of micropuncture. It requires extra steps. The catheter is not long enough so if there is a lesion nearby, you end up crossing it with the introducing guidewire, and then crossing it again with the 0.035-in. wire required for access sheath placement. If you are working with a scarred groin, a re-do groin, or a super calcified femoral artery, the catheter may not pass over the 0.018-in. guidewire. A number of tricks may be required to make up for the guidewire, which does not have the backbone to support passage through a hostile scarred area.

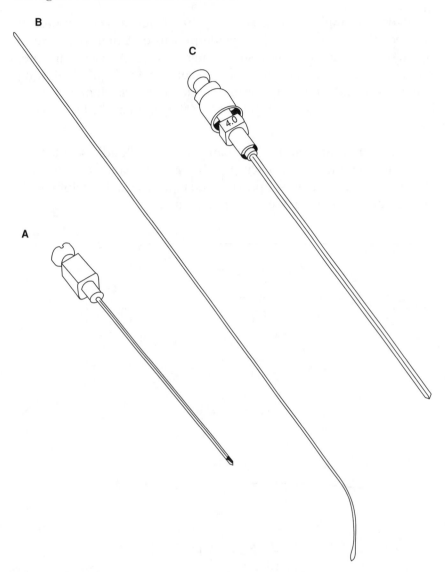

Fig. 8 The micropuncture set (Cook, Inc. Bloomington, Indiana, U.S.A.) includes (**A**) a 21-gauge needle, (**B**) a 0.018-in. floppy-tip guidewire, and (**C**) a 4-Fr short catheter with an inner 3-Fr trochar to slide over the low profile guidewire.

Percutaneous Antegrade Puncture of Femoral Artery

Antegrade femoral access permits optimal control of guidewires and catheters for infrainguinal endovascular intervention. The puncture in the skin must be proximal to the level of the inguinal ligament to allow entry of the needle into the proximal to middle common femoral artery, taking into account a 45-degree angle of approach (Fig. 9). Often a steep approach angle of the needle works best for antegrade puncture. A high puncture in the distal external iliac artery may result in hemorrhage. A distal puncture, which is too near the femoral bifurcation, results in inadequate working room to selectively catheterize the origin of the superficial femoral artery and may also be in an area where it cannot be safely compressed to achieve hemostasis.

In patients with a large abdominal pannus, wide silk adhesive tape is used as a truss to hold the pannus back (Fig. 10). A huge pannus is a relative contraindication to the antegrade approach. The tape job can be helpful with either a retrograde or an antegrade femoral puncture.

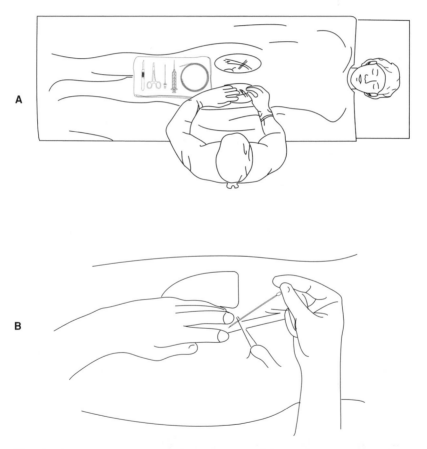

Fig. 9 Percutaneous antegrade puncture of femoral artery. (**A**) The right-handed operator stands on the patient's left side to permit a forehand approach, and a towel is placed on the patient's lap with the tools needed for arterial puncture. (**B**) The common femoral artery is trapped between the forefinger and third finger of the nondominant hand. The intended arterial puncture site is at the proximal to middle common femoral artery with the needle approach at 45 degrees. The skin puncture site is proximal to the inguinal ligament.

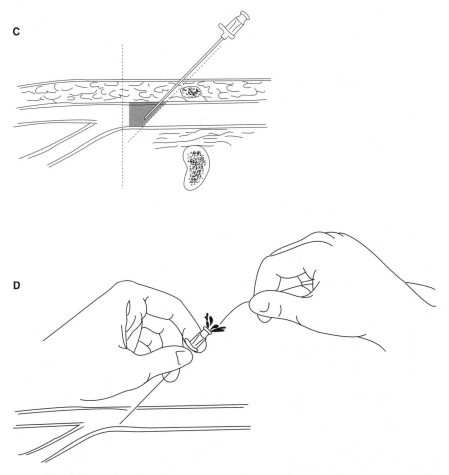

Fig. 9 Continued (**C**) The common femoral artery available for antegrade puncture is limited. Puncture above the inguinal ligament must be avoided because of the risk of hemorrhage. Puncture near the common femoral artery bifurcation leaves inadequate working room for cannulation of the superficial femoral artery. (**D**) After the needle tip enters the artery, the position of the nondominant hand is modified to hold the needle rather than trap the artery. The forefinger is placed over the hub to stop backbleeding, and the guidewire is advanced with the dominant hand.

The right-handed operator stands on the patient's left side for forehand delivery of the needle and guidewire. The image intensifier should hover over the patient from the side opposite the operator. This arrangement may be a problem in an angiographic suite where the C-arm unit is mounted on ceiling rails or on the floor. The left or nondominant hand is used to trap the common femoral artery between the forefinger and the third finger in the same way as for a retrograde femoral artery puncture. The proposed arterial puncture site is visualized in juxtaposition to the location of the inguinal ligament. The skin puncture site is then chosen and infiltrated with 1% plain lidocaine. The angiographic entry needle is advanced at an angle of

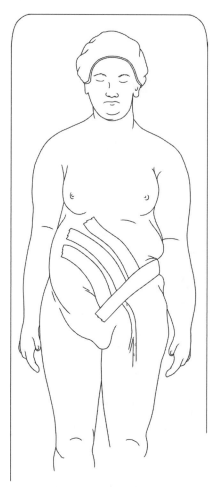

Fig. 10 The abdominal pannus can be taped up during the procedure to better expose the femoral areas.

45 degrees or steeper toward the pulse, which is trapped between the forefinger and third finger. When pulsatile backbleeding is achieved, the needle is held steady by the dominant hand momentarily. The nondominant hand position over the artery is relinquished. The nondominant hand rests on the patient on its ulnar side and takes over the needle in its intra-arterial position. The dominant hand reaches for the guidewire and inserts the guidewire into the needle hub. The guidewire is advanced with the dominant hand.

Since the superficial femoral artery is on the level plane and the deep femoral artery proceeds posteriorly from the bifurcation, the guidewire usually enters the deep artery preferentially following antegrade puncture. The guidewire must be redirected into the origin of the superficial femoral artery (see chap. 9 for a detailed discussion of selective catheterization). Working distance between the antegrade puncture site in the common femoral artery and the femoral artery bifurcation is limited. Any previously performed arteriography should be assessed to determine the level of the femoral bifurcation. Even if only contralateral lower extremity films are available, evidence of an unusually high femoral bifurcation may alter puncture site choice. Prior to performing antegrade femoral artery puncture, any previous arteriograms should be checked for the location of the deep femoral artery origin and the length of the common femoral artery. Duplex evaluation and marking of the common femoral artery bifurcation may also be performed before proceeding with antegrade puncture. The micropuncture approach works well for an antegrade puncture. The puncture is small and can be directed under fluoroscopy or ultrasound. The guidewire is relatively steerable and can be rolled between the fingers and twirled into the superficial femoral artery.

PLAN OF ATTACK: HOW DO YOU ENTER THE PROXIMAL FEMORAL ARTERY DURING ANTEGRADE FEMORAL PUNCTURE?

1. It is best when performing an antegrade approach to enter the proximal common femoral artery to maximize working distance between the puncture site and the femoral bifurcation.
2. Use micropuncture set, which has a guidewire that is somewhat steerable.
3. Under fluoroscopy, aim to hit the artery even with the very proximal part of the head of the femur, just inferior to the level of the bony cortex. Go at a sharp angle from the skin down toward the artery if you need to. Put the needle down close to where you think the artery is and then use fluoroscopy to get confirmation of appropriateness of location.
4. Once the guidewire is in the artery, guide the catheter down over the guidewire by pushing on the subcutaneous tissue with a free hand to keep the wire straight and avoid kinking under the skin.

Percutaneous Puncture of Pulseless Femoral Artery

The clinical situation that requires puncture of a pulseless femoral artery usually includes plans for iliac artery reconstruction or recanalization, rather than simple arteriography. Aortoiliac duplex scanning is valuable in this setting to assess the severity, location, and length of the lesion. The location of the femoral artery is marked after duplex evaluation. The patent but pulseless femoral artery is cannulated using a combination of several techniques (Fig. 11). The artery itself is often palpable, even when there is no pulse. The common femoral artery almost always passes over the medial half of

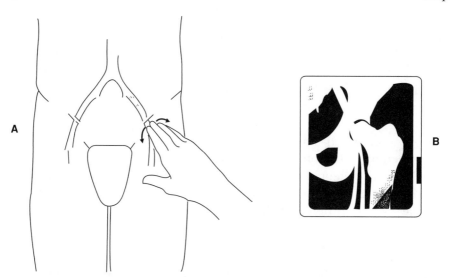

Fig. 11 Percutaneous puncture of pulseless femoral artery. (**A**) The patent but pulseless femoral artery can often be palpated. (**B**) A review of previous arteriograms shows the location of the artery relative to the femoral head. It usually passes over the medial half of the femoral head. (**C**) Fluoroscopy may reveal vascular calcification and help guide puncture. (**D**) An arteriographic catheter placed through another entry site (either contralateral femoral or proximal approach) can be used to administer contrast and road map the location of the artery. Puncture of the pulseless artery is performed using the road map as the guide.

the femoral head. Its location may be revealed by a previous arteriogram or is identifiable by vascular calcification using fluoroscopy. A blood pressure cuff placed on the ipsilateral thigh can increase peripheral resistance and enhance a diminished pulse. A catheter can be placed through another access site, either on the contralateral side or the proximal side, and contrast can be injected to road map the femoral artery. Delayed filming is required.

ANGIO CONSULT: HOW TO PERFORM FLUOROSCOPICALLY GUIDED FEMORAL ACCESS?

1. Mark out anatomic landmarks by palpation. Identify the approximate location of the inguinal ligament. Place a maker, either the needle or a clamp tip over the location that estimates the correct place to puncture the artery.
2. Perform fluoroscopy of the femoral area. Often the femoral artery is visible on plain fluoroscopy due to calcification. Check the proximal SFA for calcification because this will tell the trajectory of the common femoral artery.
3. If the artery is vaguely visible over the femoral head but you are not sure, use an oblique projection to see if the longitudinal image

of the common femoral artery moves with respect to the femoral head. (Because the common femoral artery passes within 1- to 3-cm anterior to the very sizeable femoral head, completely separating the images of the two structures is almost impossible.) (To separate the image of the two structures requires a very steep oblique, almost lateral projection. At this angle, contralateral structures contaminate the image.)

4. Anesthetize the skin. Advance the needle down toward the artery. If it is really close, the needle will be bobbing with the pulsation of the artery.

5. Do not put the image intensifier too close to the field, so you can work under it. You must be able to see the blood return from the micropuncture needle. Position the image intensifier so that the field does not include your hands. Also, there is a lot of scatter in this position so do not do it for longer than you must.

6. When the needle hits the artery, the artery often moves back and forth a bit and becomes a lot more obvious to see on fluoroscopy. If the artery is really rolling back and forth, the other hand can press from the side to provide a little back pressure.

7. A common tendency when starting out with this task is to use fluoroscopy continuously during this task and to use it much more than is necessary. There is also a tendency to place the needle at too oblique an angle and end up with the tip of the needle much more proximal along the artery than intended. In addition, fluoroscopically guided puncture is often chosen because the artery is calcified. In this situation, a more direct (not quite straight down, but almost that steep) trajectory works best for puncturing the artery.

Proximal Access

Most arteriography and endovascular procedures are performed through the femoral arteries. When this is not possible, proximal access is another option to consider. Proximal access may be secured through percutaneous or open approaches to the brachial or axillary arteries (Fig. 12). Axillary artery puncture was used in the past for arteriorphy but this is rarely done now. It is much more common to use the brachial artery for access. The brachial artery may be punctured and managed percutaneously or using an open exposure. Another option is to enter the artery percutaneously, and if there is any problem, take the sheath out using open exposure. Diagnostic studies and the occasional therapeutic procedure may be performed through the radial artery. This has been developed primarily for coronary intervention, where the caliber and distance requirements are fairly standardized.

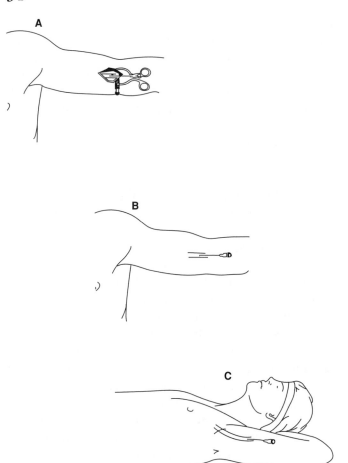

Fig. 12 Proximal access. Brachial or axillary artery entry is usually performed on the left side. (**A**) Brachial artery cutdown is performed just proximal to the antecubital crease. (**B**) Brachial artery puncture may be performed at the same location. (**C**) Axillary artery puncture (as it is commonly labeled) is performed just lateral to the axilla and is actually a high brachial artery puncture.

The advantages to the proximal approach include the following. It provides an alternative to the transfemoral approach when the femoral puncture sites are hostile or when the pathway between the groin and the pathology is blocked or when the femoral approach is not possible for some reason, it provides an opposite approach for crossing some lesions in certain arteries, There are several disadvantages to a proximal approach. Although percutaneous puncture can be safely performed, the complication rate is higher and the complications are generally worse when they occur. The arteries of the upper extremity are smaller, less forgiving, and more prone to spasm than arteries of the lower extremity. A constrictive fascial sheath encircles the artery and nerves in the upper arm, and a small hematoma may be enough to cause a brachial plexopathy. Passage of larger endovascular devices for performance of procedures any more complex than arteriography is accompanied by a proportionately greater risk of puncture site complications. The extra distance from the proximal access site to the infrarenal vasculature requires longer guidewires and catheters that are more cumbersome and less responsive to manipulation.

Percutaneous Puncture of Brachial Artery

The most common location for brachial artery puncture is just proximal to the antecubital crease. The left side is the first choice since the carotid artery origin may be avoided. In average-sized patients, sheaths up to 6 Fr may be placed without major risk of puncture site hemorrhage or thrombosis. Open access should be considered for larger devices or in smaller individuals.

The patient's arm is abducted and placed on an armboard (Fig. 13). A circumferential preparation of the arm is performed. The brachial artery pulse is palpated just proximal to the antecubital crease where the bicep has generally thinned to its tendinous portion. The artery is trapped between the forefinger and the third finger of the nondominant hand. The tips of the two fingers are held at enough distance to allow the artery to pass underneath without compressing it significantly. The 21-gauge micropuncture needle is advanced at a 45-degree angle by the dominant hand. The goal is for the needle tip to enter the anterior wall of the artery in the space between the two fingers. When backbleeding occurs, the short 0.018-in.-diameter guidewire is passed. Backbleeding through the micropuncture needle is usually not pulsatile because of its small caliber. The needle must be moved and manipulated slowly and any backbleeding carefully assessed. Heparin is administered to prevent thrombosis. Intra-arterial nitroglycerine or papaverine may be required if spasm of the upper extremity arteries occurs.

Percutaneous Puncture of Bypass Grafts

Substantial scar tissue may surround a prosthetic graft, especially in an area where an extensive open arterial exposure was performed. This is most common in the femoral area. Antibiotics are administered prior to puncture. Positioning of the patient is the same as for standard, retrograde femoral artery puncture. The position of needle entry should be proximal to the anastomosis with the native artery so that anastomotic sutures and/or thrombi are not disrupted. Dacron grafts have a tightly knitted fabric matrix that may be challenging to puncture. Considerable force may be required to push the needle through the anterior wall of the prosthetic graft. Care should be taken

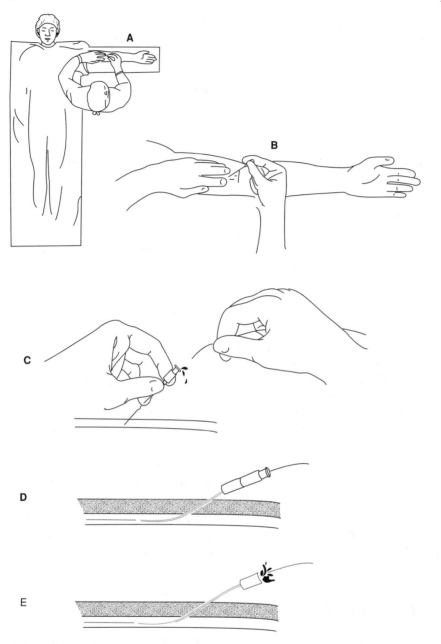

Fig. 13 Percutaneous puncture of brachial artery. Percutaneous puncture of the brachial artery should be considered for interventions requiring a sheath of 6 Fr or less. (**A**) The left arm is fully abducted. (**B**) The brachial artery is trapped between the forefinger and third finger just proximal to the antecubital crease. A 21-gauge micropuncture needle is advanced into the artery. (**C**) A 0.018-in. guidewire is advanced through the needle. (**D**) A coaxial dilator system is advanced over the guidewire. The inner dilator and the guidewire are removed and exchanged for a 0.035-in. guidewire that passes through the remaining (5 Fr) outer dilator. (**E**) After the 0.018-in. guidewire and the inner 3-Fr trochar are removed, the 4-Fr catheter may be used to introduce the desired guidewire for the case.

to avoid pushing the needle through the back wall of the graft, especially if the graft is not yet well incorporated. Once the needle is in place, a steel starter guidewire should be used to enter the artery. Slight enlargement of the tract with a 4- or 5-Fr dilator is usually advisable before attempting to pass the catheter. If the scar tissue prevents advance of the dilator, place the guidewire well inside the vasculature and have the assistant gently and gradually withdraw the guidewire as the operator advances the catheter. Occasionally, a larger-diameter (6 Fr), but stiffer, dilator will be required to follow the guidewire.

Percutaneous puncture may also be performed on a prosthetic graft that is immediately subcutaneous. The most common situation that calls for this is evaluation of a dialysis access graft. Occasionally, an axillofemoral, femoral–femoral or infrainguinal bypass graft requires direct puncture. Local anesthetic is injected into the skin and subcutaneous tissue over the graft. No skin incision is made. The needle tip is used to puncture the skin and to travel several millimeters in the subcutaneous tissue parallel to the graft. The needle hub is then tipped away from the skin so that the needle is at a 45-degree angle to the graft. The tip of the needle is then inserted into the graft. This maneuver creates a short subcutaneous tract that will help protect the graft from infection. The needle should be introduced at 45 degrees or more to avoid a larger, oval-shaped, or skiving type of puncture site hole in the graft, which may be more difficult to control. After the guidewire is placed, introduce the smallest-caliber catheter that is adequate for the intended purpose. Since these puncture sites are usually away from anastomoses, they are less subject to extensive scarring around the graft.

Occasionally, a femoral artery that serves as inflow for an autogenous infrainguinal bypass graft requires puncture. Aim for the hood of the graft or more proximally along the artery. The hood of the graft is usually where the pulse is felt most easily. Use clips and femoral calcification seen on fluoroscopy as landmarks.

Puncture Guidance with Ultrasound

Assistance with a difficult access can often be obtained using ultrasound. Portable ultrasound machines are being marketed for vascular access and are becoming more widely and readily available. This is not useful for every access. It is more equipment and more variables and may slow things down, and it is more steps. Ultrasound works well for venous puncture since they are larger and compressible and can be enlarged by manipulating the patient's position, but have no pulse that can guide the operator that is using external landmarks to guide the puncture. Often the artery is difficult to find using the portable ultrasound machine and can be located by finding the vein first. Find the vein with the probe in the transverse orientation. After

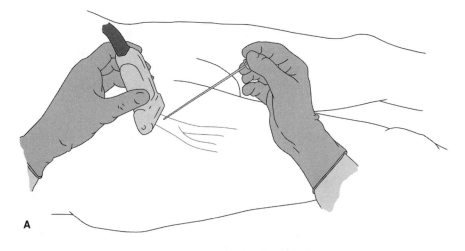

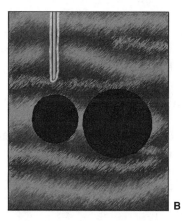

Fig. 14 Ultrasound-guided puncture can facilitate access under challenging circumstances.

Table 2 Complications of Femoral Artery Puncture and Catheterization

Complication	Frequency (%)[a]	SCVIR complication threshold (%)[b]
Minor bleeding or hematoma	6.0–10.0	
Major bleeding or hematoma (requiring transfusion, surgery, or delayed discharge)	1.0–2.4	3.0
Pseudoaneurysm	0.5–5.0	0.5
Arteriovenous fistula	0.01–0.1	0.1
Occlusion (thrombosis or dissection)	0.3–1.0	0.5
Perforation	<0.5	
Distal embolization	<0.5	
Infection	<0.1	

[a] From Valji, 1999 and Brown et al., 1997.
[b] From Spies et al., 1993.

Table 3 Comparison of Puncture Site Options

Puncture	Usefulness	Technical difficulty	Overall risk of significant complication[a]	Comments
Retrograde femoral	Most useful	Simplest	1.7%	More than 90% of cases may be performed transfemorally. It is the simplest and has the lowest complication rate.
Antegrade femoral	Useful for ipsilateral infrainguinal arteriogram or intervention	Entering the origin of the SFA can be challenging		A relatively safe but challenging approach. Especially useful for infrainguinal catheterization in patients who have a contraindication to crossing the aortic bifurcation.
Axillary	When femoral access not possible, provides alternative access for arteriography but not intervention	Challenging, blind stick	3.3%	Larger than brachial artery but also deeper. Less useful for intervention since it is difficult for patient to keep arm fully abducted with hand behind head for extended period of time.
Brachial	Useful for arteriography and/or intervention when femoral access not possible	More challenging than femoral puncture but simpler than axillary	7.0%	Smaller artery with tighter neurovascular sheath. Higher risk of neurologic complications or distal/hand ischemia. Consider open exposure for sheath $\geq$ 6 Fr.
Previously placed graft	Useful in patients whose anatomy is altered by previous surgical reconstruction	Perigraft scar tissue can make catheter passage difficult		Administer prophylactic antibiotics if graft is prosthetic.

[a] From La Berge et al., 2000.

locating the vein, orientation of the probe as to medial and lateral is checked, and this gives clues as to where the artery should be anatomically next to the vein. The artery can usually be seen to be pulsatile and noncompressible or minimally compressible, and quite a bit smaller than the vein. The dynamic presentation of the artery on ultrasound may change depending upon flow conditions. Evaluating the vascular sheath in cross section (transverse), the vein is larger, thin walled, and compressible while the artery is smaller in caliber, thick walled, and pulsatile (Fig. 14).

Place the middle of the probe over the intended puncture site in the artery. Advance the needle at an angle with the intention of having the needle hit the vessel directly under the probe. Needles create a shadow when the sound waves reflect off them and when it is in the field of the ultrasound beam is usually readily identified. Needles are also available that have scuffed up tips and are even more visible on ultrasound. (Fig. 14).

Puncture Site Complications

The most common type of complication in endovascular care is related to access. Complications of arterial puncture are listed in Table 2. The rates presented were accumulated using various techniques but do not include those who have undergone closure procedures at the puncture sites.

Summary of Puncture Site Options

Puncture site options and their relative rates of risk are summarized in Table 3. The retrograde femoral puncture is by far the most common and the most useful approach. Antegrade femoral puncture is limited in its use to the ipsilateral infrainguinal arteries. Proximal puncture sites in the brachial or axillary arteries are used when there is no adequate femoral puncture site.

Selected Readings

Brown MA, Nemcek AA, Vogelgang RL. Interventional Radiology Procedure Manual. New York: Churchill Livingstone, 1997:68.

Kiernan TJ, Ajani AE, Yan BP. Management of access site and systemic complications of percutaneous coronary and peripheral interventions. J Invasive Cardiol 2008; 20(9):463–469.

La Berge JM, Golden RL, Kerlan RK, et al. Interventional Radiology Essentials. Philadelphia, PA: Lippincott Williams & Wilkins, 2000.

Montero-Baker M, Schmidt A, Bräunlich S, et al. Retrograde approach for complex popliteal and tibioperoneal occlusions. J Endovasc Ther 2008; 15(5):594–604.

Seldinger S. Catheter replacement of the needle in percutaneous arteriography. Acta Radiol 1953; 39:368–376.

Spies J, Bakal C, Burke D, et al. Standards for arteriography in adults. J Vasc Intervent Radiol 1993; 4:385–395.

Valji K. Standard angiographic and interventional techniques. In: Valji K, ed. Vascular and Interventional Radiology. Philadelphia, PA: W. B. Saunders, 1999:12–17.

4

Basic Sheath Access

At the initiation of every case, access must be secured. The basic sheath provides access for medication and contrast, is advanced over a guidewire, may or may not have a radiopaque tip, secures the access site, prevents bleeding during the procedure, and is a place where diagnostic catheters can be introduced. Chapter 3 offers some advice about choosing an access site and making it safe. After the site is chosen, the access needle is placed in the artery, and the initial guidewire choice is introduced, then what?The usual situation is to proceed with placement of a standard access sheath, and then arteriography. A guiding sheath or guiding catheter is typically placed when the decision is made to treat a specific disease segment. Access for endovascular therapy is covered in chapter 14. A sheath is used on every case, from diagnostic arteriography to complex interventions. As soon as the needle is in the blood vessel, you will be ready to place a wire. This chapter includes the steps you need to take between when the needle is in the artery and when the access is secure.

Basic Access Site Step-by-Step

Chapter 5 includes guidewires. The guidewire you introduce initially through the access needle in the artery is a compromise. It must be stiff enough to serve as an initial rail for initial sheath passage. The tip of the guidewire must be atraumatic, so that if pathology is encountered, it is not disrupted. The guidewire must be inserted up to a long enough distance so that the anchoring is secure in the vascular system for sheath advancement. If tortuosity of disease is encountered, a steerable guidewire is sometimes necessary. Access is performed with 0.035-in. diameter guidewires. In general, steerable guidewires in this platform, such as the Glidewire, do not have much shaft strength for sheath placement. A Bentson or Newton or Starter guidewire is usually adequate for initial atraumatic guidewire placement. If there is a lot of scar or disease in the groin, a Rosen might a better choice, but the tip is stiffer and a little more traumatic. If a Glidewire is needed, I usually exchange it out using a 4-Fr dilator and place a stiffer guidewire for sheath placement.

As soon as guidewire is in, a basic access sheath must be handy. An arteriogram through a 4- or 5-Fr catheter requires a 4- or 5-Fr sheath, respectively. If an intervention is already planned and the anatomy already examined, prepare and deploy a sheath through which to perform therapy. This is faster and smoother than placing a small caliber sheath and upsizing later. If there is much of a chance that a therapy may be precluded by some anatomic detail that will be revealed during the study, then go with a smaller sheath initially so that a minimally sized puncture site is created.

Intial Maneuvers to Secure the Access

After the guidewire is in place, some operators use dilators on a regular basis and some do not. Dilators are discussed in a section below. Hold pressure on the groin when the guidewire is alone across the arteriotomy. This helps to prevent blood from accumulating under the skin and around the puncture site in between dilator or catheter exchanges. When the needle is in the artery with the guidewire going through it, do not hold pressure. The needle is rigid and pushing on it may cause it to dislodge or the tip to injure the artery.

After the guidewire is in the artery, it is advanced away from the entry site. The guidewire must be advanced through the entry needle and into the artery at least far enough so that the floppy-tip portion of the guidewire has cleared the entry site. Fluoroscopy is initiated and the guidewire is advanced into the desired location. Pressure at the puncture site is held as the needle is removed. The guidewire is wiped with heparin–saline–soaked gauze or Telfa.

A dilator is placed. If a skin incision is desired, it is best to perform the incision directly over the dilator (Fig. 1).The dilator is a hard material and will be discarded after the access is achieved. The surgical blade can be placed directly on the dilator and the dilator over the guidewire may be used as a rail. This way the incision may be minimized. When the incision is performed over the guidewire itself, it is usually done blindly since blood comes out of the access site and pools at this location. When the puncture site incision is made over shaft of the sheath, the blade can easily cut the thin-walled sheath and it will leak until it is replaced.

When you use dilators, go to the same Fr number size as that of the sheath (this is a dilator that is one size OD smaller than the sheath) or one size larger than the sheath (this is a dilator that is the same size OD as the sheath). If it is a scarred groin, use a dilator with OD the same size as the sheath (one number size larger).

How Do You Place a Sheath?

After the sheath is selected, the dilator for the sheath and the sheath itself are each flushed and wiped with heparinized saline. The stopcock on the sidearm is turned to the "off" position. Before placing the sheath, double-check that you have the desired size in hand. Lock the dilator hub in place so that the dilator does not back out while the sheath is being advanced. Check the skin insertion site to see if the skin incision needs to be enlarged slightly. Confirm that the guidewire in place is one that is stiff enough to facilitate sheath placement. Sheaths can usually be placed using starting guidewires. If the sheath is large or long or passing through a scarred groin, consider a stiffer guidewire. Make sure that whichever guidewire is in place has been

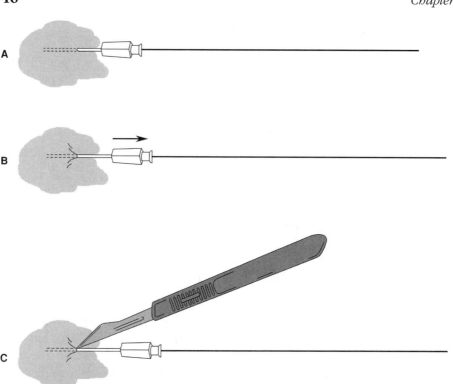

Fig. 1 Making a skin incision at the entry site. It is important to minimize the size of the incision to just what is needed for the case. (A) After the guidewire is placed and confirmed to be in the artery, a 4 or 5 Fr dilator is advanced over the guidewire. (B) When the dilator is withdrawn slightly, it 'tents' up the skin and draws out the tissue immediately surrounding the puncture site. (C) The scalpel is used to incise the skin directly over the dilator. The dilator will be discarded and it is much more resistant to a scalpel cut than a usual sheath.

advanced far enough so that the floppy tip is well inside the patient and that the artery entry site is crossed with the stiffer portion of the shaft of the guidewire.

Gradual, stepwise enlargement of the tract and artery entry site with dilators is not always required but is the cleanest way to place a sheath (Fig. 2). If the sheath is upsized by two French sizes or more, dilators should be used. When planning sheath placement through a difficult entry site (e.g., a scarred groin or a previously placed bypass graft), a series of vascular dilators should be used to predilate the entry site to one French size larger than the label on the sheath. This eases placement and helps prevent a buckle at the tip of the sheath that can damage the arteriotomy site and unnecessarily enlarge it. In between passing each dilator and eventually the passage of the sheath, pressure should always be held at the puncture site to prevent bleeding.

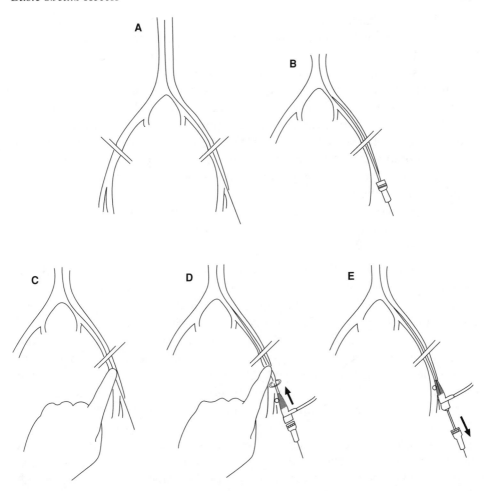

Fig. 2 Sheath placement. When multiple guidewire or catheter exchanges are anticipated, sheath placement permits safer, simpler, and more hemostatic access. (**A**) A
guidewire is placed in the infrarenal aorta. (**B**) The femoral arteriotomy is dilated
using the dilator appropriate to the sheath intended for placement. (**C**) Digital pressure is maintained over the arteriotomy to prevent hemorrhage after the dilator is
removed. (**D**) The dilator is placed within its sheath and the dilator–sheath combination is advanced over the guidewire. Slight pressure at the puncture site prevents
buckling of the sheath. The sheath–dilator apparatus can be rotated as it is advanced.
(**E**) After sheath placement, the dilator is removed.

The sheath is loaded onto the guidewire by an assistant and advanced
all the way to the entry site. The guidewire is pinned by the assistant. The
operator maintains gentle manual pressure with one hand at the access site
and with the other hand advances the sheath over the guidewire, through
the skin, and into the artery. Pressure is maintained at the puncture site until
the tip of the dilator or the sheath is inside the artery to tamponade the
arteriotomy. The sheath is advanced by holding it along its shaft near its tip
so that it does not buckle going through the skin. Sometimes it is helpful to

rotate the sheath back and forth to get through the subcutaneous tissue. Place the sidearm port in a convenient orientation, usually toward the operator. Occasionally, when the sheath is advanced, the dilator loosens at the hub and begins to back out. If this occurs, the open end of the sheath will be pushing bluntly into the tissues and will be damaged itself and may damage the artery. The sheath should be monitored visually during placement to pick this up if it occurs. Pressure is maintained on the arteriotomy with the free hand until the sheath can be felt going into the artery. This helps to avoid subcutaneous blood accumulation. After the tip of the sheath clears the arteriotomy, there is usually minimal resistance during advancement. The hand advancing the sheath can usually sense a "give" in the progress of the sheath, after which the sheath advances smoothly and easily. If there is resistance, something may be wrong. Use fluoroscopy to evaluate. Advance the sheath to its hub.

After the sheath is placed, take out the dilator that comes with the sheath, aspirate through the sidearm port, and flush with heparinized saline. After you administer contrast through the sheath, it should always be flushed. The sheath should also be flushed intermittently throughout any case. Occasionally, a continuous slow infusion of heparinized saline using a pressure bag is required to keep the sheath clear. If there is bleeding around a sheath during the case, apply gentle pressure. If that does not work, upsize the sheath to tamponade the tract. If the sheath is withdrawn at all to advance it any further, its dilator should be replaced before it is advanced. If the soft edges of the sheath tip have become frayed during a placement attempt, place a different one to avoid irregular tears at the arteriotomy site. When a sheath is placed in a patient with large and tortuous arteries, it tends to slide in and out. It is often worthwhile to secure the sheath with a stitch in the skin and around the hub to avoid spontaneous sliding. If a catheter is placed through the sheath that is labeled the same as the sheath size (i.e., a 5-Fr catheter in a 5-Fr sheath), it will not be possible to administer contrast or heparinized saline through the sidearm since the catheter completely fills the sheath. When performing interventions, you must know where the sheath tip is located to avoid performing balloon angioplasty or deploying a stent within the sheath.

Fluoroscopy is initiated as the catheter is advanced over the guidewire past the sheath. When lesions are encountered on the initial guidewire pass, it is usually best to stop the guidewire advance and secure the access site before crossing. If the guidewire is not far enough inside the artery to secure the access, a careful attempt should be made to cross the lesion. Guidewire and catheter exchanges are difficult in this position, with the guidewire barely inside the artery. Enough guidewire must be advanced into the artery so that the stiffer part of the body of the guidewire is in the arteriotomy, in order to support the advancement of a dilator. When a lesion is encountered in the iliac artery and the guidewire does not cross it, sometimes the guidewire can be looped on itself distal to the lesion in order to get enough guidewire length inside the artery to allow the stiffer part of the guidewire to be at the arteriotomy site.

When the access femoral artery is heavily calcified or there is a lot of surrounding scar tissue, the guidewire may well go in the artery but there may be significant difficulty in passing a dilator or sheath over it. In this case, the tip of the dilator may bounce off the diseased artery and the whole system, guidewire and sheath, may begin to buckle in the subcutaneous tissue. When the artery is scarred in an obese patient, this scenario is even more likely to occur. The operator can push in a more downward direction to pass the dilator, as if pushing toward the floor, so the dilator approaches the artery at nearly a 90-degree angle. The operator also guides the dilator and straightens the guidewire in the subcutaneous tissue using the nondominant hand (Fig. 3). After the initial dilator placement, the guidewire may be replaced if a different one is required for negotiation of lesions or if a stiffer one is needed over which to advance the sheath.

When is a Dilator Needed?

The use of dilators is unlikely to hurt anything, and in some cases may help a lot. A 4- or 5-Fr sheath can usually be passed without difficulty. If there is a lot of periarterial scar or the artery is heavily calcified, even a 4- or 5-Fr sheath may require use of a dilator. Make sure the guidewire is still straight using fluoroscopy and not twisted in the subcutaneous tissue. A dilator may then be advanced to secure the entry site and slightly dilate the tract. When the operator is concerned about the size of the sheath intended for placement or the quality of the access site, it is appropriate to initiate sheath placement using a dilator or even a series of dilators. When endovascular therapy is planned, the arterial access site may require substantial enlargement, from 4 or 5 Fr to 10 Fr or larger. This is done by passing progressively larger dilators over the guidewire (e.g., 6-, 8-, 10-Fr dilators) until the site is adequately sized to accept the intended therapeutic device. Since dilators are sized by outside diameter and sheaths are sized by inside diameter, a 7-Fr dilator is used to prepare the tract for a 6-Fr sheath. Occasionally, in a very scarred access site, it is necessary to place a dilator that is one size larger than the intended sheath. For example, an 8-Fr dilator may be required to prepare the tract for a 6-Fr sheath. During the sheath placement, if the tip of the sheath hits significant resistance as it is being passed into the artery, it is usually better to back off and take out the sheath and place the dilator to prepare the way. Be sure and inspect the tip of the sheath if the advancement is aborted. Occasionally, the initial pass into the subcutaneous tissue will result in tearing of the tip of the sheath. Keep in mind that the dilators are usually intended to prepare the tract and the arteriotomy, and usually do not need to be advanced to the hub. Occasionally, dilators are used to "sound" the artery,

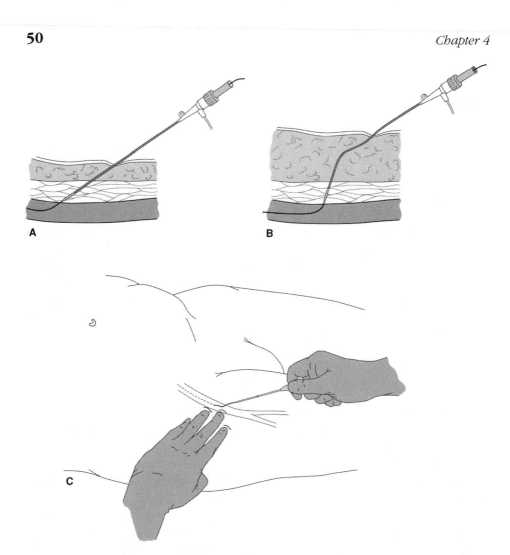

Fig. 3 Placement of the sheath in a calcified, thickened, or scarred artery. (A) After guidewire placement and enlargement of the subcutaneous tract, the sheath is advanced. (B) When the artery is calcified or thick-walled, or there is surrounding scar tissue, the tip of the dilator will sometimes bounce off the artery, instead of enter it. (C) The non-dominant hand can be used to press the tissues around the guidewire and to guide the tip of the sheath into the artery.

gently stretch the artery, or to dotter a diffusely diseased segment. This is a common maneuver in obtaining access for larger vascular devices such as stent–graft delivery catheters for treatment of abdominal aortic aneurysm. In this case, the dilator is usually advanced all the way into the artery.

Basic Sizing Issues

The sizing issues are confusing but they should be considered prior to the case. The therapeutic cases, especially the complex ones, may be a challenge with respect to sizing. In this discussion, some of the initial sizing issues are presented. In chapter 14 on Access for Endovascular Therapy, there is more detail about sizing. When referring to sizing, the discussion is usually about caliber. The length of each device is also important and is discussed in multiple venues throughout this text. Sizing, that is caliber consderations, determines what can be used and whether it may even be entered into the vascular system.

Guidewire diameter or caliber is measured in inches. The number "035" refers to a guidewire that is 0.035 in. in diameter. Guidewires are described in chapters 5 and 6. Available guidewire sizes are 0.010, 0.014, 0.018, 0.025, 0.035, and 0.038 in. in diameter. Each guidewire caliber has associated catheter sizes that are appropriate for use with it. The most commonly used guidewires are "014" and "035."

Dilator and catheter sizes are described using the French system. This system can be confusing until one gets used to it. This system is really a description of the circumference of the catheter. The French caliber measuring system is based on pi (3.14), the number of times that the diameter of a circle goes around the outside of the circle to make up the circumference. To convert from French measurement to the diameter of the catheter or sheath, one must be divided by pi or approximately 3. For example, the diameter of a 6-Fr sheath is approximately 2 mm, or 6 divided by 3. The diameter of a 24-Fr sheath is approximately 8 mm, or 24 divided by 3. To convert a Fr size, divide by 3, and that is how big the hole in the artery will be in millimeters.

Dilators and catheters are described by their outside diameter (OD) and sheaths are sized by their inside diameter (ID). A sheath is described by what will fit through it. This is appropriate since they serve as conduits and their function is to introduce other devices into the vascular system. A 6-Fr catheter has about a 2-mm OD and so on. When a catheter is placed percutaneously, it must always be exchanged for a catheter that is the same Fr size or larger so that the artery does not bleed around it.

When to Use Fluoroscopy

Fluoroscopy–eye–hand coordination is a developmental skill that must be gained by endovascular specialists. Surgeons learned a long time ago that surgical electrocautery is most efficient when the foot is not required as an intermediary in the process. Nevertheless, virtually all modern fluoroscopic equipment uses foot pedal controls. This introduces the potential for overuse and inefficiency since plantarflexion and dorsiflexion are required intermittently throughout the case.

Fluoroscopy is occasionally useful in planning the puncture (see chap. 3). This is especially true for the pulseless femoral artery or for antegrade femoral puncture. In performing an antegrade femoral puncture, where the accuracy of position is very sensitive, fluoroscopy can be very helpful for orientation. Fluoroscopy is not usually required during the actual puncture. Occasionally, when there is blood return from the puncture needle but the guidewire cannot be advanced, a fluoroscopy spot check of the guidewire position is warranted.

Soon after the guidewire has been placed into the artery after a routine puncture, fluoroscopy should be initiated. Fluoroscopy may be continuous or may be intermittent but frequent. If there is any resistance to guidewire advancement on the first pass, the operator should stop and check the guidewire's progress with fluoroscopy. The guidewire may have turned into the iliac circumflex vessel or another collateral route or may have encountered a lesion close to the puncture site. Any encounters with lesions must be observed using fluoroscopy. After the guidewire is in place, the catheter is then observed with fluoroscopy as it is passed over the guidewire.

About Access Sheaths

A hemostatic sheath provides protection of the arteriotomy from the irregular edges of endovascular devices. Multiple guidewire or catheter exchanges are made simpler and safer with a sheath in place. A sheath reduces the friction encountered at the access site when manipulating a selective catheter into a branch. An access sheath has a one way hemostatic valve, a dilator to stiffen it during placement, and a sidearm port that is used for the administration of medication or contrast. The sheath is advanced only with the accompanying dilator in place to avoid uncontrolled endarterectomy by the hollow sheath tip. The operator must be cognizant of the location of the tip of the sheath. Any angiographic or balloon catheter must clear the tip of the sheath to function properly. If there is a lesion intended for treatment near the puncture site, use a sheath with a radiopaque tip so that the tip of the sheath is easily identified. Sheaths are sized according to the largest-diameter catheter the sheath will accept (see the preceding section on sizing considerations). After the sheath is placed, the seal of the hemostatic valve can be opened for guidewire insertion by placing the tip of the dilator through the valve.

TECHNIQUE: HANDLING ACCESS SHEATHS

1. Flush and wipe the sheath and its dilator with heparinized saline.
2. Turn stopcock on sidearm to "off" position.
3. Double-check sheath size.
4. Lock or snug-fit the dilator into the hub of the sheath.
5. Enlarge the skin entry site.
6. Check guidewire type and position.

7. Use arterial dilators to prepare the tract.
8. Hold pressure at entry site during exchanges.
9. Assistant advances sheath–dilator combination to the skin entry site.
10. Assistant pins the guidewire.
11. Insert sheath by holding along its shaft.
12. Rotate sheath slightly to pass through the subcutaneous tissue.
13. Hold pressure at arteriotomy until tip of sheath is in the artery.
14. Orient the sidearm toward the operator.
15. Monitor sheath's dilator to make certain it does not back out.
16. If there is significant resistance in the artery, stop and evaluate.
17. Advance sheath to its hub.
18. After placement, remove dilator, aspirate, and flush.
19. Upsize the sheath if there is bleeding around it.
20. Don't advance sheath without dilator in place.
21. Replace sheath if tip is damaged or irregular.
22. Secure the sheath with a stitch if it tends to slide out (not usually necessary).
23. Do not inject through sidearm if sheath is filled with equally sized catheter.
24. Know where the tip of the sheath is located prior to an intervention.

5

Guidewire–Catheter Skills

Guidewire–Catheter Skills are the Basis of Endovascular Surgery

Guidewires and catheters comprise the foundation of endovascular intervention, both technically and conceptually. Guidewire–catheter skills are not necessarily intuitive but must be developed. Once acquired, these skills permit a different way of considering and treating vascular problems. Guidewires and catheters are useless without each other. However, the guidewire–catheter apparatus plays a role similar to that of the arterial clamp. It provides control and permits access to the vasculature. Although understanding the various types of guidewires and catheters is important, the specific function of each does not ring true until the clinician handles the apparatus and puts it to use. Although there are many correct choices, the wrong choice of a guidewire–catheter apparatus may become painfully obvious, often at the worst time, and may threaten the success of the procedure. This chapter provides an introduction to guidewires and catheters. Guidewires and catheters must be learned together. The manner in which these tools are manipulated is loosely called guidewire–catheter skills. As facility with these instruments grows, the guidewire–catheter combination becomes the best method of producing success in endovascular techniques.

Mastering Guidewires

Guidewires are the simplest tool available in the vascular specialist's workshop and nothing can happen without them. Mastering guidewires involves developing facility and understanding in guidewire choices, guidewire-handling techniques, and guidewire–lesion interactions.

GUIDEWIRE CHOICES

Successful guidewire deployment requires knowledge of choices. The goal is to choose the most appropriate guidewire first as often as possible and to know what to do next if the first choice turns out to be a bust. There are a full range of guidewires available. Rather than using them all, most vascular specialists develop a quiver of guidewires, which works for them in most situations. There are several standardized platforms and these are composed of different guidewire calibers. This was briefly discussed in the earlier chapter. Most of the time, basic and advanced access for sheaths placed outside the heart is with 0.035- or 0.038-in. diameter guidewires. 0.014-based devices are being used increasingly outside the heart for treating disease in branches and small vessels.In the next chapter, 014 guidewires and smaller platforms are discussed in detail.

GUIDEWIRE-HANDLING TECHNIQUES

Mastering the use of guidewires requires learning specific maneuvers. The facility and speed with which the specialist manipulates guidewires often determines the pace and success of the case. Understanding when to speed up, when to slow down, how firmly to grasp the wire, how hard to push, how to recognize tension in the guidewire, when to pull and when to push, and when to try a different approach when the chosen guidewire is not doing the job.

GUIDEWIRE–LESION INTERACTIONS

An essential step in the process of mastering guidewires is to understand the interaction between the guidewire's leading edge and the lesion with fluoroscopic imaging as the intermediary (Fig. 1). Observation of guidewire behavior in vivo requires patience. As the operator gains experience, the guidewire–lesion interaction becomes more predictable and a large proportion of these interactions are predictable. Because the fluoroscopic image provides a two-dimensional image of a three-dimensional process, the tip of the guidewire may easily trip on a portion of the lesion or another obstacle and appear stuck, sometimes repeatedly. These situations occasionally require a second or third choice of guidewire and/or the use of selective catheters. As the guidewire passes through lesions or around turns, the responsiveness of the guidewire tip becomes progressively less. One major advantage of the lower profile 0.014 guidewire (it is only 2/7 of the diameter of an 0.035) is that it is less likely to be unresponsive after passing through a tight lesion.

Figure 1 demonstrates the many ways that a guidewire may interact with a stenosis. Different types of guidewires may behave quite differently and when a catheter is added to support the guidewire and optimal imaging is used, it is rare to be unable to cross a stenosis with the guidewire. Most occlusions can also be crossed and treated with various guidewires supported by certain catheters and other devices using specialized techniques. There is more about crossing and treating various kinds of occlusions in Part III of this book.

What Makes Guidewires Different from Each Other?

Basic construction affects handling characteristics and makes each guidewire unique. Guidewires differ with respect to length, diameter, stiffness, coating, tip shape, and special features.

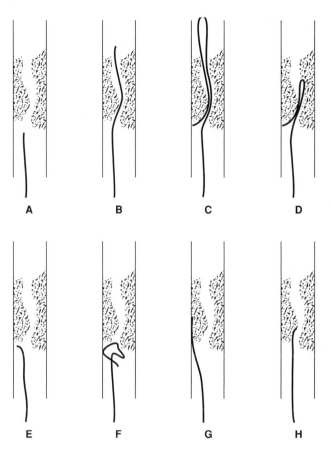

Fig. 1 Guidewire–lesion interactions. Several possible outcomes may result from interaction between the tip of the guidewire and an occlusive lesion. (**A**) A guidewire tip approaches a lesion. (**B**) The guidewire traverses the lesion on its first pass. (**C**) The guidewire's leading edge catches on the proximal end of the stenosis. The floppy-tip buckles allowing an elbow of guidewire to traverse the lesion. (**D**) The floppy tip begins to buckle but catches on a ledge of plaque and is unable to cross the lesion. (**E**) The guidewire tip hits plaque and is unable to find the eccentric lumen. (**F**) The guidewire piles up proximal to the lesion. (**G**) The guidewire finds a subintimal plane. (**H**) The guidewire disrupts plaque, which results in embolization of atherosclerotic material.

LENGTH

The operator must be certain that guidewire length is adequate to cover the cumulative distance required, both inside and outside the patient. The length inside the patient includes the distance from the access site to well beyond the lesion, so that access across the lesion will not be lost when catheter exchanges are made during the procedure. The length outside the patient includes the distance required to support the longest catheter intended for usage (most are between 65 and 145 cm in length) and permits the guidewire to extend beyond the end of the catheter so that hand control of the guidewire is always maintained (Fig. 2). Guidewire lengths vary from 145 to 300 cm, or even longer in special cases. One advantage of the mono-rail or rapid exchange system is that the length of guidewire required outside the patient is less than the coaxial system. This is because the guidewire is embedded in the catheter for only a short distance, usually 20 to 30 cm, not the entire catheter length.

DIAMETER

Vascular catheters are designed with a guidewire port of a specific diameter, and the diameter of the chosen guidewire must reflect this specification. The size (caliber or diameter) of the guidewire determines which "platform" is being used. Most operators are just thinking in terms of "large" or "small" platform. Many procedures can be performed with guidewires that are 0.035 in. in diameter, often referred to as O35 guidewires. Large devices, such as aortic stent–graft carriers, may require 0.038-in. guidewires. Medium- and small-diameter vessels may be treated with 0.018- or 0.014-in. guidewires. The 0.014 system is being used increasingly for branch vessel work in the noncoronary arteries. There is also a 0.025-in. system that has been used for a variety of devices, but much less commonly. A larger platform device can usually be passed over a smaller platform guidewire, but obviously the reverse is not true. If the guidewire is too big to fit in the guidewire lumen of the catheter, you are stuck.

STIFFNESS

Most guidewires have a tightly wound inner steel core that confers differing magnitudes of stiffness on the body of the guidewire. A surrounding wrap of lighter, more flexible wire helps prevent fracture and fragmentation while the guidewire is in use. Each platform, whether small or large caliber, has guidewires with varying levels of stiffness. The tip strength is measured for 0.014 guidewires as the weight in grams that it takes to bend the tip of the guidewire to a certain angle.

COATING

The coefficient of friction may be reduced by coating the guidewire with a layer of Teflon or silicone. This may affect many handling properties and will alter how much tenacity must be used to pin the guidewire during exchanges.

TIP SHAPE

The shape of the guidewire tip reveals a lot about what a guidewire is best used for. A starting guidewire (used to start the case) has a floppy tip.

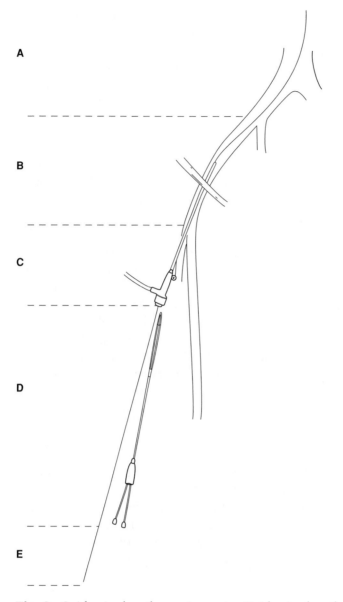

Fig. 2 Guidewire length requirements. Guidewire length requirements are represented in diagrammatic form. The length of guidewire required includes (**A**) the
distance beyond the lesion to secure access across the intended site of intervention,
(**B**) the distance from the arterial access site to the lesion, (**C**) the distance from the
hub of the sheath to the puncture site, (**D**) the length of the catheter intended for
use, and (**E**) the length of guidewire beyond the end of the catheter so that hand
control may be maintained.

A floppy-tip guidewire, which has no inner core in its tip and is therefore flexible, reduces the potential for endoluminal injury by buckling when it encounters resistance. A guidewire used for selective cannulation is curved or angled and may be steered into a desired location. Some guidewires have tips that may be hand shaped into a bend or a curve prior to insertion.

SPECIAL FEATURES

Some special features of guidewire construction include varying lengths of the floppy tip, antithrombotic surfacing, steerability with a high torque 1:1 ratio between the shaft and the tip, and varying degrees of stiffness of the shaft.

Guidewire Types in Practice

Although many features differentiate guidewires, most endovascular procedures may be accomplished using only a few types (Table 1). Starting guidewires, selective guidewires, and exchange guidewires are the three general types of guidewires that are employed in endovascular intervention. There are also a few specialty guidewires designed for specific tasks.

There are numerous starting guidewires available. These are floppy-tipped, general usage guidewires that are useful for catheter introduction and some interventional procedures and are intended to be atraumatic. The Bentson guidewire (Cook, Inc., Bloomington, Indiana, U.S.A.) is a reasonable choice. It has a floppy tip, steel construction, and a 0.035-in. diameter and it is relatively inexpensive. Most routine arteriography and angioplasty can be performed with this guidewire. The standard length is 145 cm and longer ones are available if needed. There are other guidewires that accomplish the same purpose such as the Starterwire (Meditech) and the Newton guidewire (Cook).

Selective guidewires are employed in cannulating side branches for selective catheterization or crossing critical lesions. These guidewires are steerable and some have hydrophilic coating. This class of guidewire includes the Glidewire, which is widely used in many practices. For crossing tight stenoses or highly irregular arterial segments, a hydrophilic-coated guidewire (i.e., Glidewire; Terumo) is useful since it seeks the path of the blood (liquid). These guidewires can be obtained with a straight tip or a steerable, angled tip. The straight tip is best as a backup for crossing occluded arteries. The steerable tip is useful for selective cannulation of side branches or critical stenoses. The steerable or angled-tip hydrophilic guidewire is the most widely used and for many specialists this is the first- or second-choice guidewire for a critically stenotic lesion. However, the hydrophilic-coated guidewire is so slick when it is wet that the operator often has the

Table 1 Guidewires for General Endovascular Practice

Guidewire type	Guidewire	Function	Features	Length (cm)	Diameter (in.)	Comments
Starting	Bentson[a]	General use, start the case	20-cm flexible tip, 6-cm distal floppy segment, straight, standard steel, TFE-coated	145, 180	0.035	Inexpensive, widely useful, good way to start the case
	Newton[a]	General use, start the case	10–15 cm flexible tip, 0–15 mm J-curved tip, standard steel, TFE coated	145, 180	0.035	
Selective	Wholey[b]	Selective catheterization	Floppy tip, shapeable curve, standard steel, steerable	150	0.035	Useful for catheterizing the superficial femoral artery after antegrade femoral approach
	Glidewire[c]	Crossing critical lesions, selective catheterization	Angled-tip, hydrophilic coating, steerable, regular, or stiff shaft	150, 180, 260	0.018, 0.025, 0.035	Best choice for most selective catheterizations and crossing critical lesions. Once across a lesion or a branch it does not provide much support
Exchange	Rosen	Exchange around major turns (e.g., aortic bifurcation)	J tip, not as stiff as Amplatz	180, 260	0.035	Useful for passing up and over sheath

	Name	Use	Description	Length	Diameter	Comments
	Amplatz SuperStiff[a,c]	Standard exchange, passing devices, support for endovascular interventions	1-cm flexible tip, straight	180, 260	0.035, 0.038	Best general exchange guidewire
	Lunderquist[a] exchange	Stiffest exchange	Straight, stainless steel shaft, resembles coat hanger.	260	0.035, 0.038	Used for stent–grafts in tortuous arteries
Specialty	J-guidewire[a,d]	Cross stents	Fixed-core, 5–10 cm flexible tip	145	0.025, 0.035	
	TAD[b]	Renal	36-cm tapered-tip extension available	145, 200	0.035→ tapers to 0.018	
	Magic Torque[c]	Renal	Flexible tip, cm markers	180	0.035	
	Roadrunner[a]	Crossing critical lesions, cerebral	Angled-tip, platinum spring coil tip, steerable TFE coating, 5-cm flexible tip	180, 300	0.018	

[a] Cook, Inc., Bloomington, IN.
[b] Mallinckrodt, Inc. St. Louis, MO.
[c] Boston Scientific, Natick, MA.
[d] Cordis, Miami, FL.
Abbreviations: TFE, tetrafluoroethylene.

impression that the guidewire is being advanced when, in fact, it is stationary. Occasionally, the guidewire may be withdrawn from the lesion without the operator realizing that this movement has taken place. If multiple catheter exchanges are required for treatment of a lesion that has been crossed with a hydrophilic-coated guidewire, it is often best to exchange this guidewire for a stiffer, less mobile one. In addition, because of the hydrophilic coating, the guidewire can slide easily along a dissection plane, which can be a problem if undetected, especially if a larger endovascular device is passed over it.

Standard construction, noncoated, metal guidewires may be curved at the tip. Simple manipulation of the end of the guidewire with a clamp adjusts the degree of curvature on the steerable tip (Fig. 3). Steerable guidewires come with a torque device that is locked onto the shaft of the catheter to provide a 1:1 turning ratio.

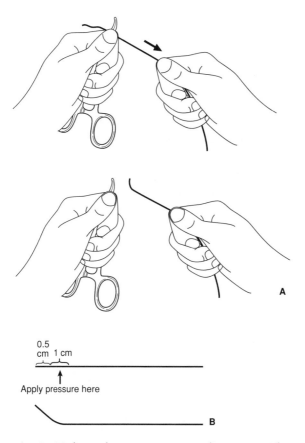

Fig. 3 Tighten the curve on a guidewire tip. The steerable guidewire is useful for selective catheterization and crossing irregular stenoses and occlusions. The amount of curvature at the tip of the guidewire can be adjusted using a simple maneuver. (**A**) The tip of the guidewire is trapped between the thumb and the edge of a hemostat. (**B**) The guidewire is pulled so that the metal edge of the clamp runs along the guidewire, which results in a tighter curvature at the tip. This is an especially helpful maneuver when using 0.014 guidewires.

Table 2 Guidewire Length Requirements

Length (cm)	Purpose
50–80	Catheterization of dialysis access. Retrograde femoral catheterization for ipsilateral femoral arteriogram
145–150	General arteriography and catheterization of the abdominal aorta and its branches, aortoiliac interventions, antegrade approach to infrainguinal arteries
180–210	Arch and carotid arteriography, renal and visceral interventions, contralateral infrainguinal interventions, subclavian interventions
200–300	Carotid intervention, exchange guidewire for aortic stent–graft placement

Exchange guidewires are stiffer than other guidewires and have a firm inner core. Once a guidewire has been appropriately placed (into a side branch, across a lesion, etc.), the security of that control may be enhanced by exchanging the initial guidewire for an exchange guidewire. If the intended path for the endovascular device is tortuous or the device is large, an exchange guidewire should be considered. The increased strength of the body of the guidewire makes it easier to pass devices over it and to maintain control across tortuous or distant passages. Some of the available exchange guidewires are the Amplatz (Cook or Boston Scientific Corp., Medi-Tech Division, Natick, Massachusetts, U.S.A.), the Rosen (Medi-Tech), and the Lunderquist (Cook). The stiff guidewire should not be used as the lead passage device or for initial entry through a lesion because it can cause damage. During complicated endovascular procedures, such as a complex, multistent reconstruction or stent–graft placement, a stiff guidewire is very useful.

J-tip guidewires are useful for passage through an occlusion or a previously stented arterial segment. The curved J tip is less likely to pass through the struts of a stent or create a false passage. Standard guidewire lengths are 145 to 300 cm. A guidewire length of 145 cm is adequate for catheter passage when performing general arteriography (Table 2). A 180-cm-length guidewire may be required for passage over the aortic bifurcation if the catheter is advanced into the contralateral superficial femoral artery (SFA). A 260-cm guidewire may be required for arch aortography or carotid arteriography, especially in a tall individual. A 260-cm guidewire, or sometimes even 300 cm, is required for long distances within the vasculature (e.g., brachial artery access to the lower extremity) or if the device intended for passage is particularly long (e.g., aortic stent–graft; Fig. 2).

TECHNIQUE: GUIDEWIRE HANDLING

Although choosing the appropriate initial guidewire is the most important decision to ensure success, facility with specific maneuvers makes the guidewire knowledge clinically applicable.

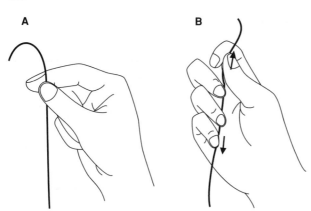

Fig. 4 Stiffen the floppy tip of the guidewire. (**A**) Floppy-tip entry guidewires (i.e., the Bentson) are relatively atraumatic to the endoluminal surface, but the tip is very flexible and sometimes difficult to handle. (**B**) The floppy tip of the guidewire can be stiffened by applying one-handed traction to pass it more easily through the hub of the needle or catheter. The guidewire is grasped with the thumb and forefinger near its leading edge and the third, fourth, and fifth fingers pin the guidewire against the palm. Applying traction causes the tip to stiffen and straighten.

1. Wet the guidewire with heparin–saline solution. All guidewires function better when wet, and hydrophilic-coated guidewires must be wet to function at all.
2. Stiffen the floppy tip of the starting guidewire (Fig. 4) so that it will pass through the entry needle hub and into the arterial access site.
3. Seek alternatives if the guidewire won't pass through the needle (see chap. 2 for plan of attack if the guidewire won't pass through the needle).
4. Always use fluoroscopic guidance, especially when encountering a lesion. Blind passage is random and may cause harm. Start fluoroscopic guidance soon after the tip of the guidewire passes the end of the needle in the access artery.
5. Don't give up hand control of the guidewire outside the patient until you are sure it is secure.
6. Don't force the guidewire.
7. Advance the guidewire in increments of a few centimeters (Fig. 5). Many small pushes are required. If there is too much length between the operator's hand position and the guidewire entry site, the guidewire kinks. Once a guidewire has a kink in it, it may be difficult to pass anything over it and the guidewire must be exchanged.
8. Take precautions when the guidewire tip encounters the lesion (Fig. 6) (see chap. 11 for a detailed discussion of crossing lesions).
9. Shape the guidewire tip. The standard, nonfloppy guidewire can be made more curved at the tip by running a metal clamp over the

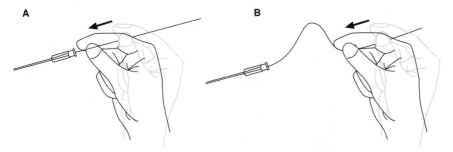

Fig. 5 Advance the guidewire incrementally. (**A**) The guidewire must be advanced a few centimeters at a time. (**B**) If there is too much length between the catheter hub and the location where the guidewire is grasped, the guidewire kinks.

> guidewire tip while holding the guidewire between the clamp and the thumb (Fig. 3). This is the same maneuver used to curl ribbon.
>
> 10. Have a torque device available whenever a steerable guidewire is used (Fig. 7). The torque device permits the operator to take advantage of the 1:1 turning ratio of the steerable guidewire.
> 11. Pin the guidewire during exchanges (Fig. 8). As a catheter is advanced over the guidewire, pin the guidewire without slack in

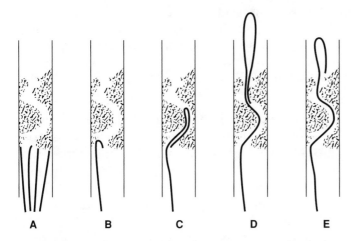

Fig. 6 Buckle the guidewire to cross a lesion. The leading edge of the guidewire may not be able to traverse an eccentric stenosis. If the guidewire begins to buckle, follow it and allow the elbow of buckled guidewire to become the leading edge. (**A**) The tip of the guidewire probes an eccentric lesion. (**B**), The leading edge of the guidewire does not enter the lumen of the lesion but the floppy tip begins to buckle. (**C**) The floppy tip forms an atraumatic elbow of guidewire. The guidewire is pushed as long as the elbow advances easily. (**D**) The elbow of the floppy tip emerges from the other end of the lesion. (**E**) After the end of the guidewire comes through the lesion, the buckle can be removed. This buckling technique is only good for moderately diseased arterial segments. If the lesion intended for crossing is critical or preocclusive in severity, the loop created by buckling may go subintimal.

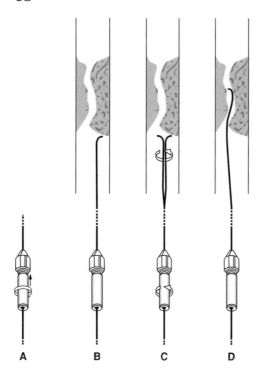

Fig. 7 Use a torque device with a steerable guidewire. (**A**) A torque device is placed on a steerable guidewire by holding the head of the torque device steady and turning its handle. (**B**) The steerable guidewire has a 1:1 turning ratio between the shaft and the tip. The guidewire tip approaches an eccentric stenosis. (**C**) The torque device turns the guidewire tip toward the lumen. (**D**) The steerable tip crosses the lesion.

it somewhere outside the patient. If the tip of the guidewire is near a lesion that should not yet be crossed, use intermittent fluoroscopy to ensure that the guidewire tip is not migrating and hitting the lesion. When removing a catheter over the guidewire, use the pin and pull technique.

12. Wipe the guidewire with heparin–saline solution-soaked gauze or Telfa after each exchange.

13. Confirm the intraluminal position of the guidewire before passing any endovascular devices over it.

14. Handle a hydrophilic-coated wire with the pincer grasp (between the thumb and the forefinger). Otherwise it will slide either too far in or out.

15. Rewind or put back in its case any guidewire that has been removed so that your back table work area does not degenerate into a confusing tangle.

16. Place a towel over the end of the guidewire outside the patient so it cannot flop around or fall of the table (Fig. 9). Some operators use a shodded clamp to secure the guidewire. When using a

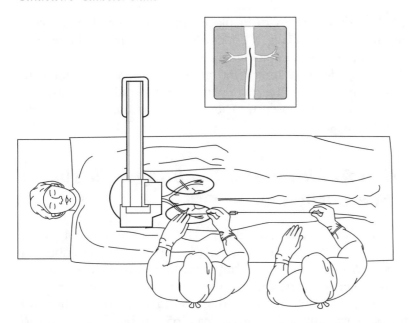

Fig. 8 Pin the guidewire. As the catheter is advanced, the guidewire is pinned so that it cannot advance simultaneously with the catheter. During catheter exchanges, the location of the tip is confirmed intermittently with fluoroscopy (inset).

buddy wire technique (two different guidewires going into the same access sheath), place a shod on one as an identifying marker. If a guidewire is contaminated, the procedure must begin again with a new guidewire. Sometimes the contaminated end of the guidewire can be removed by using a wire cutter and still maintain guidewire position.

17. Alter the qualities of a guidewire by placing a catheter or sheath over it for support. This may confer additional stiffness or body to the guidewire, which increases pushability.

18. Exchange a kinked or bent guidewire.

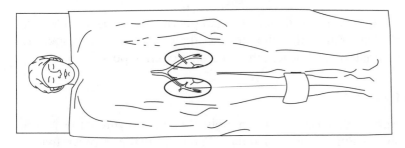

Fig. 9 Secure the guidewire. The segment of guidewire outside the patient is often quite lengthy and must be secured. A folded towel can be placed over the guidewire to prevent it from falling off the table. A contaminated guidewire must be cut off and exchanged.

19. Always leave the guidewire in place until the procedure is com-
    pletely finished, especially if endovascular therapy has been per-
    formed. Do not give up guidewire access!
20. Handle the guidewires. Important factors for successful guidewire
    placement are the way the guidewire feels as it advances and the
    appearance using fluoroscopy. These can be learned only by han-
    dling guidewires.

Introduction to Catheters: Exchange, Flush, and Selective Catheters

The simplest catheter is a vascular dilator. This is a short (12–15 cm),
slightly firm catheter with a single hole in the end and is described in
the earlier chapter. A dilator is most often used to secure vascular access
or to enlarge a percutaneous arteriotomy. Occasionally, it is appropriate to
perform arteriography through a dilator (e.g., femoral arteriography). An
exchange catheter is straight and long (at least 65 cm but may be up to
150 cm) and is used to exchange one type of guidewire for another. An
exchange catheter may also be used for interval arteriography to assess the
results of an endovascular procedure. A flush catheter is used for general
arteriography. It has an end hole and multiple side holes for high flow
administration of contrast. Flush catheter lengths vary from 65 to 100 cm.
The shape of the catheter head is usually rounded and promotes contrast
administration in multiple directions to create a blush appearance during
angiography. Selective catheters have a multitude of head shapes since
they are used to direct a guidewire into a specific location. Some selective catheters were designed with specific arteries in mind (e.g., carotid,
visceral).

Which Angiographic Catheter Should I Use?

Working with angiographic catheters is marked by the pleasant dilemma
of too many choices, rather than too few. Catheters differ with respect to
construction material, diameter, length, head shape, and special features.

CONSTRUCTION

Angiographic catheters are constructed of polyethylene, polyurethane, nylon,
Teflon, or a combination of these materials. Catheters made of polyethylene
have a low coefficient of friction and they are pliable, have good shape memory, can be torqued, and are useful for selective catheterization. Polyurethane
catheters are softer and more pliable and follow guidewires more easily, but
they have a higher coefficient of friction. Nylon catheters, which are stiffer

Table 3 Catheter Length Requirements

Length (cm)	Purpose
15–20	Dilator
65	Abdominal aortography with lower-extremity runoff
65–80	Selective renal and visceral catheterization
90	Arch aortography thoracic aortography
100	Selective cerebral catheters

and tolerate higher flow rates, are useful for aortography and general arteriography. Teflon is the stiffest material and is used mainly for dilators and sheaths.

DIAMETER

The diameter of the catheter should be as small as possible to accomplish the task at hand. Most angiography is performed with 4- or 5-Fr catheters over 0.035-in. guidewires.

LENGTH

The catheter must be long enough to reach the target site and still have enough length outside the patient for appropriate manipulations. Most commonly used catheters range from 65 to 100 cm in length but shorter and longer catheters are available for specific purposes. In general, use the shortest catheter that will perform the task (Table 3).

HEAD SHAPE

Catheter head shape determines function.

SPECIAL FEATURES

Some special features of catheters include various coatings, radiopaque tips, and graduated measurement markers.

Catheter Head Shape Determines Function

The potential for constructing different catheter head shapes is unlimited. Although hundreds are currently being marketed, most endovascular practice is based on the consistent and well-developed use of just a few types in most individual practices. Each specialist has functional favorites. Flush and selective catheters have divergent purposes and substantially different appearances. General catheter types are shown in Figure 10. These include

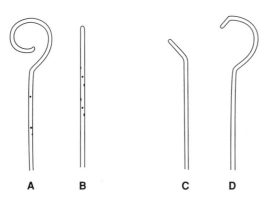

Fig. 10 Catheter head shape determines function: flush, exchange, simple-curve selective, and complex-curve selective catheters. Representative examples of the major categories of catheters as detailed in Table 4. (**A**) Flush catheters are used for aortography. They have an end hole and multiple side holes for high-pressure, high-volume contrast administration. This flush catheter example is a tennis racket catheter. (**B**) The straight catheter is used as an exchange catheter, to place a different guidewire into the artery. (**C**) Selective catheters have an end hole and a specially shaped tip. Selective catheters may have a simple curve, for directing a guidewire, as this Teg-T catheter. (**D**) Selective catheters may also have a complex curve, as this C2 Cobra. These catheters have a larger head which must be reformed in the aorta before using it to cannulate an artery. These catheters have specifically designed shapes and are used to enter aortic side branches such as carotid or renal arteries.

flush, exchange, and selective catheters. The selective catheters may have either a simple curve or a complex curve. Some catheters commonly used in endovascular practice are listed in Table 4.

Flush arteriographic catheters such as the pigtail are useful for high-pressure injection (up to 1200 psi) performed while minimizing a jet effect that might destabilize arterial plaque or thrombus. Most aortography and some peripheral arteriography can be performed with these catheters. The rounded catheter head can be converted to a hook shape by position-ing a guidewire partially into the head of the catheter. Most aortography begins with one of these flush catheters. The shape of the catheter head may be altered dramatically, depending upon the location of a guidewire placed within it. Although this is true for all catheters that are not straight, catheters with significant curve may assume the widest variety of configura-tions depending upon the location of the guidewire (Fig. 11). It is not unusual to have momentary but irritating challenge in removing a flush catheter over a guidewire. This is because the flush catheter usually has a head shape that makes the passing guidewire form a 180-degree loop with the guidewire tip coming back toward the operator. When the firmer segment of the guidewire reaches the catheter head, the catheter head flips up straight. If the catheter head is in a location that is too small in diameter to handle this maneuver, or there is disease nearby that could be dislodged by the flipping catheter head,

Table 4 Catheters for General Endovascular Practice

Catheter type	Catheter	Function	Length (cm)	Caliber (Fr)	Comments
Flush	Pigtail	Aortography	65, 90, 100	4, 5	
	Tennis racket	Aortography		5	
	Omni-Flush	Aortography: select aortic bifurcation, select renal artery	65	4, 5	
Exchange	Straight	Exchange guidewires, general arteriography	70, 90, 100	4, 5	
Selective: simple curve					
Short bent tip	Teg-T	Direct guidewire through lesion or into branch (30°)	70, 100	5	
	Kumpe	More angled than Teg-T (45°)	40, 65	5	Other examples: Berenstein, vert, DAV
Long bent tip	Multipurpose A	Direct guidewire, longer tip (45°)	65, 100	5	
	Multipurpose B	More angled than MPA (70°)	100	5	
Hook shape	RIM	Tight curve	65	5	Other examples: Hook, celiac Chuang A,B,D,E, Shepherd Hook
Selective: complex curve					
Cerebral	Simmons	Reshape to enter difficult arch branches, direct guide	100	5	Other examples: see table 2 in chapter 6
	Vitek	Reshape to enter difficult arch branches	100, 125	5	
Renal	C2 Cobra	Directs guidewire into side branch at 90° angle	65, 80	4, 5	Other examples: Sos-Omni 2, C3 Cobra
	Renal double curve	Directs guidewire laterally and inferiorly acute angle	80	5	Other examples: renal curve, and renal curve 2

Abbreviations: MPA, Multipurpose A; RIM, Right internal mammary artery.

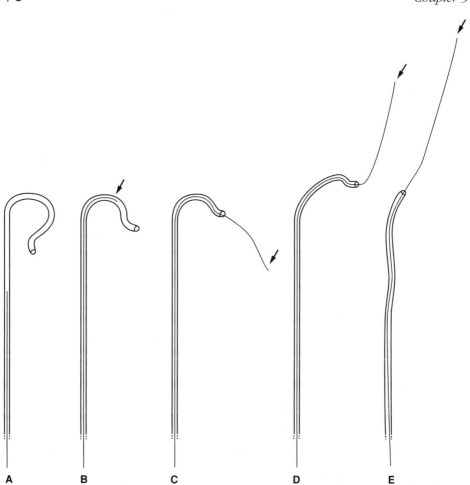

Fig. 11 Catheter head shape depends on guidewire position. The shape of the catheter head can be significantly modified by the position of the guidewire. This is especially true for flush catheters and complex-curve selective catheters. (**A**) A guidewire is present within the shaft of a hook-shaped visceral catheter. (**B**) The hook of the catheters head splays out as the guidewire enters the curve. (**C**) As the floppy part of the guidewire tip exits the catheter, the head of the catheter splays further. (**D**) The catheter straightens as the firm portion of the guidewire shaft occupies the curved portion of the catheter head. (**E**) As the firm portion of the guidewire exits the catheter head, the catheter straightens out completely.

consider taking another approach. Another option is to pass the guidewire through the catheter head but leave the catheter head curved. Go ahead and pull the catheter back over the guidewire and the curves at the head of the catheter should straighten. Do not let go of the guidewire as you walk down the wire doing the pin and pull. Sometimes if you let go of the wire, the loop in the catheter head maintains itself and actually pulls the guidewire back with it.

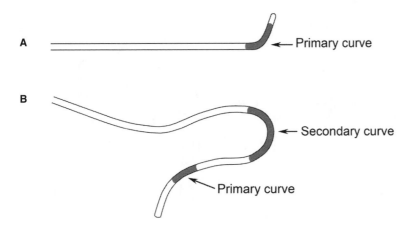

Fig. 12 Comparison of simple curve and complex curve catheters. (A) Simple curve catheters have only a primary curve that determines how they function. (B) Complex curve catheters have a primary curve and a secondary curve and sometimes more.

The straight catheter is useful as a general exchange tool, for interval arteriography, and to measure pressure proximal and distal to a lesion. It can add stiffness to a guidewire to allow it to pass or probe a lesion more easily or uncoil a guidewire that has piled up proximal to an unpassable lesion.

Selective catheters have either a simple or complex curved head shape. Figure 12 demonstrates the difference between a simple curve and a complex curve catheter. Every shaped catheter has a primary curve. When a catheter has only a single curve (primary curve) near its tip, it is a simple curve catheter. This is a "hockey stick" shape and it provides an angle of trajectory for a guidewire tip passed through the catheter that may be anywhere from just a few degrees to almost 90 degrees from the shaft of the catheter itself [Figs. 12 and 13(B)]. A complex curve catheter has a primary curve and also a secondary curve, and occasionally a tertiary curve. A complex curve catheter head needs to be reshaped inside the arterial system before it can be used to selectively cannulate a side branch [Figs. 12 and 13(E)]. The complex curve catheter head assumes a relatively straight configuration while it is being passed over the guidewire. When it arrives at its destination, the guidewire is withdrawn and the complex curve catheter attempts to shape itself. Specific maneuvers must be performed to achieve the correct shape. This is discussed in detail in chapter 9.

The bent-tip Berenstein catheter (Boston Scientific Corp., Medi-Tech Division, Natick, Massachusetts, U.S.A.) is a simple-curve selective catheter, but it can be used simultaneously for general applications. This catheter is useful for directing a guidewire through a critical lesion or into a branch

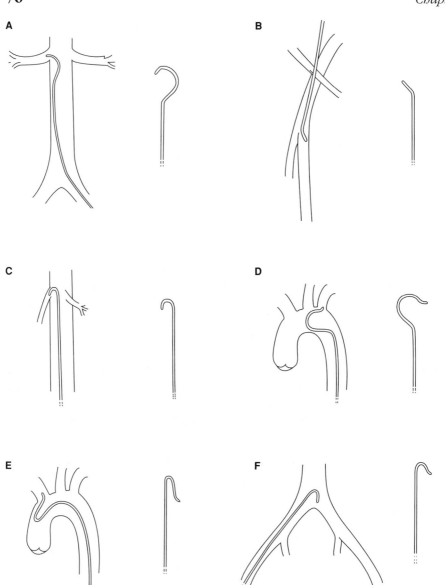

Fig. 13 Selective catheters in action. (**A**) A cobra catheter is used for renal artery catheterization. (**B**) A Berenstein catheter is used for cannulation of the superficial femoral artery. (**C**) A tightly curved hook-shaped catheter is used for catheterization of the visceral arteries. (**D**) A headhunter catheter can be used to enter the branches of the aortic arch. (**E**) A Simmons catheter is used to cannulate the carotid and innominate arteries. (**F**) A shepherd's hook catheter is used to cross the aortic bifurcation.

Table 5 Contrast Media Flow Through Catheters[a]

Type	Caliber (Fr)	Length (cm)	Maximum flow route (ml/sec)[b]
Flush (multiple side holes)	4	65	19
	4	100	15
	5	65	32
	5	100	27
Selective (end hole)	5	65	15
	5	100	11

[a] Data from Cook, Inc. (Bloomington, IN) using 100% Oxilan 350 at 25°C.
[b] Maximum pressure = 1200 psi.

vessel. The bend at the tip of the catheter confers directionality to the guidewire tip. Hook-shaped catheter heads are useful for turning an acute angle at a tight corner. Complex-curve catheter heads have a curve in one direction, then back in the other direction. These are used primarily to select out aortic side branches for cannulation. Examples include the Simmons and the H3 Headhunter cerebral catheters. Many head shape configurations have been designed for selective catheterization, each with a different purpose (see chap. 9 for a detailed discussion of selective catheterization).

The rate at which contrast may be administered through a catheter varies with the catheter caliber, its length, and the number of side holes (Table 5).

LINGO: CATHETER TALK

Trackability. The ability of the catheter to follow the guidewire through tortuous vessels and around corners without pulling the wire out of its intended location.

Pushability. The description of how a force applied by the operator at the hub of the catheter relates to the forward movement of the tip (the leading edge) of the catheter.

Crossability. The facility with which a catheter follows the guidewire across a lesion or through a diseased arterial segment.

Steerability. The steering responsiveness of the catheter tip to handling maneuvers performed at the hub.

French. The scale used to size catheters (1 Fr = 0.33 mm).

Handling Catheters

After the guidewire has been placed into the major flow stream of the arterial segment of interest, the next challenge is to pass the catheter into the correct location. The catheter should be suitable for the diameter sizing of the guidewire. In general, the catheter will follow the guidewire when it is advanced incrementally and the guidewire is pinned to ensure that it does not also advance. Don't advance the catheter unless the guidewire is pinned. If working over a hydrophilic guidewire, the guidewire must be pinned with a pincer grasp so that it is not accidentally advanced with the push forward on the catheter. The catheter is advanced by grasping it a certain distance from the hub of the sheath and giving it a push. Don't advance the catheter by grasping on the catheter hub. If the fingers are too far from the place where the catheter goes into the sheath, the catheter and guidewire will just bend. Each catheter and guidewire combination has a certain body to it based on the overall stiffness and strength of the combined structures. The stiffer the guidewire–catheter combination is, the farther down the catheter may be grasped with each incremental garb and push by the operator. An innate sense will be developed for this after doing many cases. If the catheter is grasped too far down the shaft, the whole thing will bend instead of advance. If it is grasped in increments that are too small, this easy part of the case will make it take all day.

The catheter won't advance very well over the floppy-tip portion of the guidewire (Fig. 14). When the catheter reaches the floppy portion of the

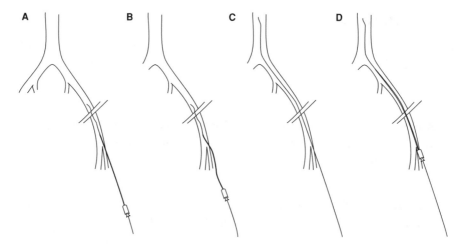

Fig. 14 Advance the catheter over the stiff portion of the guidewire. (**A**) The catheter is advanced into the arterial entry site over the floppy portion of the guidewire, which lacks the shaft strength to support guidewire advancement. (**B**) The catheter buckles and advancement stalls. (**C**) The guidewire is advanced so that the floppy portion is well inside the vasculature. (**D**) The catheter is advanced over the stiffer portion of the guidewire.

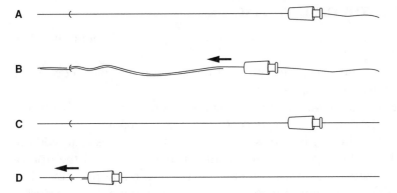

Fig. 15 Use stiffer guidewire if catheter buckles at entry site. If the catheter will not advance through the entry site over the firm portion of the guidewire, exchange for a stiffer guidewire. (**A**) Catheter tip attempts advance over standard guidewire. (**B**) The catheter tip advances a short distance beyond the entry site, but then begins to buckle. (**C**) A 4- or 5-Fr arterial dilator is passed to dilate the entry site and exchanged for a stiffer guidewire, such as an Amplatz Super-stiff guidewire. (**D**) The catheter is passed over the stiffer guidewire.

wire, the catheter head begins to take its shape and pushability is dramatically decreased. The guidewire may be advanced to ensure that a firm segment of the guidewire is available for the catheter to advance.

If the catheter cannot be advanced through the arterial entry site over the firm portion of the guidewire, an arterial dilator should be passed to predilate the entry site or a stiffer guidewire should be used to give additional support to the catheter (Fig. 15).

If pushability is lost after the vasculature has been entered, a stiffer guidewire should be considered. If the catheter cannot be advanced over the guidewire through a lesion, the lesion itself may be providing the resistance; either the stenosis is so severe that the guidewire itself occludes the residual lumen or the guidewire is subintimal.

When the catheter cannot be advanced into position because of significant vessel tortuosity or because of the long distance between the catheter head and the entry site, a steady and gentle withdrawal of the guidewire while the catheter is advanced decreases friction at the level of the catheter head and usually accomplishes the requisite advancement, if it is not too far. This is the "push-pull" technique. The risk of using this maneuver is potentially losing guidewire access. Do not advance the catheter beyond the end of the guidewire or allow the catheter head to reform during advancement. If the catheter and guidewire combination tends to buckle freely, the operator can choose to insert a stiffer guidewire. Another option is to leave the guidewire in place, remove the catheter, insert a long sheath to decrease friction, and reinsert the catheter through the sheath.

TECHNIQUE: CATHETER HANDLING

1. Prepare the catheter by flushing and wiping with heparin–saline solution.
2. Choose catheter size, length, and head shape that will most easily accomplish the proposed task.
3. Place the guidewire in the correct location. This is probably the most important factor in successful catheter placement.
4. Whenever the guidewire is in place across the access site without a catheter, hold pressure at the arterial entry site until the appropriate dilator, sheath, or catheter is passed to tamponade bleeding from the arteriotomy. Bleeding into the subcutaneous tissue during exchanges leads to postprocedure ecchymosis. Pressure in the right place helps to minimize the likelihood of hematoma formation.
5. Use mosquito clamp to dilate skin entry site to the appropriate size for the intended sheath or catheter.
6. Pass the sheath or catheter through the skin and soft tissue over the stiff portion of the guidewire, not on the floppy segment (Fig. 14).
7. Consider using sequential arterial dilators, a stiffer guidewire, or a hemostatic access sheath if the catheter cannot be advanced across the entry site.
8. Advance the catheter incrementally, a few centimeters at a time.
9. Handle the catheter near its entry site when advancing and at its hub when steering.
10. Maintain hand control of the guidewire. An assistant should pin the guidewire so that it does not simultaneously advance (Fig. 8).
11. If the catheter won't cross a lesion and arteriography is the goal, use a different approach and don't force it. If therapy is the goal (e.g., balloon angioplasty), make sure the guidewire is in the correct location across the lesion. Then predilate the lesion with a small-diameter angioplasty balloon.
12. If the catheter won't advance because of long distance and/or multiple turns from the leading edge to the operator's hand, and there is plenty of guidewire in place ahead of the catheter tip, gently and steadily withdraw the guidewire while advancing the catheter to reduce friction. Continuous fluoroscopy is required during this maneuver to ensure that the guidewire is not withdrawn too far.
13. If the catheter has a longer distance to travel and cannot be advanced, it is usually due to accumulated friction. Place a long sheath to decrease friction, use a stiffer guidewire, or choose an alternative entry site.
14. After the catheter is in place, aspirate and flush with heparin–saline solution. Do not inject anything unless there is appropriate blood return.
15. Puff contrast to verify placement and ensure that the catheter tip is in a safe position before high-pressure injection is performed.

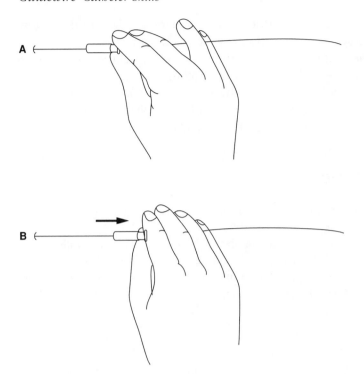

Fig. 16 "Walk along" the guidewire to remove catheter. When a catheter is exchanged, the guidewire position is maintained while the catheter is removed. (**A**) The catheter hub is grasped between the thumb and the forefinger and the guidewire is grasped between the fourth and fifth fingers of the same hand. (**B**) The catheter hub is withdrawn while the guidewire position is held constant. The fourth and fifth fingers then grasp the guidewire again at the further distance along its length and the maneuver is repeated. This creates the appearance of the hand "walking along" the guidewire.

16. When removing or exchanging the catheter, maintain guidewire placement by "walking along" the guidewire while the catheter is being pulled (Fig. 16). Intermittent fluoroscopy checks should be performed to ensure that guidewire position is maintained.
17. If the end of the catheter becomes knotted, pass a stiff guidewire into the catheter to untangle it.
18. If there is any doubt about the location of the catheter, make sure it is intraluminal. Check for blood return. Twirl the catheter and visualize the catheter head moving using fluoroscopy to be certain that it moves freely. Puff contrast to see that it rapidly enters the flow stream rather than staining the wall of the artery or remaining stagnant.
19. It is common to have difficulty identifying the catheter as it is being placed. Consider using a catheter with a radiopaque tip. When advancing any catheter over a guidewire, there is a slight bend of

the guidewire at the location of the catheter head and this imprint can be monitored fluoroscopically as it is advanced.

20. Remove the catheter over a guidewire to straighten the catheter head. This prevents injury to the endoluminal surface.
21. After the guidewire has been removed, if there is uncertainty about the location of the catheter head, add a milliliter of contrast to fill the catheter and it may be better visualized.

Selected Readings

Neequaye SK, Aggarwal R, Van Herzeele I, et al. Endovascular skills training and assessment. J Vasc Surg 2007; 46(5):1055–1064.

Tedesco MM, Pak JJ, Harris EJ Jr, et al. Simulation-based endovascular skills assessment: The future of credentialing? J Vasc Surg 2008; 47(5):1008–1011.

Verzini F, De Rango P, Parlani G, et al. Carotid artery stenting: Technical issues and role of operators' experience. Perspect Vasc Surg Endovasc Ther 2008; 20(3):247–257.

6

Small Platform Guidewires and Monorail Systems

The Development of Small Platform Guidewires and Monorail Systems

Small platform guidewires with 0.014-in. diameters were developed to manage the smaller diameter arteries of the coronary vasculature. Coronary arteries range in size from less than 1 to 4 mm in diameter. Using higher caliber 0.035-in. diameter guidewires and 4- or 5-Fr catheters would be severely limiting in the coronary circulation. The routine use of 0.014-in. platforms in the coronary circulation has been standard for many years and more recently has been adapted for use in carotid, renal, and infrainguinal systems. The coronary system, in addition to being small diameter, is remote from major arterial access sites, such as femoral and upper extremity arteries. The monorail system or so-called "rapid exchange" system help to make long distance passage of devices faster and delivery more stable. Figure 1 demonstrates how a monorail system works.

How Do Monorail Systems Differ from Coaxial Systems?

The coaxial system has been the standard in the noncoronary vasculature for decades. The coaxial system is one in which there is a channel in the catheter for the guidewire and that channel is present along the whole length of the catheter. The guidewire goes into a lumen that is visible on the tip of the catheter, and the guidewire emerges from the catheter on the other end. This is a relatively stable situation because the presence of the guidewire along the whole length of the catheter confers a certain stiffness and support to the catheter. During a therapeutic procedure, such as balloon angioplasty or stenting, the position of the sheath tip need not be close to the target lesion for treatment because the coaxial nature of the guidewire is usually sufficient to maintain stability. The disadvantages of the coaxial system are as follows. The presence of the guidewire over the whole length of the catheter causes a lot more friction since the catheter and guidewire are in direct contact with each other over a long distance. The need for the internal position of the guidewire within the catheter also raises the profile of the catheter, making it just a little larger in caliber.

In the monorail system, the channel in the catheter in which the guidewire is placed is along a much shorter distance and is present only at the leading end or tip of the catheter. The guidewire goes into a lumen that is visible on the tip of the catheter, and the guidewire emerges from the side of the catheter. The guidewire channel may be 5 to 30 cm in length, and much less than the total length of the catheter. Monorail and coaxial systems can be used with either 0.014-in. guidewires or 0.035-in. guidewires. Guidewires that are 0.014 in. in diameter are usually employed with monorail

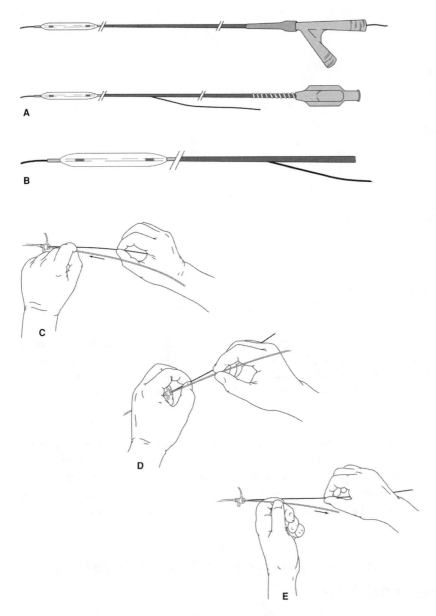

Fig. 1 Comparison of coaxial and monorail systems. (**A**) The coaxial balloon angioplasty catheter (top) has a guidewire lumen that is present for the whole length of the catheter. The monorail balloon angioplasty catheter has a guidewire lumen that is present for only part of the length of the catheter. (**B**) Close up of the monorail balloon angioplasty catheter shows that the lumen for the guidewire begins at the tip of the catheter and exits along the shaft. (**C**) The monorail catheter may be inserted with one hand and the operator is also able to pin the guidewire with the other hand. (**D**) After the front end of the monorail catheter is inserted in the sheath and the catheter and guidewire are separate as they exit the sheath, the left hand is used to hold the guidewire steady, while the right hand is used to advance the catheter. The reverse of this maneuver can be used to remove the catheter. The catheter may be removed for most of its length by holding the guidewire steady with the left hand and withdrawing the catheter with the right hand. (**E**) When the catheter has been removed to the point where the guidewire and catheter are joined together, the two-handed technique is used t remove the remainder of the catheter.

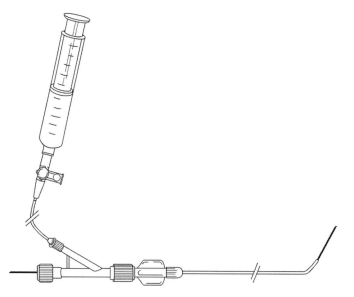

Fig. 2 Advantage of the 014 system. The 014 guidewires are low profile and may be placed through a 4 or 5 Fr angiographic catheter and this leaves space to administer contrast or medication and still maintain guidewire access. A Tuohy-Borst adaptor is used to secure the system, prevent backbleeding, and permit contrast administration.

systems, and guidewires that are 0.035 in. in diameter are usually employed with coaxial systems. This apparent exclusivity is not a structural requirement and is probably more procedural habit and manufacturing convenience than anything else. Some of the devices for lower extremity and carotid revascularization that are 014 compatible are also coaxial in design (Fig. 2).

What are the Advantages and Disadvantages of Monorail Systems?

The monorail system gives the operator more control over the guidewire and makes it stable. The monorail system has less friction, so pushability of catheters is faster and smoother. Catheter insertion can be done more independently since the operator can pin the guidewire without help from an assistant. Catheter removal is faster since most the catheter can be removed in a single long pull without any guidewire manipulation. The "pin and pull" segment of the catheter that takes longer to remove is much shorter. The guidewires used for monorail systems may be shorter. The guidewire length required outside the patient is not the whole length of the catheter, but is only the length of the monorail segment along the catheter. An example of how this works is in carotid stenting: with monorail systems, a 180-cm guidewire is used and if a coaxial system is required, a 300-cm guidewire is used. The sheath tip must be close to the target lesion; this permits the monorail catheter and guidewire to be close together and to be directed into the target lesion. If the sheath tip cannot be placed close to the lesion, as is sometimes the case with infrainguinal interventions, the catheter may not follow the guidewire after it passes out of the end of the sheath.

The coaxial systems are meant to travel over any distance, even long distances, with the guidewire as support. These tend to be stable systems, as mentioned earlier. When a stiff 0.035 guidewire is used, or even a 0.038 guidewire, the system is more stable. The challenge comes with the amount of friction generated by having the guidewire channel take up the length of the catheter. Pushability is diminished. The amount of force and effort required to insert and remove the catheter over the guidewire is increased. When the catheter is removed, the operator must perform the "pin and pull" technique, gradually removing the catheter from the patient and taking great care to avoid removing the guidewire or losing guidewire position. If it is a long catheter, the "pin and pull" maneuver over a long distance brings the operator further away from the monitor and the patient.

Principles for Use of Rapid Exchange Systems

The monorail system is demonstrated in Figure 1. After the 0.014-in. guidewire is in its desired location, the catheter is placed on the guidewire and advanced to the hub of the sheath. The operator is able to reach and pin the guidewire with one hand and advance the catheter with the other hand. Once the catheter is in far enough that the monorail segment of the catheter is inside the sheath, the guidewire and the catheter will each be exiting the hub of the sheath separately. The operator can then use one hand to hold the guidewire, usually stabilizing the sheath at the same time. The other hand is used to advance the catheter. After therapy is complete, the catheter is removed by reversing the order of events. One hand rests on the hub of the sheath and pins the guidewire between thumb and forefinger. The other hand retracts the catheter until the location where the guidewire and catheter join starts to emerge from the hub of the sheath. After that, a short distance of "pin and pull" is required. There are many ways to perform the "pin and pull" maneuver. The key is to find one comfortable for you so it is quick and smooth.

Which Platform Is Best for Each Task?

Coronary interventions are performed using guidewires that are 0.014 in. in diameter. This is less than half the caliber of the 0.035-in. guidewires that

Table 1 Preferred Platform for Different Endovascular Procedures

Intervention	Platform
Carotid stent	014
Common carotid, innominate stent	014 or 035
Subclavian stent	014 or 035
Thoracic aortic stent–graft	035 or 038
Abdominal aortic stent–graft	035
Aortoiliac stent	035
Renal or visceral stent	014 or 035
Femoro-popliteal intervention	014 or 035
Tibial intervention	014

have generally provided the platform for most noncoronary interventions over the years. In general, aortic and iliac procedures are performed with "035" systems (Table 1). Branch arteries such as carotid, renal, visceral, and infrainguinal may be treated using either platform. However, the majority of procedures are moving toward "014" for all branch artery reconstructions. The lower profile, the simplicity of the monorail systems, and the ability to place the guiding sheath close to the lesion all favor use of small platform monorail systems for these branch artery interventions.

7

Guidewire and Catheter Passage

The Goal of the Procedure Determines the Course of the Guidewire–Catheter Apparatus

The guidewire–catheter apparatus is the endovascular workhorse. Before you go to any trouble, be as deliberate as possible about establishing the goal of the procedure and anticipating the likely scope of the arteriogram or intervention. The operator must decide what it should be composed of in any given case and decide how to get it into position. After percutaneous access has been achieved (chap. 3) and guidewires and catheters have become familiar tools (chap. 5), the next step is guidewire and catheter passage to the desired location. The goal of the intended procedure should be well proscribed prior to the puncture. Whether an arteriogram or a therapeutic intervention is planned will influence the puncture site choice and the approach. Options should be considered for converting the procedure from a strategic one to a therapeutic one if the need should arise. Access for endovascular therapy is discussed in chapter 14.

When arteriography is the goal, the smallest acceptable access sheath should be placed. Angiographic catheter head placement at specific locations is required for visualization of the desired anatomic area. Selective catheterization for arteriography or therapy requires specific steps, which are discussed in chapter 9. Crossing lesions with guidewires and catheters prior to endovascular therapy is presented in chapter 11. Other details of catheter head placement for arteriography are discussed in chapter 10. These maneuvers have been separated into a stepwise approach for illustrative purposes. As the operator gains facility, one step leads to the next in a seamless flow of events that lead toward the goal of the procedure.

INITIAL CATHETER PLACEMENT

Bony landmarks or other anatomic signs are usually adequate to establish the correct location for catheter head placement (Fig. 1). The catheter head may be advanced or withdrawn slightly without reintroducing the guidewire. Hand-powered injection of contrast to establish the position is usually worthless through a 5-Fr catheter into the aorta. Hand-powered contrast injection may be used to visualize smaller, lower-flow arteries. After the catheter is in place, aspirate, remove bubbles, flush with heparin–saline, and connect to the injector, meniscus to meniscus. Then have the technician aspirate through the injector and inspect the line for air bubbles.

FLUOROSCOPY FOR CATHETER PLACEMENT

Table 1 summarizes some general concepts about when to use fluoroscopy for guidewire and catheter placement. The guidewire should be advanced so that its floppy portion extends beyond the location desired for catheter

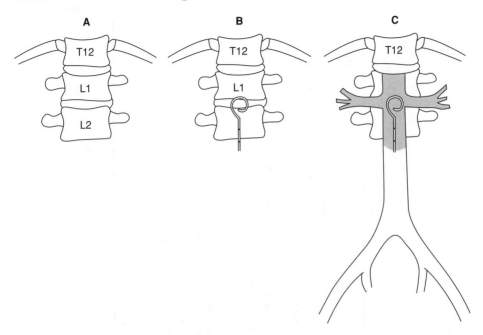

Fig. 1 Use landmarks to assist with catheter positioning. Bony landmarks are used to help place the arteriographic catheter. (**A**) The renal arteries are usually located near the junction of the first and second lumbar vertebral bodies. The twelfth thoracic vertebral body is identified by its attached ribs and the operator counts down. (**B**) The catheter head is placed near the L1–L2 junction so that a high-pressure injection of contrast will reflux a few centimeters above that level. (**C**) The aortogram demonstrates the origins of the renal arteries.

head placement. After the guidewire is appropriately placed, fluoroscopy stops while the catheter is prepared and advanced over the guidewire outside the patient. Fluoroscopy is initiated again when the catheter is in the artery. The progress of the catheter is monitored using fluoroscopy until it is in the desired location. Fluoroscopy is used as the guidewire is withdrawn to ensure that the head of the flush catheter assumes its proper shape (Fig. 2). As the guidewire is removed from the curved-head shape of the flush catheter, the catheter head which has been straightened onto the guidewire assumes its shape which shortens the overall length of the catheter. Therefore, the catheter is usually advanced a little further into the artery than appears necessary. After the guidewire is removed, it is useful to twirl the catheter to ensure its tip is free within the flow stream. It is usually best to avoid unguided interactions between the catheter and any lesions along the way. The position and behavior of the catheter is helpful in determining whether the catheter is in a safe position. If there is doubt about that, hand administration of a small amount of contrast will solve the issue. In general, intermittent fluoroscopy can be performed to provide adequate information to guide the case but minimize the radiation required.

Table 1 When to Use Fluoroscopy During Guidewire and Catheter Passage

Task	When?	Purpose	How Often Is It Necessary?
Planning puncture	Prior to arterial puncture	Identify anatomy when there is no pulse or poor pulse; locate proximal femoral artery for antegrade puncture	Occasional Usually
Guidewire passage through entry site	Guidewire won't pass	Guidewire passes through needle but won't advance into artery; check guidewire position/direction with fluoroscopy	Occasional
Advancing guidewire into position	Soon after guidewire enters the artery	Observe guidewire progress, avoid endoluminal injury, avoid passing the guidewire into the wrong place	Always
Advancing catheter through entry site	Catheter won't advance through entry site	Check to see if catheter is coiling in the subcutaneous tissue; check to see if guidewire is bent	Rare
Advancing catheter into position	Soon after catheter enters the artery	Observe catheter progress; monitor position	Always
Removing guidewire	As guidewire is withdrawn from catheter head	Observe appropriate formation and final position of catheter head	Always

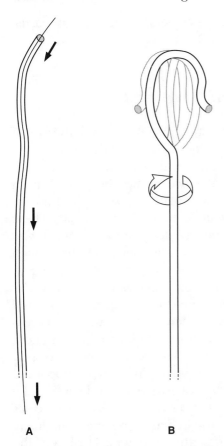

A   **B**

Fig. 2 Evaluate the catheter head to ensure that it has reached its appropriate shape and location. (**A**) As the guidewire is removed, the catheter head can be observed to take its preformed shape. (**B**) The catheter may be twirled to make certain that the catheter head is not stuck against the wall of the artery.

Guidewire and Catheter Combinations

There are many correct guidewire and catheter choices. But if the one you have chosen is not working, move on. The goal of the procedure, whether strategic or therapeutic, determines the order and range of choices of guidewires and catheters. The guidewire is chosen first for routine arteriography. If a guiding sheath is needed to treat a lesion, a stiffer guidewire is required for sheath placement. If crossing lesions is required to set up a therapeutic procedure, a different guidewire may be required. If the initial guidewire choice is not successful, a catheter may be placed over it to alter the handling characteristics of the guidewire. A catheter may add stiffness, steering, and pushing strength to a guidewire. When the goal is selective catheterization of a branch artery before the lesion is encountered, the catheter is selected first. When a selective catheter is required, the usual guidewire choice is hydrophilic (low friction) and steerable (directionality).

Passing Through Diseased Arteries

As a general rule, lesions are only crossed just prior to performing therapy, if at all possible (chap. 11). Occasionally, arteries may be so diffusely diseased that there is no approach through relatively healthy segments for arteriographic catheter placement. In addition, a puncture may be placed in an artery with a relatively normal pulse, and there may be a severe but unsuspected stenosis just upstream or downstream from the puncture site. These factors indicate that fluoroscopy should be initiated early after guidewire insertion. The guidewire should be advanced steadily but carefully through diseased segments. If the guidewire forms a leading elbow, continue to advance the guidewire but do not force it. You don't want the guidewire to become a loop stripper. When the guidewire does not cross the desired arterial segment, place a dilator over the guidewire to secure the access site and remove the initial choice guidewire. If the guidewire has formed a loop, use the catheter to pull the guidewire back to remove the loop. Puff contrast to ensure intraluminal position and to obtain information about the diseased segment. The catheter is used in this case to guide and support the guidewire. A hydrophilic-coated guidewire may cross the artery with greater ease. Use a steerable guidewire and probe the lumen of the artery gradually as the guidewire is advanced (Fig. 3). After the guidewire is placed, the catheter is advanced over it and is continuously observed using fluoroscopy. If the arterial segment that has been crossed is severely diseased, the passage of the guidewire and catheter may stop flow or slow it down. Consider anticoagulation to avoid generating thrombus and also consider whether the arterial segment should be treated right away.

PLAN OF ATTACK: CATHETER WON'T FOLLOW GUIDEWIRE

1. Use gentle catheter manipulations to assess the exact location where the catheter fails to pass. Where is the hang-up? Is it at a location of disease or tortuosity? Is the guidewire at that location stiff enough or is that segment too floppy?

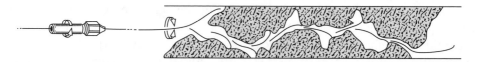

Fig. 3 Passing through severely diseased arterial segments can be challenging. A steerable guidewire may be used to make multiple turns in attempting to cross a lengthy critical lesion. The guidewire tip may be used to probe the lesion.

2. Is the guidewire kinked? A seemingly minor kink may be very difficult to pass with the catheter. Use a magnified view to study the guidewire. Withdraw the guidewire a few centimeters and pass the catheter again.

3. Is the guidewire subintimal? Does the guidewire itself move freely within the artery? Usually, when the guidewire is in a dissection plane, it will not advance beyond a certain point and it will appear tethered at the point of subintimal passage. Is the guidewire in a small collateral or side branch?

4. Is the lesion so critical that the guidewire itself has interrupted flow and there is not enough residual lumen to pass a catheter? In this case, heparin should be given. Immediate plans should be made for either treating the lesion or withdrawing from it.

5. In these situations, consider passing a smaller (4 Fr) straight catheter with side holes. After the tip of the straight catheter is passed just beyond the point of obstruction, the guidewire may be withdrawn and a puff of contrast should clarify the situation and an appropriate guidewire may be placed.

Negotiating Tortuous Arteries

There are two issues: advancing the guidewire through a tortuous passage and advancing the catheter over the guidewire. Sometimes the guidewire will go but the catheter won't go over it. Sometimes the guidewire will not advance unless it is supported by a sheath and possibly also a catheter. Tortuous arteries place constrictions upon guidewires and catheters that may not be immediately obvious under the two-dimensional representation available with fluoroscopy. Anatomic segments such as iliac vessels and branches of the aorta may exhibit tortuosity, kinks, and loops. Despite a widely patent lumen, forces upon the guidewire–catheter apparatus may be such that they are prevented from advancing after passing through multiple turns. Each turn in a tortuous system restricts the forward movement and the steerability of the catheter as it approaches the next turn. Oblique views of the tortuous segments are useful to identify the true angles followed by the arteries. A steerable, hydrophilic guidewire helps to negotiate the turns. A straight or angled-tip catheter may be passed over the guidewire to help straighten some of the initial curves and provide support for the guidewire as it goes into its next turn. A sheath may also be placed at the entry site. This may be very useful for decreasing friction, even if it only reaches through the first major turn the guidewire has to make. After the guidewire and catheter have been passed, consider exchanging the guidewire for a stiffer one before initiating therapy. When the forward motion of the catheter stalls, the options are as follows: place the guidewire further into the system, place a stiffer guidewire, exchange for a longer access sheath to support the guidewire–catheter apparatus and straighten some of the initial tortuosity, and use a softer, more hydrophilic catheter.

Going the Distance: The Very Remote Puncture Site

A very remote puncture site may occasionally be required by a variety of circumstances. An example of this includes infrainguinal intervention through a brachial approach when a femoral approach is contraindicated by anatomy, infection, previous surgery, or other conditions. The approach required for arteriography is different from that required for treatment. Arteriography requires catheter positioning upstream from the lesion, whereas therapy requires guidewire and catheter placement across the remote lesion at a distance where guidewire control may be poor. The operator must be prepared to undertake multiple maneuvers to reach the intended destination several vascular beds away from the entry site. In general, the closer the tip of the sheath can be placed to the target lesion, the more efficient and safe the control of the intervention.

In the example mentioned above, selective arteriography would necessitate catheter placement at the groin or just distal to it. The guidewire is introduced into the brachial artery and advanced retrograde into the subclavian artery. A catheter and a steerable-tip guidewire are used to advance into the aortic arch and avoid entering branches. The angle of takeoff of the subclavian artery from the aorta determines whether the guidewire will preferentially enter the arch or the descending aorta but it usually enters the ascending aorta preferentially. A curved-tip catheter, such as an omni-flush, is often required to direct the guidewire inferiorly into the descending aorta. The guidewire is advanced into the distal descending aorta, and the catheter may be advanced over it. If a longer guidewire is required, it may be exchanged at this point. Usually a 260-cm angled-tip Glidewire is a reasonable choice. The guidewire is advanced into the femoral artery using the steerable tip and using the catheter for support. After the catheter has reached the infrainguinal area, the guidewire is withdrawn and the arteriogram is performed.

If endovascular therapy is appropriate, the guidewire is replaced and a long (90 cm) 6- or 7-Fr sheath is placed over the guidewire. The patient is heparinized to protect the brachial access site from thrombosis and prevent thrombus formation along the lengthy sheath. The steerable Glidewire is advanced antegrade into the infrainguinal arteries. The long sheath provides extra support for the guidewire and helps to maintain its pushability and steerability. Consider passing an angled-tip catheter through the sheath to assist in directing the guidewire across the lesion.

PLAN OF ATTACK: GUIDEWIRE–CATHETER BUCKLING

A catheter–guidewire combination that buckles when the catheter is advanced (Fig. 4) has lost its pushability. This is usually because of distance

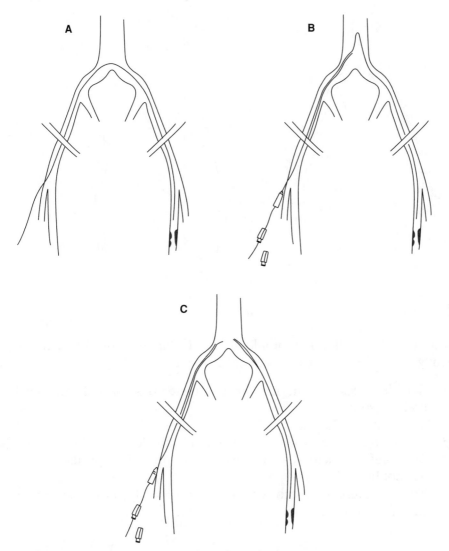

Fig. 4 Guidewire–catheter buckling. (**A**) A contralateral approach is selected for treatment of a proximal superficial femoral artery stenosis. (**B**) Advancement of the balloon catheter results in buckling of the guidewire and catheter into the distal aorta. The guidewire–catheter combination often buckles when the approach to the target is lengthy or tortuous. (**C**) The standard guidewire is exchanged for a stiffer guidewire so that the catheter tracks over it. (**D**) A long, curved sheath (Cook, Inc. Bloomington, Indiana, U.S.A.) can be placed over the aortic bifurcation to reduce tortuosity and friction and deliver the catheter antegrade into the iliac artery. (**E**) The contralateral access approach can be abandoned in favor of an ipsilateral antegrade femoral artery puncture.

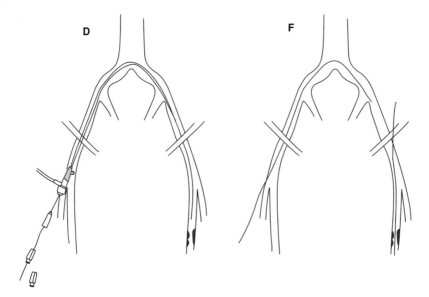

Fig. 4 Continued.

or tortuosity. The particular example shown in Figure 4 used to happen frequently before longer sheaths were available.

1. Double check that the guidewire–catheter position is intraluminal and not subintimal.
2. Try a stiffer guidewire (e.g., Amplatz Super-stiff).
3. Use a long sheath to decrease friction over the length of the catheter.
4. Try a stiffer catheter (e.g., nylon) if catheter head shape alternatives are not limited.
5. Try a different approach with a shorter or straighter course, rather than force one that is not going to work.

Passing Through Aneurysms

The development of stent–graft treatment of abdominal aortic aneurysms has resulted in aggressive catheterization of aneurysms. Passing catheters through aneurysms is associated with a risk of embolization of the compacted thrombus in the aneurysm sac. Associated occlusive disease that involves the neck of the aneurysm tends to be friable, and embolization is an even higher risk when this material is present. The usual approach is retrograde through the common femoral artery. Passing through aneurysms involves crossing the iliac arteries, which may also be aneurysmal, and then getting through the abdominal aortic aneurysm.

Tortuosity of the iliac arteries may make the approach challenging, especially if there is associated occlusive disease. Because occlusive disease and calcification causes an iliac segment to become stiffer than adjoining segments, relatively fixed in configuration and less pliable, the angle of curvature is more extreme in the more compliant, juxtaposed segments. Unfortunately, this causes the occlusive lesions to be present at either end of a tortuous segment. Therefore, the operator must be prepared to use steerable guidewires and selective catheters to cross the aneurysm. Sometimes tortuosity is severe enough that the loops formed as the guidewire crosses the tortuous segments create significant tension. As the forward progress of the guidewire bogs down, the back pressure by the vessel system on the wire tries to "spit out" or force back the guidewire. When this happens, reconsider the approach. If significant tortuosity occurs in an aneurysmal common iliac artery, the guidewire may want to "pile up" inside the iliac aneurysm and the neck may be difficult to find since it is not a straight shot.

Passage of a guidewire through a large abdominal aortic aneurysm can be difficult if the neck is hard to find. High-pressure contrast injection into the aneurysm to define anatomy is contraindicated. Puffing contrast in the iliac arteries may be useful but in the aneurysm it is useless since there is tremendous mixing with nonopacified blood. Multiple attempts at passage are sometimes required. The guidewire should not be placed so redundantly into the aneurysm that it curls up within the sac. It is a counterproductive maneuver and may result in embolization of aneurysm contents or tangling of the guidewire.

It is usually best to pass a starting guidewire from the femoral artery using fluoroscopy. Often, the guidewire will pass without specific direction, despite tortuosity and nearly blind sacs. If it does not pass, place an angled-tip catheter over it, such as an MPB or a Berenstein or a Teg-T. Exchange for a steerable guidewire and advance carefully. Puff contrast into the iliac arteries if necessary. If a CT scan or other imaging study is available, refer to that for clues about what to expect. After entering the aneurysm from

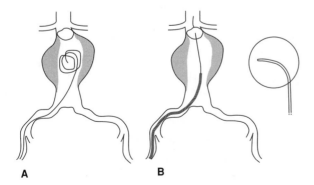

A　　　　　**B**

Fig. 5　Crossing an aneurysm. (**A**) The guidewire tends to pile up in the aorta when crossing an aneurysm. (**B**) A multipurpose, simple-curve selective catheter, such as an MPB, may be used to direct the guidewire past tortuous iliac and aortic segments.

below, advance the angled-tip catheter over the guidewire and use it to point the guidewire toward the neck of the aneurysm (Fig. 5). Always use a floppy-tipped guidewire.

Selected Readings

Braun MA. Basic catheterization skills. In: Braun MA, Nemcek AA, Vogelzang RL, eds. Interventional Radiology Procedure Manual. New York: Churchill Livingstone, 1997:23–30.

Kim D, Orron DE. Techniques and complications of angiography. In: Kim D, Orron DE, eds. Peripheral Vascular Imaging and Intervention. St. Louis, MO: Mosby, 1992:83–89.

8

Imaging: The Key to Future Success

Imaging and Best Therapy Are Intricately Linked

Imaging provides guidance for the performance of procedures with precision. Many procedures were performed with a relatively high degree of success in the past and without much guidance except for a thorough understanding of the anatomy and its variants. The occasion technical misadventure, device misplacement, or repeat procedure in an image-guided setting was considered part of standard practice. The addition of fairly routine use of complex imaging for diagnosis and for procedure guidance has become or is becoming the standard of care in most settings. Image guidance has further increased success and accuracy for many procedures with the broader use of ultrasound, CT, MRI, endoscopic, and arteriographic modalities. This evolution introduces new complexity and variables that must be managed.

Image Quality

The fluoroscopic image provides the equivalent of surgical exposure. High-quality images do not necessarily ensure a good result, but poor-quality images add to the risk of a bad one. Despite its importance, assessing image quality is an ambiguous and difficult task. How good is good enough? How do you know if there is something you are missing? The simplest way to know good imaging is to have experience with bad imaging. Two-dimensional images of three-dimensional hollow, tubular, dynamic structures might not ever be good enough to tell us everything. Seasoned vascular practitioners know that arteriography routinely and predictably underestimates the severity of disease at bifurcations (aortic bifurcation and carotid bifurcation), along posterior walls (common femoral and iliac), and when lesions are heavily calcified or tortuous. However, until some other imaging modality improves enough to take its place, fluoroscopic imaging will be required to guide vascular procedures in daily practice.

Imaging equipment must be versatile and functional so that it does not lengthen a procedure needlessly. The operator must be prepared to work within but also maximize the capabilities of the imaging equipment that has been procured. Images must be available and adequate so that strategic decisions may be made during the procedure. Digital arteriography affords the opportunity to have high-quality monitor images available for immediate decision making.

The practical determinants of image quality are listed in Table 1. The mode of image acquisition is exclusively through digital subtraction arteriography (DSA). The technology built into the imaging equipment determines its capabilities. The greater the number of pixels that contribute to the image,

Table 1 What Determines Image Quality?

Presentation of image	Monitor, Hard copy
Mode of image acquisition	Digital subtraction
Technology of imaging equipment	Pixels
	Postprocessing
	Other
Optimize X-ray settings	Kilovoltage
	Milliamperes
	Focal spot
	See Table 2
Imaging technique	Timing of administration
Contrast administration	Volume of administration
	Location of administration
Patient factors	Patient size
	Anatomy being imaged
	Motion

the higher the resolution. The higher the heating capacity, the less likely it is that the images will blur or fade during the procedure. These types of issues are under human control only at the time of purchase. The quality of the image may vary, depending upon its presentation: whether it is viewed on the television monitor or in its hard-copy form. As digital storage capabilities improve, fewer laboratories will produce any hard copy as all images will be accumulated and saved in digital format. Imaging technique is a very important factor controlled by the operator. Specific maneuvers that affect X-ray beam generation and scatter are discussed later. Contrast concentration and method of injection (automated vs. hand-powered) must be tailored to the situation. The patient's size may dramatically alter the distance from the image intensifier to the target artery and will affect the resultant images accordingly.

Generating an X-ray Image

The X-ray tube emits a prescribed energy beam that passes through the patient (Fig. 1). The level of kilovolts (usually 60–80 kV) sets the penetrability of the beam. The focal spot (0.15–1.2 mm) should be as small as possible for reasonable resolution but should still permit an adequate frame rate. The X-rays emitted from the tube (beneath the table) travel through the patient. Some of the X-rays are absorbed and some scatter. Dense objects, such as bone, contrast, and surgical clips, absorb more energy. The remaining energy strikes the image intensifier (above the patient) and is converted to an image created by contrasting varying degrees of X-ray beam absorption. Scattering of the X-ray beam can be decreased by placing the image intensifier as close to the patient as possible. The result produced by the X-ray beam that hits the

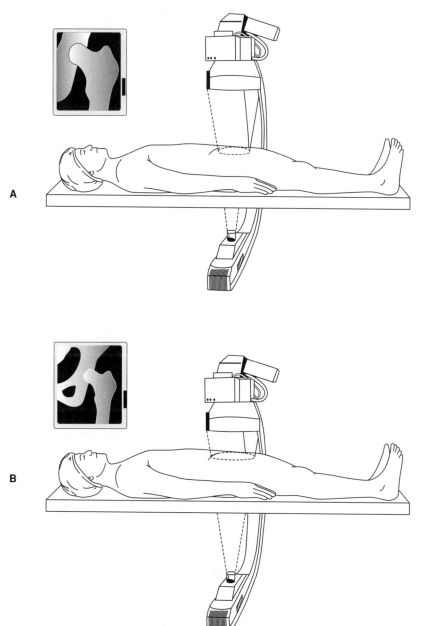

Fig. 1 Production of an X-ray image. (**A**) The X-ray tube emits an energy beam that is partially absorbed by the patient. The remainder of the beam strikes the image intensifier and is converted to an X-ray image. (**B**) Placing the image intensifier closer to the patient decreases radiation scatter and broadens the field of view.

image intensifier is transmitted to a television system that displays a moving image. Movement of the area being imaged is avoided, since the demarcated lines of differential beam absorption are blurred by movement.

Digital Subtraction Arteriography

The advantages and disadvantages of DSA are listed in Table 2. DSA is cheap, fast, easy, and simple with which to work. The past decade has included continued development of digital systems with attention to variables that improve resolution and create images that exceed what was available in the recent past. As a result, angiographic suites and endovascular operating rooms have converted to digital-only systems.

A DSA image is created by first obtaining a mask that is computerized and recorded and later subtracted from the acquired images. After the mask is subtracted, the contrast column is the primary feature of the remaining image. The digital processing system automatically divides the information transmitted from the image intensifier into a matrix, which is composed of pixels. Many systems are currently available with 1024×1024 pixels or more. The more pixels that make up a given field of view, the smaller the pixel and the better the resolution. The images are computerized and recorded in a cineradiographic format. Prior to selecting images for storage, either with digital or hard copy, the sequences of moving images are evaluated for flow pattern and rate on the control console (Fig. 2). Information that affects decision making is available more rapidly, and the study is tailored to the patient's needs without waiting for films to develop. This is hard to believe, but in the very recent past, cut film arteriography was the standard.

Table 2 Digital Subtraction Arteriography

	Digital subtraction
Advantages	Fast
	Inexpensive
	Immediate feedback
	Postimage processing
	Easy image storage
	Improving image resolution
	Contrast may be minimized
	Other contrast options may be used (CO_2)
	Continued technologic development
Disadvantages	Multiple contrast injections required
	Subject to motion artifact
	Image obstruction by metal or calcium
	Only provides two-dimensional representation
	Will eventually be replaced

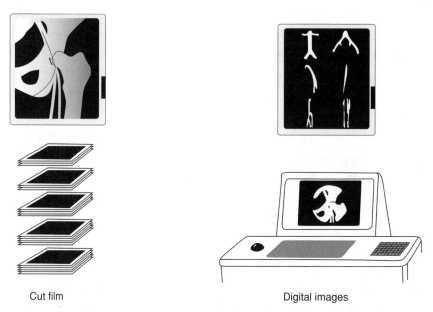

Cut film   Digital images

Fig. 2 The process and production of cut film and digital images. The processing and presentation of images varies significantly for cut film and digital sequences. In this example of an aortogram with lower-extremity runoff, the cut film sequence results in the accumulation of 20 films. A few images are recorded at each of five stations. The digital images can be reviewed on the control screen and postimage processing performed. Representative images are selected and committed to hard copy.

This has been completely replaced by DSA and is represented in Figure 2 for historical purposes.

Timing of contrast administration is usually simple with DSA. The image intensifier is placed over the desired arterial segment and image acquisition continues through the period during which the contrast passes through that segment. DSA may be performed with dilute iodinated contrast, to as little as 20%, or carbon dioxide to decrease contrast load in selected situations. DSA permits postimage processing, which helps to enhance or delineate an image further. Digital information may be accumulated at rates of up to 30 frames per second, although 2 to 4 frames per second is usually adequate, depending on whether a low-flow or high-flow bed is being imaged. The DSA field of view is specified by the diameter of the image intensifier; 16-in. image intensifiers are now available in digital angiographic suites, and 14-in. image intensifiers are available on portable digital units.

DSA requires quite a bit of effort when an entire lower extremity runoff must be obtained, unless bolus chase is available. Many digital systems require a separate mask, position, injection, and filming run for each level of the arterial tree. Bolus chase technology is also available that allows the runoff to be obtained in sequence as a single run.

Imaging Technique for Best Resolution

Imaging technique is one factor within control of the operator that significantly affects the quality of the resulting images. Specific maneuvers that improve resolution are listed in Table 3. Placing the image intensifier closer to the patient decreases X-ray scatter and increases the overall size of the field of view but also decreases magnification. Motion must be minimized by all potentially moving parts to prevent blurring of the image. Most digital imaging systems provide several differently sized fields of view (e.g., 4, 9, 11, up to 16 in.). A smaller field of view magnifies the area of interest and improves resolution but also increases radiation. The operator must balance the disparity between an adequately sized field in which to work and the degree of resolution that comes with it. Using the appropriate contrast type, concentration, and method of injection enhances imaging and also decreases patient movement since the contrast is better tolerated. Extraneous objects should be removed from the field. An X-ray of the operator's hand or arm is bad form as well. Remain focused on the area of interest until it has been adequately interrogated. Oblique views or changes in patient positioning may be required. Decreasing kilovoltage improves resolution but increases radiation. A smaller focal spot improves resolution but decreases frame rate and energy available for image production. An increase in the number of frames acquired per second during DSA not only increases radiation exposure but also improves resolution, creating a motion picture effect, and may provide a better understanding of lesions with almost real-time observation of contrast flow. Some high-flow lesions, such as arteriovenous fistulas, may only be identified and evaluated using high frame rates (up to 30 frames per second). Slow flow arterial beds, such as the ischemic lower extremity, are best evaluated using a longer run (e.g., 30 seconds) with fewer frames acquired per second (e.g., 2 or 3 per second). The object of interest should be centered in the field of view and the beam filtered to decrease scatter.

Table 3 Techniques for Enhanced Image Resolution

Center the area of interest within the field of view
Minimize the distance between image intensifier and patient to reduce scatter
Use a smaller field of view to provide magnification
Filter the unimportant parts of the image to reduce scatter
Remove extraneous objects such as leads, wires, tubes, and heating blanket
Minimize patient motion—coach breathing, use isosmolar contrast, and keep patient
  comfortable
Obtain appropriate oblique views

ANGIO CONSULT: HOW CAN I GET BETTER IMAGES?

1. Interrogate one area at a time, especially if clinically important disease is suspected.
2. Position the patient and the image intensifier before imaging is begun.
3. Use magnification to enhance detail in a specific area of interrogation. This can be achieved by changing to a smaller field of view (e.g., 4 or 6 in. instead of 9 or 12 or 16 in.).
4. Decrease the kilovoltage to increase image contrast (see chap. 24?).
5. Use the smallest possible focal spot.
6. Move the image intensifier closer to the patient to reduce scatter.
7. Increase the resolution (and radiation) of DSA by using a higher number of frames per second.
8. Minimize motion, especially with DSA. This usually requires coaching (for breath-holding during body cavity and neck or cerebral imaging and general stillness for imaging of the extremities), sedation, restraint (taping the leg to the angiography table if necessary), or a combination of these.
9. Filter the X-ray beam to reduce scatter. This is key to produce better images and also decrease radiation exposure.
10. Use of appropriate concentration of contrast. Contrast may be diluted and continue to produce adequate image quality, especially in low flow situations.
11. Use contrast that is well tolerated in the awake patient, especially when imaging an ischemic limb (low osmolality).
12. Administer contrast as close to the target site as is safe. The catheter head must be positioned to deliver an adequate bolus to the area of interest, taking into account the rate of flow in the vessel.
13. Use catheters and sheaths with radiopaque tips.
14. Initiate filming in the best projection (i.e., an oblique view) for a given artery.
15. Be as specific as possible about what information is required.

Road Mapping: How It Works and When to Use It

Road mapping is a feature of digital units that permits real-time guidewire–catheter guidance. Road mapping works by subtracting the initial noncontrast mask from the field, thus eliminating bony landmarks. Contrast is administered that opacifies the vessels in the field of interest. A new mask is digitally constructed that is added to or superimposed upon the subsequent real-time images on the monitor screen. Any moving items that are later passed into the field, such as guidewires or catheters, are seen on the monitor screen

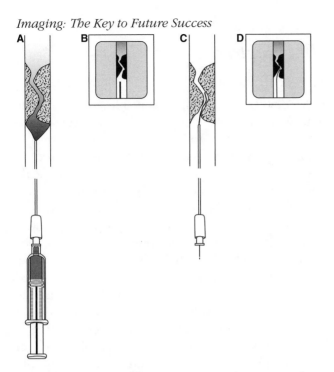

Fig. 3 Use road mapping to cross a lesion. Road mapping can be used to cross a stenosis or occlusion or assist in selective catheterization. (**A**) The tip of the arteriographic catheter is placed in proximity to the lesion. Contrast is administered and an image of the opacified lesion is digitized and recorded. (**B**) The road map is superimposed on the real-time fluoroscopic image. (**C**) The guidewire is passed through the lesion using the road map as a guide. (**D**) The guidewire is observed in real time on the monitor with the image of the lesion superimposed.

as superimposed within the framework of the initially acquired road map (Fig. 3).

Road mapping has assumed a broader role as it improves from a technical standpoint. Road mapping is useful in (1) finding and marking the vessel origin during selective catheterization, (2) passing through a critically stenotic arterial segment, (3) encountering and crossing an occlusion, (4) guiding the puncture of a pulseless artery, (5) guiding sequential maneuvers in a complex reconstruction without multiple interval arteriograms, and (6) guiding thrombectomy or embolectomy.

Road mapping is an extra step and is only worth the extra procedure time when undertaking specific tasks. Road mapping is not particularly helpful in areas where there is a high degree of mobility and also where the flow is so high that an acceptable contrast concentration cannot be reached (i.e., aortic arch). The resolution of the road-mapped images is not as good as DSA. The road map mask blurs with motion and with time so that the image quality further degrades during usage. Interval fluoroscopy or arteriography typically requires loss of the road map mode.

Automated Power Injector

When performing aortography through a 65- to 100-cm length, 4- or 5-Fr catheter, high pressure (up to 1050 psi) is required to produce an adequate bolus of contrast. The contrast must be emitted from the catheter over a short period of time against arterial pressure to create a blush of contrast in a large arterial structure. No rate of rise in pressure over time is required. In other words, the pressure may be permitted to immediately reach its peak, since there are many side holes in a flush catheter for egress of the contrast. When selective arteriography is performed using specially shaped end hole catheters, a rate a rise is required to avoid the occasional high-pressure injection into the arterial wall. Power injectors provide a pressure of up to 2000 pounds per square inch (psi). Each individual arteriographic catheter has a manufacturers' recommended limit of psi for power injection. The automated power injector may be integrated with the filming run to predetermine the timing of contrast injection or it may be controlled and times by the operator as the image acquisition is being performed. The power injector offers a constant rate and pressure of injection. Percutaneous arteriography in larger arteries, especially those with a high rate of flow, using small catheters would not be possible without a power injector (Fig. 4). Contrast administration, image acquisition, and arteriography sequences are detailed in chapter 10. The power injector also represents an additional link in the arteriographic system—more connections that may leak under high pressure, more preparation time, and more potential for a misfire during a filming run. Power injection should not be performed when the contrast jet has the potential to cause arterial injury in an aneurysm, against the arterial wall, or in a lesion (Fig. 5). Care must always be taken to avoid the inadvertent administration of air bubbles, especially during cerebral arteriography.

Power Injection vs. Contrast Administration by Hand

Contrast may be administered using an automated power injector or hand power. Table 4 provides some general guidelines about how these methods may be used. These two methods are often combined during an arteriographic procedure to complement each other. The high viscosity of contrast and the small caliber of catheters make contrast administration challenging at times.

When power injection is not mandatory, it is often faster and simpler to administer the contrast by hand, either directly or through a manifold. Hand injection can be used to puff contrast in any location and should be considered when the contrast volume required is 8 to 10 ml or less, the conduit is large (7 Fr or more), and there is lower flow (e.g., most selective arteriography or distal to a flow-limiting lesion). The smaller the syringe,

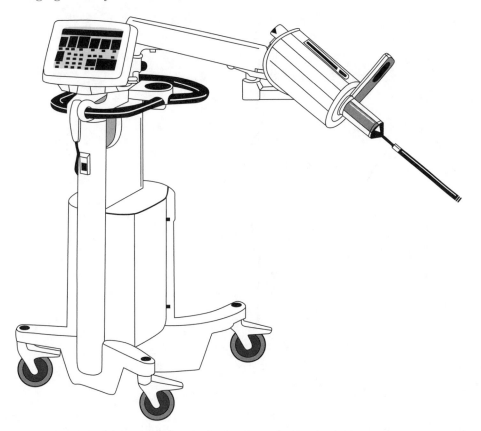

Fig. 4 Power injector. An automated power injector permits high-pressure administration of contrast. A timed bolus of contrast is delivered at a preset pressure. A rate of rise of pressure is introduced when an end hole catheter is used in a side branch.

the higher the positive pressure that can be achieved during injection. The accuracy of this method improves significantly with clinical experience.

Volume and flow rate in the aorta are usually enough to overwhelm pressure generated by hand. A power injector is required for performing aortography through a 4- or 5-Fr catheter. Under special circumstances (e.g., a combined procedure in the operating room), some limited aortic or iliac arteriography can be performed through a larger sheath with the tip placed near the site of interest and a hand-injected contrast bolus.

Selective, branch vessel arteriography and lower-extremity arteriography may be performed with either hand injection or the power injector. These situations require a smaller volume at a lower flow rate than the aorta or iliac arteries. Injection by hand may be preferable in some situations (e.g., infrapopliteal artery, vertebral artery).

Whether contrast is administered by hand power or injector, all air bubbles must be removed from the system prior to injection. This is a ritual

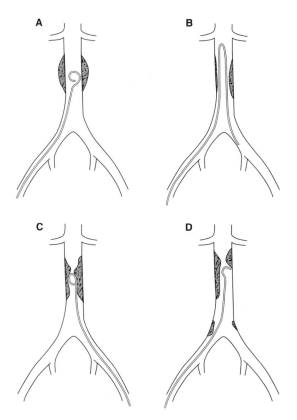

Fig. 5 Power injection is not used when an artery could be injured. (**A**) Compacted thrombus within an aneurysm may fragment as a result of high-pressure contrast administration. (**B**) Significant recoil may result from high-pressure injection. Redundancy is removed to prevent catheter whip. (**C**) The catheter head may be constrained by its position within an occlusive lesion. When the catheter head changes shape under pressure, the lesion may fragment. (**D**) The tip of the catheter may be against the aortic wall rather than free within its lumen.

that is followed multiple times per day in angiographic suites around the world. The catheter is aspirated and the injector tubing is purged. The sterile tubing is luer-locked to the catheter. The catheter is then aspirated (through the injector) until blood returns, and the clear injector tubing is inspected for bubbles. This maneuver is extremely important during cerebral and visceral arteriography, since a bubble, even a tiny one, is an embolus. Injection sequences are discussed in detail in chapter 10.

Contrast Agents

There are several factors to consider in selecting the appropriate contrast solution, including osmolality, ionic charge, cost, and complications (Table 5). Standard contrast contains iodine, which is highly absorptive of

Table 4 Contrast Administration: Automated Versus Hand Powered

Location of catheter head	Power injector	Hand power	Either
Aortic arch	X		
Innominate	X		
Subclavian artery	X (proximal)	X (distal)	
Axillary artery			X
Carotid artery			X
Thoracic aorta	X		
Visceral aorta	X		
Visceral arteries			X
Renal artery			X
Infrarenal aorta[a]	X		
Iliac artery [b]			X
Femoral artery			X
Popliteal artery			X
Tibial artery		X	
Infrainguinal graft		X	

[a]Hand-powered aortogram may be obtained using a $\geq$6-Fr sheath.
[b]Hand-powered iliac arteriography may be obtained using a $\geq$6-Fr sheath.

Table 5 Examples of Iodinated Contrast Media

	Generic name	Trade name	Iodine content (mg iodine/ml)	Osmolality (mOsm/kg H_2O)
Ionic	Sodium distrizoate	Hypaque sodium 25%	150	696
	Meglumine diatrizoate	Renograffin-60	292	1549
	Meglamine iothalamate	Conray-30	141	681
	Meglumine ioxaglate	Hexabrix	320	600
Nonionic	Iopamidol	Isovue #28	128	290
	Iohexol	Omnipaque 140	140	322
	Ioversol	Optiray 320	320	702
	Iohexol	Omnipaque 240	240	520
	Iotrolan	Visipaque[a]	320	290

[a]Author's choice. High iodine concentration increases resolution, while low osmolality decreases complications. Disadvantage is cost.

X-rays. Available contrast agents are hyperosmolar (320–1700 mOsm) in comparison to blood (approximately 300 mOsm). Many of the complications of contrast are related to its hyperosmolarity, such as pain on injection, cardiac overload, and renal toxicity. Lower osmolality contrast is the standard in most angiographic laboratories; it is better tolerated physiologically but the more expensive. Nonionic contrast has a lower incidence of common systemic complications. Life-threatening reactions, such as anaphylaxis, may occur with either ionic or nonionic contrast administration and the incidence is about the same with each. Contrast concentration must be adequate for the type of imaging selected. DSA can be performed with dilutions to 60 μg/ml (20%), depending on the vascular bed being imaged. Total contrast loads vary substantially depending upon whether a strategic or therapeutic procedure has been performed. Patients with normal renal and cardiac function usually tolerate several hundred milliliters of contrast without difficulty.

Carbon dioxide has been employed as an alternative contrast agent but has some distinct disadvantages. When CO_2 encounters occlusive disease, it tends to break up into bubbles, making images difficult to interpret. Since it is a gas, it will rise. The patient must be positioned so that the CO_2 will flow and not form an air lock. Brachiocephalic arteriography using CO_2 is contraindicated since bubbles may cause stroke. Visceral or even upper abdominal, aortic injection may result in visceral ischemia due to air lock. The major advantage of CO_2 is that it is exhaled by the lungs and has no nephrotoxicity.

ANGIO CONSULT: IS THERE ANY WAY TO LIMIT CONTRAST LOAD?

1. Keep an ongoing tally of usage. Each bottle contains 50 or 100 ml.
2. Have a clear plan for how much arteriography is required. Be specific about which information is required and which anatomic beds require delineation (see chap. 10 for a detailed discussion of strategic arteriography).
3. Use the clinical presentation, physical examination, and duplex scanning to help limit arteriography.
4. Go directly to an oblique view when treating lesions in certain areas (e.g., femoral or iliac bifurcations).
5. Dilute contrast when using DSA.
6. Use techniques discussed earlier in this chapter to improve images, thus decreasing the need for highly concentrated contrast.
7. Puff 1 to 3 ml of contrast at a time to check catheter position prior to an angiographic run, this will decrease the number of useless runs that are performed. An arteriographic sequence will be required for more detail.
8. Be specific about catheter head placement for arteriographic runs (e.g., catheter head placement for an aortogram should be at the

Table 6 How Do You Know Where You Are?

During guidewire passage
Follow guidewire progress with fluoroscopy
Road map
During catheter passage
Use catheter with radiopaque tip
Follow catheter progress with fluoroscopy
Puff contrast
Road map
Magnify field to visualize catheter head
Anytime during the case
Internal landmarks
Vascular calcification
Surgical clips
Bony structures, such as ribs, vertebral bodies, joints, pelvic landmarks, limb bones
External landmarks
Ruler
Stent-guide
Clamp

level of the renal arteries; high-pressure injection refluxes the contrast proximally despite arterial flow and if the catheter head is too high, a major portion of the contrast bolus will be lost in the visceral arteries).

How Do You Know Where You Are?

The best answer to this question is to go there often so that familiar appearances become internalized. Table 6 lists several methods of reminding yourself where your guidewire or catheter is located as you are starting out. As an endovascular operator, you get used to processing all these bits of information while gazing at a fluoroscopic image, and having a sense of where you are becomes second nature.

Radiation Safety and Occupational Health Issues

Numerous occupational health issues require vigilant attention and preventive steps (Table 7). The maximum safe occupational whole body X-ray dose per year is 5 rems. Up to 75 rems may be absorbed by the hands and 15 rems by the thyroid. Radiation exposure causes cataracts and cancer. Leaded glasses, a thyroid shield, and lead apron are recommended. Thyroid cancer, lymphoma, or impotence may result from X-ray exposure. Cervical radiculopathy and low back strain and disc problems have been reported in

Table 7 Occupational Risks of Endovascular Work

Radiation exposure
Cataracts
Thyroid cancer
Hematopoietic cancer
Skin cancers/other lesions
Other cancers
Sterility/impotence
Watching monitor
Cervical radiculopathy
Wearing lead
Back strain
Disc herniation

relationship to wearing lead aprons and extending the neck to see the image monitor.

Scatter is the main source of radiation to the operator. Exposure to scatter decreases as the inverse square of the distance from the primary X-ray beam. Scatter radiation also decreases significantly as the fluoroscopic field size is decreased. Most portable and stationary systems are designed with the image intensifier above the patient and the tube emitting X-rays below. This arrangement decreases operator exposure by half. In addition, judicious use of fluoroscopy or pulsed fluoroscopy decreases exposure proportionately. Protective devices such as a lead apron (0.5-mm lead), lead shields, leaded glasses with side shields, and thyroid collars should be used.

Radiographic Equipment

CATHODE/ANODE/X-RAY TUBE

Within the X-ray tube, the cathode is a heated tungsten filament that emits electrons. The anode is the target. This process transforms energy into X-rays. Most of the energy becomes heat and a small amount is converted to X-rays. Fluoroscopic procedures that require high-energy settings risk overheating the equipment.

GENERATOR

The generator serves as the electrical power source for the X-ray tube. One of the significant differences between portable and stationary angiographic systems is the size of the generator. Better image quality is to be expected with a more powerful generator.

IMAGE INTENSIFIER

The X-rays travel through the patient and strike the image intensifier. Differential energy absorption is converted into light images and displayed on television monitors.

C-ARM

The image intensifier and X-ray tube are usually mounted together in a C-shaped configuration, regardless of whether a portable or a stationary fluoroscopic unit is used. This is referred to as the gantry.

POWER INJECTOR

A power injector is a high-pressure contrast injector.

DIGITAL CONSOLE

The console commands the computer in which digital information is acquired and processed.

Radiographic Terms

KV

Kilovoltage is a measure of the penetrability of the X-ray beam and affects image contrast. It represents the electrical potential across the X-ray tube. The higher the voltage is across the X-ray tube, the greater the penetrating power of the beam and the better the contrast. Cerebral, thoracic, and abdominal arteriography usually require 65 to 75 kV. Extremity arteriography is performed with 55 to 65 kV.

MAS

The current (milliampere/second) required to generate the X-ray beam should be set at the highest milliamperage (to minimize image noise) for the shortest exposure time (to minimize motion artifact). The number of milliamperes determines the density of the image.

FRAME RATE

The frame rate is the number of image frames generated per second. Resolution increases with higher frame rates, but so does radiation. Images may be acquired anywhere from 1 to 30 per second. A standard DSA run usually includes frame rates of three or four images per second.

MATRIX

The digital matrix is divided into pixels. When the matrix is divided into more but smaller pixels, the resolution is better. Modern DSA units acquire 1024 × 1024 pixels per frame.

FOCAL SPOT

The focal spot is the area on the anode that receives the electrons. The smaller the focal spot size, the better the resolution. Focal spot size ranges from 0.15 to 1.2 mm. Smaller focal spots, however, limit the frame rate and the amount of energy available for generating images because of heat production.

MASK

The digital mask image is obtained before contrast is injected. It is later subtracted from the images obtained during arteriography to eliminate overlying bone and other structures.

Radiation Exposure

ALLOWABLE LIMITS

The maximum permissible dose for adults is 5 rems per year.

DOSE CALCULATION

The amount of radiation to the operator is equal to the exposure rate multiplied by the time. Radiation exposure decreases proportionally to the square of the distance from the beam.

X-RAY TUBE POSITION

Scatter radiation is decreased by turning the X-ray tube away from the operator and by placing it under the patient (rather than above).

ORGAN SUSCEPTIBILITY

Skin and soft tissue are less susceptible to radiation damage than the eye, thyroid, gonads, and hematopoietic system.

PROTECTIVE GEAR

A leaded apron, thyroid shield, gloves, and glasses reduce radiation exposure but are cumbersome. Aprons decrease radiation exposure by 75% to 90%.

LIMITING EXPOSURE

A radiation dosimeter is worn to ensure that exposure remains below allowable limits. The image intensifier is placed close to the patient to reduce the scatter of X-ray beams. The image intensifier is turned away from the area in which the operator is working. Exposure time is shortened by using fluoroscopy intermittently rather than continuously. The frame rate is decreased. The beam is collimated to reduce scatter. Maximum distance from the beam is maintained. A ceiling- or floor-mounted shield may be used in addition to leaded apparel.

Selected Readings

Ahn SS, Obrand DI. Radiation safety and principles. In: Ahn SS, Obrand DI, eds. Handbook of Endovascular Surgery. Austin, TX: Landes Bioscience, 1997:1–6.

Hiatt MD, Fleischmann D, Hellinger JC, et al. Angiographic imaging of the lower extremities with multidetector CT. Radiol Clin North Am 2005; 43(6):1119–127.

Kashyap VS, Pavkov ML, Bishop PD, et al. Angiography underestimates peripheral atherosclerosis: Lumenography revisited. J Endovasc Ther 2008; 15(1):117–125.

Pavlovic C, Futamatsu H, Angiolillo DJ, et al. Quantitative contrast enhanced magnetic resonance imaging for the evaluation of peripheral arterial disease: A comparative study versus standard digital angiography. Int J Cardiovasc Imaging 2007; 23(2):225–232.

Slonim SM, Wexler L. Image production and visualization systems: angiography, US, CT, and MRI. In: White RA, Fogarty TJ, eds. Peripheral Endovascular Interventions. St. Louis, MO: Mosby, 1996:140–157.

9

Selective Catheterization

Too Many Catheter Choices

Selective catheterization is a basic tool that permits focused arteriography and delivery of therapeutic devices. It is a key skill that forces the operator to choose a course, assess its pitfalls, pick the correct tools, and get there without harming anything along the way. Selective catheterization is facilitated by taking a direct approach and by gaining facility with a couple of catheter choices for each application. Table 1 details options for approaching selective catheterization of various arteries. Table 2 provides an example of top catheter choices for each task.

Endovascular intervention is only rarely limited by the technical ability to arrive at a remote vascular location. This is a result of improving technology that enables catheter placement in almost any location. A byproduct of this improvement in technology is a broad array of selective catheter choices with confusing names and slight variations in shape from one to another. Some of these catheters are tremendously useful, and others were an opportunity for someone in a dimly lit laboratory somewhere to get their name on

Table 1 Approaches to Selective Catheterization and Arteriography

Destination vascular bed	Approach: first choice	Alternative approach
Brachiocephalic		
Carotid	Either femoral	Left brachial (when femoral approach contraindicated)
Subclavian	Either femoral	Ipsilateral brachial (for endovascular therapy in some patients or when femoral approach is contraindicated)
Visceral		
Celiac/SMA	Either femoral	Left brachial (for endovascular therapy in some patients)
Renal	Either femoral	Left brachial (for endovascular therapy when renal artery origin is at an acute angle or when there is severe aortoiliac disease)
Aortoiliac		
Infrarenal aorta	Either femoral	Left brachial (when femoral approach is contraindicated)
Common iliac	Contralateral femoral	Ipsilateral femoral when endovascular therapy is planned near aortic bifurcation.
Internal iliac	Contralateral femoral	Left brachial (when contralateral femoral approach is contraindicated)
External iliac	Contralateral femoral	Ipsilateral femoral (when contralateral femoral approach is contraindicated)
Destination vascular bed	Approach: first choice	Alternative approach
Infrainguinal		
Femoral	Contralateral femoral	Ipsilateral antegrade femoral (when there is no inflow disease and endovascular therapy is planned, especially in distal tibial segments)
Popliteal		
Tibial Pedal		

Table 2 Catheter Options for Selective Catheterization

	First choice	Second choice	Third choice
Brachiocephalic Innominate/right carotid	H1	Simmons	Vitek
Left carotid	Angled Glidecath	vert	Simmons
Left subclavian	Angled Glidecath	vert	Simmons or H3
Visceral			
Celiac/SMA	RIM	Chuang-C	Chuang-3
Renal	C2 cobra	Renal double curve	Sos-Omni
Aortoiliac			
Aortic bifurcation	Omni-flush	RIM	C2 cobra
Infrainguinal			
SFA	Berenstein	Kumpe	Vertebral
Tibial	Teg-T	Kumpe	Vertebral

Abbreviation: RIM, Right internal mammary artery.

a piece of plastic. Nevertheless, each specialist must find what works best in his or her hands and then add additional shapes as specific needs arise. Selective catheterization adds time and risk to any procedure and should be reserved for necessary strategic arteriography and/or endovascular treatment.

ANGIO CONSULT: WHAT IS YOUR STRATEGY FOR SELECTIVE CATHETERIZATION?

1. Complications increase with higher degrees of selectivity (e.g., embolization, occlusion, dissection). How important is the information? Is there another way to obtain the information?
2. If the anticipated catheter time is lengthy (more than 15 or 20 min) or if the catheter is passed into a small-caliber or low-flow vascular bed, heparin administration should be considered.
3. An understanding of what the different catheter heads can do is an important determinant of selective catheterization.
4. Catheter head shape may be modified in situ by passing the guidewire varying distances into the catheter head.
5. After the vessel is cannulated, the guidewire should be advanced past that point as far as possible ("bury the guidewire") to prevent it from becoming dislodged during catheter advancement. This provides stable support for the advancing catheter.
6. Crossing lesions should be avoided unless treatment is planned.
7. When endovascular therapy is planned, a stiffer guidewire and delivery sheath should be placed. This enhances control of the lesion intended for treatment. If a long sheath cannot be placed, but additional support is needed, a guiding catheter (e.g., renal) should be considered (chap. 14).

8. The shape of the directional catheter that is being used for selective catheterization will change shape as the guidewire is advanced into the catheter head. This shape change can be used to the operator's advantage but must be anticipated.

9. When tortuosity or juxtaposed disease make selective catheterization more challenging, use a guiding sheath to stabilize the platform before cannulating the branch in question.

10. If placement of the selective catheter has a demonstrable effect of flow and perfusion to the organ in question is reduced, administer anticoagulation, such as heparin. Low-flow states that persist for too long become no-flow states and this rapidly progresses to resemble a three alarm fire.

PLAN OF ATTACK: SHOULD I LEAD WITH THE GUIDEWIRE OR WITH THE CATHETER?

1. Selective catheterization usually involves branches of the aorta and making turns into those branches. Selective catheterization can be performed by leading with either the guidewire or the catheter. Either of these options is acceptable in nondiseased vessels. When significant disease is present, take the least risky option.

2. When the aorta and the branch origins are without significant degenerative disease, it is usually safe and fast to lead with the catheter. An example of this is catheterization of the branches of the aortic arch or the visceral and renal branches when there is little or no arterial disease.

3. The tighter the turn into the branch and the more remote it is from the puncture site (operator has less control), the more sense it makes to have specific and complex catheter shapes that do the work of selective catheterization. In this case, one usually leads with the catheter. The best example of this is the branches of the aortic arch when the arch configuration is tortuous. Special shapes for arch catheterization, such as the Simmons or the Vitek, become very helpful.

4. The more disease that is located in the branch artery and the closer it is to the origin where the turn into the branch is also located, the more it makes sense to lead with the guidewire. An example of this would be a complex lesion at the renal artery origin. In this case, a "no touch" technique may be considered. The guiding sheath or guide catheter is stabilized by placing an exchange guidewire through it. Along next to the exchange guidewire and through the sheath, a low-profile, steerable guidewire is advanced and used to steer across the lesion.

5. When crossing a long, diseased conduit artery, lead deliberately with the guidewire. An example of this is crossing a lengthy,

diseased segment of superficial femoral artery (SFA) to get to the infrapopliteal vessels.

6. When using a 0.014-in. system, the guidewire and catheter may be used alternatively to lead; one and then the other alternating. Over a 0.014-in. steerable guidewire, a selective catheter is placed. A Tuohy-Borst adapter is placed over the guidewire and fastened to the hub of the catheter. Contrast may be administered through the side arm of the adapter to help guide the way. The guidewire is advanced, then the catheter, then the guidewire again.

Selective Catheterization of the Brachiocephalic Arteries

The brachiocephalic arteries are usually approached using femoral artery access. Alternatives to this are the left brachial artery, and lastly the right brachial artery. The femoral artery approach requires guidewires and catheters of adequate length to reach the arch branches from the groin. Cerebral catheters are 90 to 100 cm in length. A standard retrograde femoral puncture is performed and a pigtail catheter (90 cm) is placed in the ascending aorta. A 30- to 45-degree left anterior oblique (LAO) projection is performed of the arch and an arch aortogram is obtained (Fig. 1). This angled view separates the aortic arch branch origins since the aorta courses posteriorly as it moves to the patient's left. The arch branches may be cannulated by using local landmarks. When diffuse or shaggy disease is present in the roof of the aortic arch, selective catheterization of the arch branches may be contraindicated. Systemic heparin is administered prior to selective catheterization of

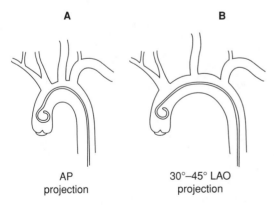

A   **B**

AP
projection

30°–45° LAO
projection

Fig. 1 Arch aortogram using AP or LAO projections. (**A**) The flush catheter is placed in the ascending aorta in preparation for an arch aortogram. (**B**) Since the aortic arch travels posteriorly as it moves from right to left, a 30-degree to 45-degree LAO projection is required to "open up" the arch and separate the origins of the arch branches.

the arch branches. Based upon the vessel planned for catheterization and the angle of its origin from the arch, a selective cerebral catheter is chosen and exchanged for the pigtail. During catheter exchanges, extra care must be taken to avoid guidewire or catheter thrombus and to avoid passing any bubbles through the catheter. Guidewires are removed slowly and steadily, rather than whipped out, to avoid generating microbubbles along the inner surface of the catheter lumen. Because of the risk of stroke with routine cerebral arteriography, some operators advise withdrawing the catheter head to a position distal to the left subclavian artery origin prior to making catheter exchanges over a guidewire. When a critical stenosis or highly irregular plaque formation is present at the origin of the branch artery, selective cannulation may be unwise. This must be considered on a vessel-by-vessel basis. In the discussion that follows, normal arch branch anatomy is given. When significant anomalies or unfavorable anatomy occur, additional maneuvers are required.

SELECTIVE CEREBRAL CATHETERS

There are a myriad of catheter shapes used for selective cerebral arteriography (Fig. 2). Most operators develop their quiver of favorites and use two or three catheters routinely for most of the cases they do. The pigtail catheter used for arch aortography has an end hole and multiple side holes for large-volume contrast injection, allowing a blush of contrast to be created in the large volume arch in only two seconds. The selective catheters have only an end hole for passing the guidewire and administering contrast after the guidewire has been removed. When a vessel origin is cannulated with the tip

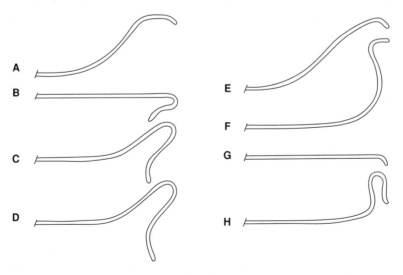

Fig. 2 Selective cerebral catheters. A few of the many examples of specially shaped selective cerebral catheters. These include (**A**) H1 Headhunter, (**B**) Simmons 1, (**C**) Simmons 2, (**D**) Simmons 3, (**E**) JB 1, (**F**) JB 2, (**G**) Vert, and (**H**) Vitek.

of a selective catheter, contrast may be puffed into the branch vessel without losing contrast into the aortic arch through side holes. Care must be taken to assure that the tip of the selective catheter is free of the artery wall and distant from unstable lesions prior to any pressure injection, since the only outlet for the contrast is the end hole and any jet effect may cause damage (chap. 10). These selective cerebral catheters are generally 100 cm in length, but some are available up to 125 cm length, most notably the Vertebral catheter (vert), the Vitek, and the angled Glidecath. The guidewire length required to make an exchange with a catheter length of 100 cm or more is 260 cm.

Although there are an overwhelming number of differently shaped catheters for selective cerebral use, there are really only two major categories: (1) simple-curve catheters, which have an angled or bent tip, and (2) complex-curve catheters, which must be reshaped or reformed in the wide diameter aorta for the catheter head to assume its intended shape. The curve at the tip of a simple-curve catheter is the primary curve, and this angulation may vary anywhere from 90 degrees to only a few degrees of curvature. Commonly used simple-curve catheters include the angled-taper Glidecath (Medi-Tech), H1 Headhunter, the JB1, Dav, and vertebral catheters. This type of catheter is placed into the arch just proximal to the origin of the artery of interest and rotated toward the orifice as it is being withdrawn slightly. Complex-curve catheters have a primary curve at the tip of the catheter and in also have a secondary curve along the distal shaft of the catheter that redirects the tip of the catheter, usually 90 degrees or more. The two or more curves on a complex-curve catheter shape work together to achieve a desired configuration that conforms to tortuous or challenging anatomy. Complex-curve cerebral catheters include the Simmons (1, 2, and 3) the H3 Headhunter, the JB2, and the Vitek catheters. These catheters have a head that must be reshaped in either the ascending or descending aorta, where there is minimal wall disease and a large enough diameter to allow the whole catheter head to take its shape. The catheter head is placed proximal to the branch vessel origin, and the catheter is simultaneously withdrawn and rotated.

AORTIC ARCH BRANCHES

The image intensifier remains in the LAO position after the arch aortogram and the approximate location of the vessel origin for cannulation is identified using bony landmarks. For example, the location of the origin of the left common carotid artery may be juxtaposed in the LAO projection to the location of the head of the clavicle. The best position for the image intensifier during arch aortography is a placement in which the field of view includes the area from the mid-ascending aorta to the mandible. This area will visualize the origin of the innominate artery and also the carotid bifurcation. The angled Glidecath or the H1 or other simple-curve catheter is passed over the guidewire to the location in the arch just inferior and proximal to the vessel

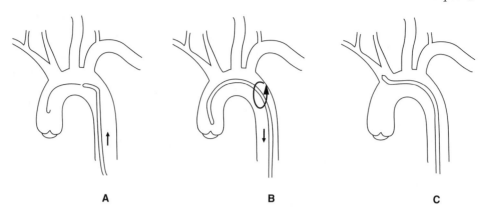

A B C

Fig. 3 Selective catheterization using a simple-curve cerebral catheter. (**A**) A guidewire is introduced into the ascending aorta and a simple-curve selective cerebral catheter is advanced over it. (**B**) The guidewire is removed, allowing the catheter head to take its shape. The catheter is gently withdrawn and rotated clockwise. (**C**) The tip of the catheter pops into the arch branch and the guidewire is advanced to secure access.

origin (Fig. 3). The guidewire is withdrawn and the catheter tip takes its shape. The guidewire is withdrawn into the shaft of the catheter to allow the head of the catheter to function freely and so that the catheterization is performed by leading with the catheter tip. The simple-curve catheter is rotated and withdrawn slightly so that its tip approaches the origin of the arch branch vessel. The tip of the catheter must be visualized using fluoroscopy and magnified views. The tip of the selective catheter tends to pop into the origin. The catheter may be rocked gently from side to side to allow the tip to seed more securely at the artery origin. An angled-tip, steerable Glidewire, usually 260 cm in length, is advanced into the artery. As the guidewire approaches the tip of the catheter along the shaft, slow down the advancement and observe carefully. Sometimes the guidewire itself will change the catheter shape enough so that the catheter will pop out of the artery of interest. After the guidewire has been advanced a few centimeters into the artery, nudge the catheter gently to follow the guidewire without popping out of the artery. Care must be taken to avoid advancing the guidewire tip into the bifurcation or across a lesion. Although this maneuver would add more purchase on the vessel for the catheter to enter the artery, it increases the risk of embolization. The placement of the bifurcation is available to the operator if the arch aortogram was performed with optimal placement of the image intensifier. Watch the catheter as it is being advanced. If the guidewire does not have enough purchase within the branch artery, the catheter and guidewire together will flip out of the artery. As the catheter is following the guidewire, if any of the curves are becoming tighter or more angulated, that is a sign that the guidewire will not follow to its intended destination. When too much tension builds in the guidewire–catheter apparatus, especially when traversing tortuous anatomy, a sudden jump of the catheter may occur. When the catheter follows the guidewire into the artery, it tends to gather up guidewire slack, eventually straighten out, and advance the guidewire forward. Care must be taken to avoid an undesired advancement of the guidewire. Refer back to the LAO arch aortogram to estimate the approximate location of the carotid bifurcation.

The innominate artery has the largest diameter of all the arch branches but it is placed in the most right-sided position on the arch. In addition, once the catheter is in the innominate, the guidewire does not always naturally go where it is intended. The innominate can often be catheterized with a simple-curve catheter, but if the arch is tortuous, a complex-curve catheter may be required. If the guidewire goes into the right common carotid artery, be careful to avoid passing the guidewire into the bifurcation. In some projections, the guidewire may appear to be in the right common carotid artery but may actually be in the right vertebral artery. Follow the projection of the guidewire. If it is heading into the vertebral foramina, it may be in the vertebral artery. Alternatively, the guidewire may be steered into the proximal right subclavian artery. The catheter is advanced over the guidewire and into the right subclavian artery. Cannulation of the right common carotid artery is performed by withdrawing the catheter head while administering contrast and slowly pulling the catheter into the innominate artery. The best projection for this, to see the innominate artery bifurcation, is a right anterior oblique. There is usually a small but perceptible jump inferiorly by the catheter tip as it is withdrawn from the origin of the right subclavian artery. The catheter head is rotated medially toward the origin of the right common carotid artery, and the steerable guidewire is advanced. Care must be taken to avoid advancing the guidewire into the bifurcation or across a lesion. The catheter is passed over the guidewire and into the right common carotid artery. If the guidewire will not enter the right common carotid artery, consider an innominate arteriogram in the right anterior oblique projection to show the innominate bifurcation. This is a location where distal innominate or proximal right subclavian artery stenosis may hide when it is only seen in the LAO projection. After the catheter is advanced into the appropriate position, the guidewire is removed steadily, the catheter is aspirated, and a few milliliters of contrast are puffed to check the position of the catheter tip before pressure injection is performed.

The left common carotid artery and left subclavian artery are cannulated in a similar manner; leading with the catheter, seeding it in the artery origin, then advancing the guidewire. The distance along the aortic arch from the origin of one branch to the next may be short, and it is occasionally a challenge to recognize which vessel has been entered. If it is not clear which artery has been entered, advance the guidewire and see where it is headed, which side of the neck. The catheter is placed so that its tip is just proximal to the left common carotid or left subclavian arteries. The catheter is withdrawn slightly and rotated. When the catheter tip pops into the artery, the guidewire is advanced using the same principles as outlined previously. In general, the simple-curve catheter functions well for cannulation of the left subclavian and left common carotid arteries since the angle of approach is usually less severe for these vessels than for the innominate artery. One exception to this is when the left common carotid artery is retroflexed or when it arises from a bovine configuration. In these cases, a complex-curve catheter may be required.

The complex-curve catheter may be used to cannulate any of the branch vessels but is most useful when the angle of origin of the arch branch is acute. This is often the case with the innominate artery. The multiple curvatures of the catheter head shape give these catheters a width that must be achieved prior to approaching the vessel. The catheter head must be reshaped to its intended configuration after the guidewire is removed and before it can be used for selective catheterization. The aorta is the only vessel large enough for this task. A complex-curve catheter head may be reshaped in the ascending aorta. The catheter is passed over the guidewire into the ascending aorta or into the proximal descending aorta (Fig. 4). The guidewire is withdrawn and the catheter is advanced slightly, permitting the catheter head to take its shape. In the example shown in Figure 4, the guidewire has been bounced off the aortic valve, creating a curve that can be followed by the catheter. When the guidewire is removed, the secondary curve is formed.

The reformed catheter head shape is advanced into the ascending aorta. The catheter is simultaneously withdrawn and rotated so that its tip lands in the branch vessel origin. Aortic arch disease is a contraindication to this maneuver. The catheter tip is visualized using fluoroscopy as it pops into the vessel origin. The guidewire is advanced into the artery. Gently withdrawing the catheter does two things: it removes some of the catheter's redundancy in the aortic arch, and the tip of the catheter tends to advance further into the selected artery as the distance of catheter distal to the secondary curve straightens out.

The catheter may also be reshaped using the distal aortic arch and the left subclavian artery (Fig. 5). A guidewire is placed into the left subclavian artery using a simple-curve catheter, such as Vert catheter. A complex-curve catheter, such as a Simmons 2, is placed over the guidewire. The secondary curve of the catheter is placed so that it is mostly left in the arch, with only the tip of catheter hanging into the left subclavian artery. The guidewire is withdrawn to the location of the origin of the artery. Without guidewire in the distal portion of the catheter, the head begins to take shape, and the tip of the catheter becomes much softer. The catheter is withdrawn slightly until the large elbow of the secondary takes shape in the arch. As the secondary curve takes shape, the catheter is advanced into the proximal arch.

The subclavian artery may be approached antegrade through a femoral artery access or retrograde through a brachial artery puncture. Through the

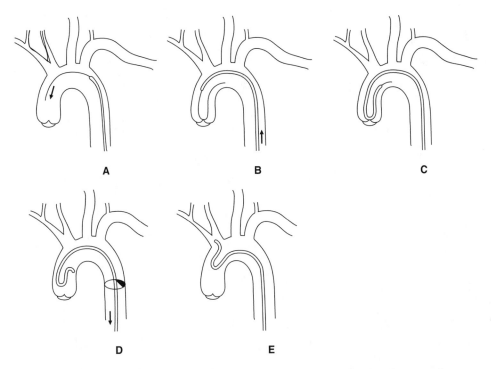

Fig. 4 Selective catheterization using a complex-curve cerebral catheter: reforming a Simmons catheter in the ascending aorta. (**A**) A guidewire is introduced into the ascending aorta and a complex-curve (Simmons) selective cerebral catheter is advanced over it. (**B**) The guidewire is allowed to bounce off the aortic valve and come back on itself antegrade in the aortic arch. The catheter is advanced into the ascending aorta. (**C**) The catheter follows the guidewire antegrade into the aortic arch. (**D**) The guidewire is removed and the catheter head has reformed in the ascending aorta. The catheter is gently withdrawn and rotated clockwise. (**E**) The tip of the catheter engages the origin of the arch branch as the tip spins superiorly.

aortic arch, the left subclavian artery may be cannulated using a simple- or complex-curve catheter (Figs. 6 and 7). The guidewire is advanced after the catheter tip is placed in the artery origin. The guidewire usually follows the characteristic curve of the left subclavian artery. When the catheter is advanced, consider placing the tip either well proximal or well distal to the origin of the vertebral artery to avoid injury during arteriography.

The retrograde approach is simple and direct and does not always require instrumentation of the aortic arch or its other branches. If a very large sheath is required for brachial access (8 Fr or larger), a cutdown should be considered. A floppy-tip guidewire is advanced from the brachial artery into the subclavian artery. A straight, multiple side hole arteriographic catheter is passed over the guidewire. The guidewire is removed and an arteriogram is obtained. When a subclavian artery lesion is present, contrast may be injected either distal or proximal to the lesion. High-pressure injection is

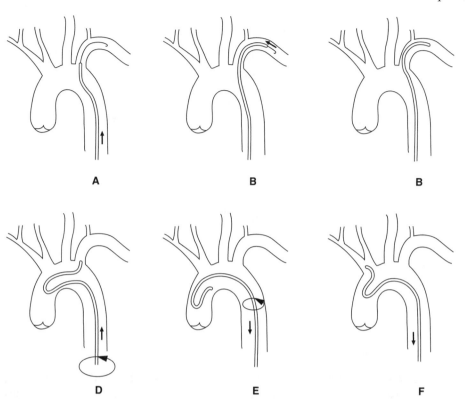

A **B** **B**

D **E** **F**

Fig. 5 Selective catheterization using a complex-curve cerebral catheter: reforming a Simmons catheter in the subclavian artery. (**A**) A simple-curve catheter is placed in the subclavian artery and exchanged for a complex-curve catheter. (**B**) As the guidewire is withdrawn, the catheter head begins to take its curved shape. (**C**) The guidewire tip is withdrawn until it is just proximal to the second curve. (**D**) Slight forward pressure on the catheter permits the head to reform in the arch. After reforming, the catheter is rotated and advanced simultaneously into the ascending aorta. (**E**) The catheter is gently withdrawn and rotated clockwise to engage the arch branches. (**F**) After the catheter tip has entered the arch branch of interest, in this case the innominate artery, slight traction on the catheter tends to advance it into the artery as the large curve begins to straighten out. Advancing the Simmons catheter tends to pull the tip of the catheter out of the artery as the large curve moves toward the aortic valve.

usually not required distal to a significant subclavian artery stenosis and is contraindicated at the origin of the vertebral artery. Contrast usually refluxes through the lesion to delineate it. If the lesion to be evaluated or treated is at the origin or proximal subclavian artery, the guidewire is passed into the aortic arch and steered inferiorly into the descending thoracic aorta using an LAO projection (Fig. 8). The guidewire usually advances into the proximal arch, so an angled-tip or hook-shaped catheter is usually required to steer the guidewire into the descending aorta. This is most important when

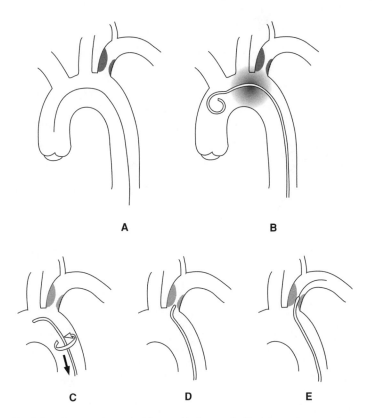

Fig. 6 Selective catheterization of the subclavian artery using a simple-curve catheter. (**A**) A guidewire is placed in the ascending aorta. (**B**) A flush catheter is placed and an arch aortogram is performed, usually in the LAO position. (**C**) After the location of the origin of the artery and the lesion are identified, the flush catheter is exchanged for a simple-curve catheter. The catheter is withdrawn slightly and rotated. (**D**) The catheter tip enters the origin of the artery. (**E**) A selective guidewire is advanced into the artery. After a substantial length of guidewire is in the artery, the catheter may also be advanced.

endovascular therapy is planned so that a satisfactory length of guidewire may be safely deployed distal to the lesion. Injections in the aortic arch must be performed with a pressure injector. The location and detail of the left subclavian artery origin are usually difficult to visualize through a retrograde subclavian injection. High flow in the arch rapidly carries away any contrast, which refluxes into the arch. Forward flow into the subclavian artery may be minimal, and residual lumen is partially occupied by the catheter which has been passed retrograde through it. Use of a radiopaque-tipped catheter helps to identify the subclavian artery origin with fluoroscopy. The vertebral artery is protected somewhat when there is reversed flow. If the subclavian

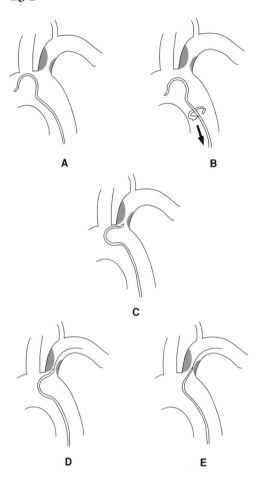

Fig. 7 Selective catheterization of the subclavian artery using a complex-curve catheter. (**A**) The catheter, in this example an H3 Headhunter, is placed in the aortic arch proximal to the subclavian artery. (**B**) The catheter is simultaneously withdrawn and rotated. (**C**) The tip of the catheter engages the origin of the artery. (**D**) The selective guidewire is passed into the artery. The guidewire must be advanced gently because if forward pressure is applied too vigorously the catheter will pop out of the artery. (**E**) As the guidewire passes into the artery, the catheter head straightens and the catheter may be advanced.

lesion anatomy is still unclear, a flush catheter can be placed transfemorally and an arch aortogram can be obtained.

Selective Catheterization of the Visceral and Renal Arteries

CELIAC AND SUPERIOR MESENTERIC ARTERIES

The visceral arteries may be approached through the femoral or the brachial arteries. Catheterization for arteriography is usually satisfactory using a

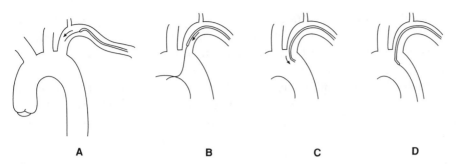

Fig. 8 Retrograde or transbrachial catheterization of the subclavian artery. (**A**) After brachial puncture using a micropuncture set, the guidewire is passed retrograde into the proximal subclavian artery and a selective catheter is placed over it. (**B**) The tendency of the guidewire when advanced into the arch is to proceed into the ascending aorta. A simple-curve or hook-shaped selective catheter is advanced into the distal arch. (**C**) The guidewire is withdrawn and the catheter is directed posterolaterally. (**D**) The guidewire is redirected into the descending aorta.

femoral approach. When therapy is indicated, a transbrachial approach should be considered, since the angle of origin of these arteries is more favorable for entry through a proximal approach. A diagnostic catheter is placed in the proximal paravisceral aorta and an anteroposterior aortogram is performed. This permits approximate localization of the arterial origins, evaluation of the integrity of the distal visceral vessels, and identification of variant anatomy. The catheter head may be adjusted slightly proximally or distally so that the side holes end at the level of the arteries' origins. The image intensifier is placed in full 90-degree lateral position and brought close to the patient's side. The arms are extended above the patient's head, which may be relatively uncomfortable for the patient. The field is magnified and filtered so that the catheter head is at the top of the field of view and the posterior portion of the vertebral column is excluded from the field. The aortogram is repeated with breath-holding technique in midinspiration. Full contraction of the diaphragm may result in impingement of the visceral artery origins in some patients, especially the celiac artery. The locations of the artery origins are identified using the vertebra as bony landmarks. A hook-shaped catheter is exchanged for the diagnostic catheter (Table 2). The guidewire is withdrawn, allowing the hook to take its shape. The catheter is withdrawn slowly as its tip is steered anteriorly. The tip of the catheter engages the origin of the artery. The catheter tip tends to pop into the orifice of the artery. The lateral profile of the aorta can often be visualized on fluoroscopy because of calcification lining the wall of the aorta. The catheter tip is seen extending anterior to the profile of the aorta, as the tip enters the branch. This is another example where leading with the catheter is usually the best approach. The catheter is gently manipulated to seed it at the artery origin and advance it slightly into the vessel origin. An angled-tip Glidewire is advanced into the artery and the catheter may be advanced. Through a transfemoral approach, the angle of advancement of the catheter as it enters the visceral artery is acute. Therefore, the guidewire must be advanced a fair distance into the artery being selected in order for the operator to have enough purchase to advance the catheter. The catheters with a more acute turn are best for cannulating the visceral arteries. However, they are not as simple to advance into the artery because it takes more guidewire length to straighten the curve of the catheter to get it to advance past the artery origin.

RENAL ARTERY

Aortography is performed with a flush catheter to evaluate the aorta, iliac arteries, and renal arteries. The catheter head is usually placed at the level of the first lumbar vertebral body. After the initial aortogram is assessed, the catheter head may be adjusted slightly so that it lies distal to the superior mesenteric artery (SMA) and is less likely to reflux a significant amount of contrast into the visceral arteries. An aortorenal arteriogram is then performed with magnification and filters. The flush aortorenal arteriogram usually demonstrates whether there is any significant stenosis at the origin of the renal artery. Occasionally, the lie of the superior mesenteric artery obscures the proximal renal artery, especially on the right side. In addition, if the aorta or renal arteries are tortuous, the proximal renal artery can be covered by the aorta itself. An ipsilateral anterior oblique projection of approximately 10 degrees is best for evaluating an orifice lesion if additional detail is required prior to selective catheterization of the artery. If there is CT imaging available from a prior study, the angle of origin of the renal artery from the aorta can be measured and the appropriate oblique projection obtained.

The arteriographic catheter is exchanged for a C2 cobra catheter and passed into the pararenal aorta (Fig. 9). After passage of the cobra catheter to a level just above the renal artery origin, the guidewire is removed and the catheter head takes shape. The tip of the cobra catheter is directed toward the posterolateral sidewall of the aorta and the catheter is slowly withdrawn. The guidewire may be maintained in the shaft of the catheter so that it can be rapidly advanced when necessary. Since the renal artery orifice is on the posterolateral wall of the aorta, other major visceral branch vessels are not encountered by the tip of the catheter but a lumbar artery may be. The tip of the catheter usually falls into the renal artery orifice with a small but perceptible jump, so that its tip appears beyond the profile of the aortic wall. The guidewire may be advanced to probe the artery. Puffed contrast confirms the location of the catheter tip and ensures that it is safe for a higher-pressure injection.

This discussion is about selective catheterization of the renal arteries as described. However, since most renal artery lesions requiring treatment

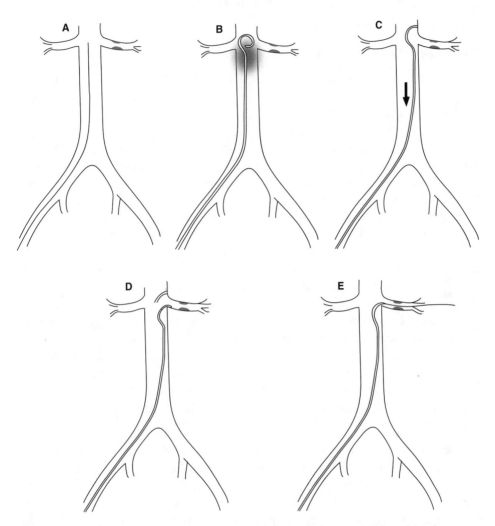

Fig. 9 Catheterization of the renal artery. (**A**) A guidewire is placed in the aorta. (**B**) An arteriographic catheter is placed and an aortogram and renal arteriogram are obtained. (**C**) The arteriographic catheter is exchanged for a cobra catheter that is advanced proximal to the renal artery. The cobra catheter is slowly withdrawn with its tip along the posterolateral aortic wall. (**D**) The tip of the cobra catheter falls into the renal artery orifice. (**E**) The guidewire is advanced through the renal artery lesion.

are at the origin of the artery, catheterization of a severely diseased artery is usually not carried out unless treatment is planned. In that case, a guiding sheath or guide catheter would be placed and a platform created so that once the guidewire is across the lesion, treatment can be performed without further exchanges.

Selective Catheterization of the Aortoiliac Arteries

PASSAGE OVER THE AORTIC BIFURCATION

An aortoiliac arteriogram is performed to evaluate aortic bifurcation disease, angle, and location. The aortic bifurcation may be localized using bony landmarks or vascular calcification. It is usually located at or near the level of the iliac crest. Vascular calcification often outlines the aortic bifurcation and serves as a road map. A hook-shaped catheter is passed into the infrarenal abdominal aorta (Fig. 10). The catheter should be a minimum of 65 cm in length. Some catheters such as the Omni-flush (Angiodynamics, Queensbury, New York, U.S.A.) are designed for aortography but also have a hook-shaped head and may be used to cross the aortic bifurcation. Aortic bifurcation cannulation may also be performed with a C2 cobra (Cook, Inc., Bloomington, Indiana, U.S.A.). In a patient with a narrow aortic bifurcation, a Rosch IMA catheter (Cook, Inc.) has a tighter hook shape and allows the guidewire to turn at a more acute angle. The catheter head is withdrawn using fluoroscopy and bony landmarks to a location within one vertebral body proximal to the bifurcation. The guidewire is withdrawn so that the catheter head takes its shape. If the catheter head is not reshaped to its usual configuration after the guidewire is withdrawn, the catheter shaft must be manipulated with fluoroscopic guidance. If the infrarenal aorta is narrow or diseased, the catheter tip may catch on the vessel wall. Give the catheter a small forward push and it usually forms the correct shape. If there is doubt, turn the catheter to be sure the head clears the sidewall without changing shape.

The catheter is slowly withdrawn and rotated until the tip of the hooked portion of the catheter head is pointing toward the contralateral iliac artery. An angled-tip Glidewire is advanced gently into the contralateral iliac artery, and the torque device is used to allow the guidewire tip to probe the proximal contralateral iliac artery. When a few centimeters of guidewire have been passed to the contralateral iliac system, the catheter may be withdrawn slightly to hang it on the flow divider at the bifurcation of the aorta. The head of the catheter assumes a slightly more splayed configuration when it is pulled into position where it is resting on the aortic flow divider. The tip of the guidewire frequently catches on plaque in the contralateral iliac artery and the torque device is used to steer the guidewire away and antegrade down the artery. The catheter head may not be safely pulled onto the flow divider if the guidewire is still caught on the plaque. If the guidewire catches on the plaque in the contralateral iliac artery and the operator does not recognize this and continues to push the guidewire, the catheter and guidewire will pop out or flip out of the iliac artery and back into the infrarenal aorta.

When the iliac arteries are tortuous, the extra turns the catheter must pass through usually make the hook of the catheter point to the ipsilateral

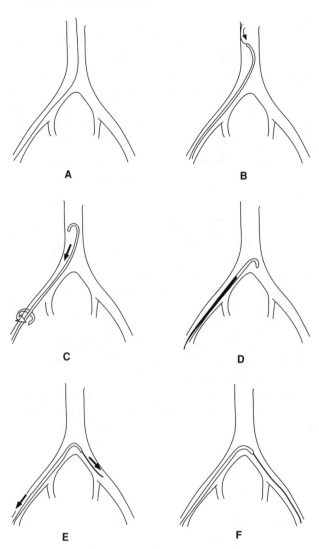

Fig. 10 Crossing the aortic bifurcation. (**A**) After an aortogram is performed to identify the location, configuration, and arterial disease burden of the bifurcation, the guidewire is placed in the infrarenal aorta. (**B**) A hook-shaped selective catheter is passed over the guidewire. The catheter and guidewire are withdrawn until the head of the catheter is just proximal to the aortic bifurcation and the guidewire is removed. (**C**) The catheter head takes its shape. The catheter is rotated toward the contralateral side and withdrawn simultaneously. (**D**) The guidewire is advanced into the catheter head. (**E**) As the guidewire passes through the catheter head, the catheter head becomesmore firm and takes a more rounded shape. The catheter can be pulled back slightly so that its curve sits directly on the flow divider. (**F**) The guidewire is then advanced from a very secure position.

side. Tortuosity also makes the catheter head less responsive to turns performed at the catheter hub. The catheter head may not rotate in response to turning the hub and then suddenly turn 360 degrees back to its original position. The operator may have to use both hands to slowly manipulate the catheter head so that it points in the correct direction and have the assistant advance the guidewire. Another option is to withdraw the catheter just as it begins to rotate so that its tip catches the contralateral iliac origin as it comes around. Crossing the aortic bifurcation is usually performed with 0.035-in. guidewires and 4- or 5-Fr catheters. If the bifurcation is very narrow, as is the case with a prosthetic graft, a 0.025-in. guidewire may be used since it has a tighter radius of curvature.

When the catheter head hangs on the aortic bifurcation, it assumes a more broadly curved shape. If a contralateral iliac arteriogram is planned from this position, a catheter without side holes should be used since the segment with side holes extends well back into the infrarenal aorta and ipsilateral iliac artery. Most often, the plan is to advance the catheter further into the contralateral iliac artery. The guidewire is advanced beyond the inguinal ligament if possible. The guidewire is pinned and the catheter is advanced. The further the guidewire is advanced, or "buried," on the contralateral side, the better purchase is obtained to permit the catheter to be advanced over the guidewire, despite the acute-angle turn at the aortic bifurcation. If the catheter is advanced by hand but the catheter tip is not advancing antegrade into the contralateral iliac system, the guidewire and catheter are usually bunching up together into the distal aorta (Fig. 11). If this is not

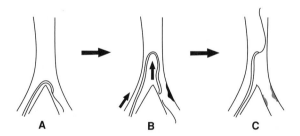

Fig. 11 Catheter pops out of contralateral iliac artery. (**A**) Guidewire is placed antegrade into contralateral iliac system and the catheter is passed over it. If the catheter engages the wall of the proximal iliac artery, it may not advance. (**B**) If continued forward motion is applied to the catheter when its tip is not advancing, the catheter begins to buckle into the infrarenal aorta. (**C**) Continued forward pressure on the catheter will cause the catheter tip to pop out of the iliac artery and drag the guidewire along with it. This scenario can usually be avoided by passing the guidewire as far as possible into the contralateral iliac system as possible before advancing the catheter. When the catheter tip is passing through the proximal contralateral iliac artery, observe it carefully, especially if the artery is diseased. If the catheter tip hangs up, stop applying forward pressure.

recognized early, continued catheter insertion will drag the guidewire out of the contralateral iliac artery and into the aorta.

When the ipsilateral iliac artery is tortuous or redundant, retrograde advancement of the catheter up the ipsilateral iliac artery over the guidewire can be challenging. With each push, the catheter and guidewire may accordion on the ipsilateral side without making progress toward the bifurcation. Other challenges arise when the aortic bifurcation has a very narrow angle, is proximally placed, or is heavily calcified. When any of these conditions are combined with a scarred or diseased femoral access site, the passage of a catheter or sheath over the aortic bifurcation can be difficult.

When the guidewire passes over the bifurcation and progresses antegrade down the contralateral iliac system, it usually enters the internal iliac artery as it is advanced. The internal iliac artery is often a straight in-line direction of advance, especially with tortuous iliac arteries (Fig. 12). In that case, the guidewire usually hangs up in a branch of the internal iliac artery or progresses into a branch far enough from the intended course that it becomes clear that the guidewire has entered the internal iliac artery. The catheter may be advanced over the bifurcation and into the contralateral common iliac artery or even the internal iliac artery. The guidewire is withdrawn. Hook-shaped catheter heads shorten substantially when the guidewire is withdrawn and they are no longer forced into a straight position. The catheter is withdrawn if necessary to make sure its tip is in the common iliac artery. The steerable guidewire is passed again. The catheter may be used to direct the guidewire anterolaterally toward the external iliac artery.

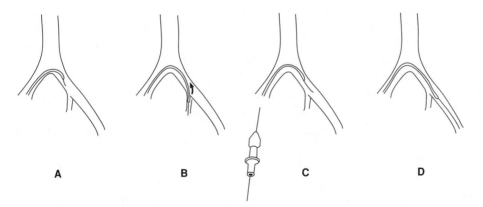

A   B   C   D

Fig. 12 Guidewire–catheter advances into the internal iliac artery. (**A**) The guidewire frequently, almost preferentially, enters the internal iliac artery as it is advanced into the contralateral iliac artery. This is especially the case when the iliac system is tortuous. (**B**) The catheter is withdrawn back toward the common iliac artery. The guidewire is pulled back to the catheter tip. (**C**) A torque device is used to steer the guidewire anterolaterally. (**D**) The guidewire is advanced into the external iliac artery and the catheter follows.

Significant occlusive or aneurysmal disease of the distal aorta or the common iliac arteries are a contraindication to crossing the aortic bifurcation. Safe passage across the aortic bifurcation is more difficult if there is occlusive disease at the bifurcation, significant iliac tortuosity, or aneurysmal degeneration near the aortic bifurcation. Occlusive disease at the aortic bifurcation is usually worse along the posterior aortic wall just proximal to and extending into the iliac arteries. The anteroposterior aortogram almost always underestimates the plaque load at this location and the operator must be wary of generating emboli. Significant tortuosity of the iliac vessel through which the catheter is passed makes the torque of the catheter much less predictable. After going through several longitudinal turns, the catheter head may be difficult to rotate. A sheath may be placed with its tip in the proximal ipsilateral iliac artery. This maneuver helps to counteract some of the impingement effect of the tortuosity upon the guidewire–catheter apparatus. Aneurysmal changes in the aorta or iliac arteries may add significant risk to this maneuver. When an infrarenal abdominal aortic aneurysm is present that does not involve the aortic bifurcation, the hook-shaped catheter head should be reshaped in the proximal ipsilateral iliac artery or very distal aorta to avoid dragging the hook through the aneurysm. Occasionally, it is safer to perform an additional contralateral femoral puncture to complete the intended catheterization than to cross a severely diseased bifurcation.

PLAN OF ATTACK: CROSSING THE AORTIC BIFURCATION

1. Evaluate the aortogram to determine that the bifurcation is relatively free of aneurysmal and occlusive disease so this will be a safe maneuver. The presence of significant disease in the proximal contralateral iliac artery may also be a contraindication to crossing the bifurcation.
2. Choose the catheter based on the appearance of the aorta. A bifurcation angle that is more acute requires a tighter hook to accomplish the task. Use a catheter with a radiopaque tip.
3. Advance the catheter over the guidewire and into the infrarenal aorta (Fig. 10).
4. Use bony landmarks to identify the location of the aortic bifurcation. The aortogram may be used as a guide to assist the operator in deciding how to maneuver the catheter into position.
5. Withdraw the guidewire a short distance to allow the catheter head to take its shape. The guidewire position is maintained in the shaft of the catheter.
6. Slowly withdraw the catheter and guidewire together as a single unit until the hook of the catheter head is just proximal to the aortic flow divider. Rotate the catheter so that its tip points into the contralateral iliac artery. Evaluate using fluoroscopy to be sure the catheter tip

does not hook a sidewall aortic plaque. Use a smaller field of view so that the catheter and guidewire are magnified.

7. Advance the guidewire into the contralateral iliac artery as far as possible and "bury" it so that the catheter can be advanced over it. After the guidewire has passed into the contralateral iliac artery for several centimeters, readjust the catheter by withdrawing it slightly. This will allow the hook of the catheter to hang on to the aortic flow divider. This is a fairly secure position for guidewire advancement.

8. Advance the catheter antegrade into the contralateral iliac system after a long segment of guidewire has been placed.

9. After the catheter has crossed the bifurcation, withdraw the guidewire for arteriography. If larger endovascular devices such as a guiding sheath are intended for passage, place a stiffer exchange guidewire.

10. Use fluoroscopy during catheter placement to inspect the tip of the guidewire to be sure it is not migrating. Spot-check the aortic bifurcation to ensure that redundant catheter is not accumulating in the distal aorta.

Selective Catheterization of the Infrainguinal Arteries

SUPERFICIAL FEMORAL AND POPLITEAL ARTERIES: UP-AND-OVER APPROACH

The selective catheter is passed up and over the aortic bifurcation as described in the earlier section (Fig. 10). A 150-cm guidewire permits catheter passage to the contralateral groin or proximal infrainguinal arteries in the average-sized adult. A longer guidewire, 180-cm or 260-cm guidewire, is required for catheter passage to the distal femoral or popliteal level. In this area, because arterial disease tends to be diffuse, the operator leads with the guidewire and then follows with the catheter. In addition, catheter pushability is severely limited in long conduit arteries, unless the guidewire is used as a rail over which to push the catheter.

A 65-cm catheter will usually reach the proximal to mid SFA. A 90-cm catheter is required to reach the distal SFA or popliteal artery levels. After the hook-shaped catheter that has been used to cross the aortic bifurcation is securely placed into the contralateral iliac artery, the guidewire may be advanced into the infrainguinal arterial segment. If it is anticipated that a longer guidewire is needed to go the distance in the contralateral lower extremity, the operator should make the exchange after the catheter has crossed the aortic bifurcation. When performing selective arteriography, the catheter itself will be left passing over the aortic bifurcation and down the lower extremity. During guidewire exchanges, the catheter must be stable enough so that the guidewire does not drag the catheter back up into the aorta. Consider using a catheter with some shaft stiffness, such as a braided catheter, to enhance stability. During intervention, a sheath is placed to use as a platform for treatment. The tip of the sheath is typically placed fairly close to the target lesion, whether in the SFA, popliteal, or tibial arteries. This is a much more stable apparatus and is covered in more detail in chapter 14.

When the guidewire is passed from the contralateral side, it tends to preferentially enter the SFA when it is pushed past the inguinal ligament. This can usually be identified under plain fluoroscopy by the path followed by the advancing guidewire. If the guidewire enters the profunda or a collateral, the operator should remove the guidewire, place the image intensifier in an ipsilateral anterior oblique position to view the femoral bifurcation, and obtain a road map. This opens the femoral bifurcation and permits the operator to localize the SFA origin. The guidewire is advanced, using a steerable tip, and the SFA origin is cannulated. If the femoral anatomy is complex or there is significant common femoral artery disease, it may be difficult to catheterize the SFA with these maneuvers. In this case, advance the guidewire as far as it will go into the profunda or into a collateral vessel. Then advance the catheter into the distal external iliac artery or proximal common femoral artery. Withdraw the guidewire into the common femoral artery and probe the origin of the SFA. This catheter positioning provides better control and improves guidewire responsiveness. If there is too much disease, one may elect to get the best angiogram possible form this location.

The guidewire is advanced into the SFA as far as possible and the catheter is advanced over it. The catheter usually follows the guidewire; however, trackability may be poor because of the long distance and the acute-angle turn at the aortic bifurcation. The guidewire is pinned and the catheter is advanced firmly by pushing on the catheter shaft near the percutaneous access site. A slight twist of the catheter while advancing may also be useful. If the catheter will not advance, a stiffer guidewire should be used. The operator may also consider removing the hook-shaped catheter used to cross the aortic bifurcation and placing a straight catheter with multiple side holes. This catheter may track the guidewire better.

SUPERFICIAL FEMORAL AND POPLITEAL ARTERIES: ANTEGRADE APPROACH

Antegrade femoral puncture is presented in detail in chapter 3. Prior to antegrade puncture, any previous arteriograms of the femoral area should be evaluated for the location of the bifurcation relative to the inguinal ligament. The femoral bifurcation may also be localized with duplex scanning. Puncturing the common femoral artery under ultrasound or fluoroscopy will help to ensure that the access is in the proximal common femoral artery and will permit working room to get into the SFA. An antegrade approach should only be considered when ipsilateral aortoiliac inflow occlusive disease has been ruled out. Consider using a micropuncture set with a 21-gauge needle and a 0.018-in. steerable guidewire to help facilitate antegrade puncture. Following antegrade puncture of the common femoral artery, a steerable-tip steel guidewire is passed through the needle (Fig. 13). Occasionally, the guidewire enters the SFA on the first pass; however, it tends to preferentially enter the orifice of the deep femoral artery after an antegrade puncture because of the angle of approach. The guidewire should be advanced far enough so that it does not fall out of the artery, usually about 10 or 15 cm. A torque device is advanced along the guidewire until it is a few centimeters from the hub of the needle. The curved-tip guidewire is directed anteriorly and medially to enter the SFA. Frequently, the SFA may be catheterized by directing the steerable guidewire directly from the puncture site. Care must be taken to avoid losing access since working room between the puncture site and the SFA origin may be only a few centimeters. If the guidewire cannot be directed into the SFA, advance the guidewire into the deep femoral artery until the firm portion of the guidewire crosses the arterial entry site at the common femoral artery. A short (40 cm), 5-Fr bent-tip catheter (C2 cobra, Berenstein, or Kumpe) is passed over the guidewire and the guidewire is removed. The catheter is gradually withdrawn using fluoroscopy while small amounts of contrast are injected by hand. As the tip of the catheter nears the femoral bifurcation, contrast refluxes into the bifurcation. When the SFA orifice is opacified by contrast administration, the tip of the catheter is rotated and directed anteriorly and medially to cannulate the SFA. The operator may also consider road mapping the femoral bifurcation.

Because working room is usually minimal, the catheter must be carefully secured. Catheter movements must be deliberate. A few millimeters of movement in either direction can pop the tip of the catheter out of the SFA orifice or even out of the common femoral artery puncture site. The guidewire is passed through the short catheter and into the SFA orifice. The guidewire is advanced into the mid or distal SFA. The selective catheter is exchanged for the appropriate arteriographic catheter. If the puncture site is so close to the bifurcation that the SFA cannot be catheterized, remove the guidewire and hold pressure until hemostasis is adequate. The anatomy of the inguinal ligament is reevaluated. Fluoroscopy is used to locate the superior aspect of the femoral head. A repeat attempt at the antegrade approach may be undertaken if it can be done safely.

TIBIAL ARTERIES

An adequate tibial and pedal arteriogram can usually be obtained by administering contrast somewhere proximal to the origin of the tibial arteries. However, when flow is impaired due to inflow or outflow disease, and especially if there is severe tibial or pedal disease, arteriography of the distal lower extremity may be very difficult to obtain. Arteriography is further discussed

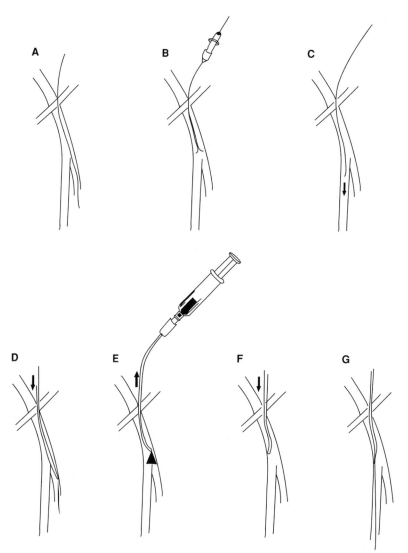

Fig. 13 Catheterization of the SFA. (**A**) After antegrade puncture of the common femoral artery, the guidewire tends to preferentially advance into the deep femoral artery. (**B**) The initial guidewire can be exchanged for a steerable Wholey guidewire. A torque device is used to redirect the guidewire tip. (**C**) The steerable guidewire rotates medially and anteriorly and advances into the SFA. (**D**) A Berenstein or cobra catheter can be passed over the guidewire in the deep femoral artery and the guidewire removed. (**E**) The selective catheter is very slowly withdrawn as contrast is puffed to identify the femoral bifurcation. (**F**) The tip of the selective catheter is rotated toward the origin of the SFA. (**G**) The guidewire is advanced through the selective catheter and into the SFA.

in chapter 10. The operator should be skilled in catheterization of the tibial arteries when needed for adequate arteriography or for intervention.

The guidewire is directed into the popliteal arteries using either an up-and-over or an antegrade approach. Advance an appropriately lengthy angled-tip catheter into the popliteal level. Perform an arteriogram of the trifurcation area and use it as a road map. Usually an AP projection or a slight anterior ipsilateral oblique is used to identify the tibial artery origins. Place a Tuohy-Borst adapter and a 0.014-in. guidewire and use this set up to enter the tibial arteries (chap. 6). Contrast is administered through the adapter to help identify the location of the tibial origin. Better control may be obtained with an antegrade approach due to the shorter distance and lack of major turns. The choice of approach is discussed further in chapter 20. If extensive catheterization of the tibial arteries is planned, continued advance of the guidewire results in cannulation of the tibioperoneal trunk and then the tibial arteries (Fig. 14). Contrast injection demonstrates the location of the orifice of each of the arteries.

INFRAINGUINAL VEIN BYPASS GRAFTS

The most important factors influencing the catheterization of lower-extremity bypass grafts are the location of the proximal anastomosis, the volume of flow within the graft, and whether the graft has been tunneled in a superficial or deep plane. Worthwhile preoperative maneuvers include a review of the original operative report and arteriograms and a current duplex map of the vein graft.

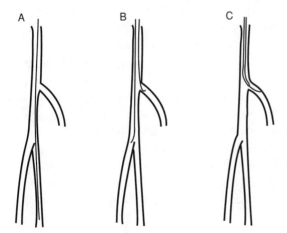

Fig. 14 Catheterization of the tibial artery. (**A**) The peroneal artery is usually the preferential course of a guidewire passed beyond the below-knee popliteal artery. (**B**) A steerable hydrophilic-coated guidewire can be used to cannulate the anterior tibial artery or posterior tibial artery. (**C**) The steerable guidewire is directed by a bent-tip Berenstein catheter to enter an anterior tibial artery with a difficult angle of origin.

The approach is based upon the location of the proximal anastomosis. Infrainguinal bypass grafts that originate from the superficial femoral artery, deep femoral artery, or popliteal artery may be approached through either an up-and-over approach or an ipsilateral antegrade femoral puncture. The ipsilateral approach provides better control of endovascular devices but it also means a puncture site proximal to the bypass graft that must be closed by holding pressure. Antegrade punctures may sometimes be closed with closure devices but this is not recommended. A graft that has its origin in the common femoral artery must be catheterized from the contralateral side by passing the guidewire over the aortic bifurcation. The volume of flow within the graft determines how readily the graft origin is identified. If the graft is patent and functioning, contrast injection with the image intensifier in the right position will show the way to catheterization. If the graft is occluded or flow is very low, look for an outpouching or nipple of contrast extending beyond the usual confines of the artery of origin that represents the location where the proximal anastomosis is located. Grafts that have been tunneled superficially may be punctured percutaneously, usually almost anywhere along the course of the graft. Use a micropuncture set for this. Noninvasive mapping to show the location of the abnormality is useful to ensure adequate working room between the puncture site and the lesion.

An anastomosis is usually created on the anterior aspect of the inflow vessel and bypass grafts have no branches. These factors are considered in identification of the graft orifice. Flow through the proximal aspect of the graft may be minimal and is usually superimposed on the artery from which it originates. As the catheter and guidewire approach the proximal anastomosis in an antegrade direction, an oblique or even lateral view of the artery is useful to assist in identifying the location of the proximal anastomosis. Look for the presence of surgical clips to define the correct radiographic field of view. A patent but low-flow infrainguinal graft that could not be visualized upon initial contrast injection will often be seen when contrast is injected closer to the graft origin and with the image intensifier in the oblique or lateral position. A bent-tip catheter, steerable guidewire, or combination of the two may be used to enter the hood of the graft. The hood is gently probed with the steerable guidewire and a magnified field of view until the guidewire falls into the graft. A 0.014-in. guidewire is useful in this situation. When a low-flow graft is catheterized, the catheter itself may stop flow. Therefore, heparin should be administered in this situation, even if intervention is not intended.

TECHNIQUE: ENTERING AN INFRAINGUINAL VEIN GRAFT

1. Find out the location of the proximal anastomosis. Hints can be found in operative notes, previous preoperative or intraoperative completion angiography, previous graft surveillance duplex studies, and fluoroscopy of surgical clips.

2. If the graft is patent, check the duplex map to see if the lesion is at or near the proximal anastomosis. It helps if the operator knows whether to expect a wide-open graft hood or a tight proximal lesion.

3. Check the graft flow rate on the duplex scan to judge the expected flow of contrast in the graft. If it is less than the adjacent native circulation, sometimes only a wisp of contrast enters the graft. Use the preoperative duplex scan to mark the location of occlusive lesions, especially if endovascular therapy is planned.

4. If the graft originates from the deep femoral artery, superficial femoral artery, or popliteal artery, consider approaching through an ipsilateral, antegrade puncture. If it originates from the common femoral artery, use a contralateral femoral approach.

5. Use an oblique view rather than an anteroposterior view since the graft origin is almost always on the anterior surface of the artery and is superimposed upon the native circulation.

6. When the tip of the arteriographic catheter is close to where the anastomosis is located, puff contrast. If the graft hood can be seen, advance the catheter closer to it, adjust the oblique angle of the image intensifier for the best view, and road map the origin of the graft.

7. Use a steerable, hydrophilic-coated guidewire to enter the origin of the graft. Consider using a 0.014-in. platform for entering the graft, especially if the lesion is very tight.

8. If the graft lesion is very tight, administer heparin because the catheter or even the guidewire alone may effectively stop flow.

9. If the graft is subcutaneous, make sure that table straps and other appliances do not impinge on the graft and impede the flow of contrast into it.

10. Manipulate and change both the leg position and the C-arm position to obtain the best views of the graft.

11. If the graft origin cannot be entered, puncture the graft directly with the assistance of real-time duplex scanning. This may be difficult in low-flow situations. If the graft is punctured and endovascular intervention does not result in improved flow, be alert to the possibility of immediate thrombosis.

Selective Catheterization of Prosthetic Bypass Grafts

Prosthetic bypass grafts may require catheterization as a strategic maneuver prior to endovascular or open revision or to evaluate end organ ischemia in the vascular bed served by the previously placed graft. Percutaneous access may be obtained by one of three methods: (1) puncture of the native artery at a site remote from the graft, (2) direct puncture of the graft near its anastomosis with the native artery, and (3) puncture of the body of the graft in a subcutaneous position. Chapter 3 includes more details about direct graft puncture for percutaneous access. In general, puncture of the native artery followed by fluoroscopic placement of a catheter into the graft is safest. Direct percutaneous, prosthetic puncture is commonly performed but is slightly more likely to be complicated by thrombosis or infection. When puncturing a prosthetic graft through a scarred groin, use a standard 18-gauge entry needle and a stiffer introduction guidewire, such as a Rosen wire. This is because the scar at the groin often makes it difficult to pass the next larger-sized device and the placement of a stiffer wire early helps with that. Antibiotics should be administered prior to the procedure. Prosthetic grafts are lined with pseudointima that may embolize or form an obstructive flap if disrupted. The lining of the prosthetic graft is less resistant to thrombus formation than that of an autologous graft. Catheterization of low-flow grafts may be followed by thrombosis, especially if holding pressure at a graft puncture after catheter removal further impedes flow.

Approaches to selective catheterization of prosthetic grafts are listed in Table 3. Brachiocephalic grafts, such as carotid-subclavian bypasses, usually originate at a 90-degree angle. This is a difficult angle to negotiate and there is a risk of cerebral embolization of pericatheter clot or pseudointima. If the graft is not adequately evaluated with a selective common carotid artery injection, consider approaching the graft retrograde through the ipsilateral brachial artery. The graft is best viewed using an anteroposterior (AP) or slight LAO projection.

Axillofemoral grafts may be catheterized through the ipsilateral subclavian-axillary arteries, through a puncture at the femoral level near the anastomosis, or along the body of the graft. Femoral–femoral grafts may be catheterized by puncturing the hood of the graft or by a percutaneous midgraft puncture. Because the hood of the graft may be difficult to localize, duplex guidance is advised. If the puncture is in the native artery just distal to the anastomosis, it may be very difficult to enter the graft rather than the native iliac artery. Anastomoses are best evaluated with steep lateral oblique views.

Aortofemoral grafts are usually punctured directly near the femoral anastomosis. These grafts offer the advantage of relatively straight limbs for maneuvering catheters. Proceeding up and over the bifurcation of a pros-thetic graft may be quite difficult due to the narrow angle of the bifurcation and the tendency for the catheter tip to catch on the fabric of the graft. When catheterizing the contralateral limb of an aortofemoral or aortoiliac bypass, use a Simmons 1 catheter and place the tip over the bifurcation to administer contrast. Iliofemoral grafts may be catheterized through direct

Table 3 Approaches to Selective Catheterization of Prosthetic Grafts Options

Bypass graft	Remote puncture	Puncture graft or native artery near anastomosis	Puncture body of graft	Comments
Carotid–subclavian	Femoral or brachial			Femoral puncture for arteriography. Brachial approach for intervention.
Axillofemoral	Brachial	Femoral	Chest or abdominal wall	Midgraft puncture is simplest.
Femoral–femoral	Brachial	Either femoral	Midgraft (over pubic area)	Can be difficult to maneuver into graft after puncture of native femoral artery.
Aortofemoral	Brachial	Either femoral		Puncture the groin opposite the side with suspected outflow problem.
Iliofemoral	Contralateral femoral (up and over)	Ipsilateral femoral		Avoid puncture of graft if possible.
Infrainguinal graft	Contralateral femoral (up and over)	Antegrade femoral (when graft originates from SFA or PFA)		Place up and over sheath if needed for better guidewire–catheter control.

Abbreviation: PFA, profunda femoris artery.

puncture in the groin or using an up-and-over approach from the contralateral groin. If an up-and-over approach is selected, the natural tendency of the guidewire passed over the aortic bifurcation is to remain in the native circulation, rather than pass into the graft. A steerable guidewire with a magnified, lateral oblique view will assist the operator in cannulating the proximal anastomosis.

There are many similarities between vein and prosthetic infrainguinal grafts, and the maneuvers in the earlier section on vein grafts are also useful for prosthetic grafts. The location of the proximal anastomosis (common femoral artery or distal to the groin) determines the approach (antegrade or up and over). Direct percutaneous puncture of infrainguinal prosthetic grafts may be performed but is more likely to be followed by graft thrombosis since these grafts tend to be low flow, especially if failing.

Selected Readings

AbuRahma AF, Elmore M, Deel J, et al. Complications of diagnostic arteriography performed by a vascular surgeon in a recent series of 558 patients. Vascular 2007; 15(2):92–97.

Braun MA. Basic catheterization skills. In: Braun MA, Nemcek AA, Vogelzang RL, eds. Interventional Radiology Procedure Manual. New York: Churchill Livingstone, 1997:23–30.

Jacobs JJ. Diagnostic neuroangiography: Basic techniques. In: Osborne AG, ed. Diagnostic Cerebral Angiography. Philadelphia, PA: Lippincott Williams & Wilkins, 1999:421–446.

10

Arteriography

Arteriography is Strategic, Not Diagnostic

Rarely does arteriography yield a new diagnosis. "Diagnostic arteriography" is a misnomer that will take a long time to disappear. This misconception is understandable since most departments performing arteriography were intended to provide assembly line style imaging, not individualized therapy. Except for an unusual case of vasculitis, most patients who undergo arteriography already have a diagnosis based upon history, physical examination, and noninvasive vascular evaluation.

Modern arteriography has two major purposes: strategic planning and guiding endovascular interventions. Arteriography presently provides much of the information used for the strategic planning of vascular reconstruction. It is still the most common strategic method with which most vascular specialists are familiar and comfortable. Arteriography permits the vascular specialist to evaluate disease patterns and the lesions that make them up and decide which should be treated with open surgery, which should undergo endovascular techniques, and which are best treated with a combination of the two. Some anatomical patterns are risky enough to treat that the whole revascularization plan is reconsidered once the arteriogram has fully delineated the morphologic features of the disease. Some of these patients may be best off with medical management, rather than intervention. When endovascular therapy has been selected as the treatment approach of choice, arteriography is the best way to guide the intervention. Intermittent periprocedural arteriography is crucial to guidewire and device passage and assessment of the results of treatment.

The Future of Arteriography

The development of duplex mapping, computed tomography (CT), angiography, and magnetic resonance arteriography (MRA) is likely to obviate the future need for much, if not most, of the strategic arteriography performed today. This will be a tremendous advance for vascular specialists and their patients for several reasons. Standard, percutaneous contrast arteriography has puncture site, end organ, and systemic complications associated with it. Among patients who avoid these complications there is obligatory cost, discomfort, and inconvenience experienced with each procedure. Over the next 5 to 10 years, arteriography will be performed less often for the purposes of identifying disease patterns and planning therapy. Standard catheter-based arteriography is likely to remain stable in terms of quality, cost, and risk while other vascular imaging modalities continue to improve.

A major drawback to the reality of decreasing need for arteriography is that several generations of vascular experts have been trained using arteriography. This training and orientation has led to much of the development

Table 1 What Do We Learn from Performing Arteriography?

Guidewire–catheter handling
Percutaneous access
Contrast management
Optimal imaging technique
Positioning of the image intensifier
Radiation safety
Guidewire manipulation, steering, advancement
Selective catheterization
Vascular flow physiology
Local perfusion phenomena
How to interpret and react to real-time arteriographic findings

of endovascular therapy. What we learn from becoming adept at performing arteriography is listed in Table 1. Going forward, these important concepts and techniques will have to be learned during therapeutic endovascular procedures. The primary current role of arteriography is in real-time guidance of therapeutic endovascular procedures. In the future, even this procedural guidance role may be replaced by other technologies.

Supplies for Arteriography

Arteriography requires that specific supplies be readily available, whether the procedure is done in the angiography suite or the operating room. These include the contents of an "arteriography pack," items to be opened at the operator's discretion, and protective gear (Table 2).

Table 2 Supplies for Arteriography

Arteriography pack	Specialist's choice	Protective gear
No. 11 scalpel blade	Starting guidewire	Leaded apron
4 × 4 gauze	Angiographic catheter	Thyroid shield
Mosquito clamp	Heparinized saline flush	Leaded eye shields
Drapes	Contrast	
Gown	Entry needle, 18-gauge orm	
Gloves	Micropuncture set	
Sterile cover for image intensifier		
Several 10- and 20-mL syringes		
Local anesthetic		
22-gauge needle		
Basin for discards		

Planning for Strategic Arteriography

Treatment strategy is developed as a result of information gained from arteriography. The role of arteriography in clinical management is determined by patient presentation: (1) the location of symptoms (which vascular bed is involved), (2) the severity of symptoms, (3) probable etiologic factors, and (4) comorbid medical conditions. Arteriography is most efficient and successful when its purpose and scope are determined prior to the procedure and driven by an understanding of the patient's presentation and spectrum of treatment options.

LOCATION OF SYMPTOMS

The vascular bed involved determines the type of arteriogram required and to some extent the degree of selectivity involved.

SEVERITY OF SYMPTOMS

This factor influences the urgency of the study, the degree of detail required, and it may prompt additional views. Patients with claudication and patients with gangrene require different degrees of filming detail.

ETIOLOGY

Embolic, thrombotic, aneurysmal, and chronic occlusive disease each requires some modification of the approach to angiography. Oblique views and additional runs are required to find a source if embolic disease is suspected. Acute thrombotic occlusive disease requires enhanced images of the site of the lesion and the operator may consider converting the procedure to a therapeutic one for the delivery of thrombolytic agents. Evaluation of patients with aneurysms focuses upon the integrity of the arteries proximal and distal to the aneurysm where suture lines or stent may be placed. Other vascular beds may require evaluation for associated aneurysms. The integrity of the inflow and the quality of the distal target site are the main concerns in patients with chronic occlusive disease.

COMORBID MEDICAL CONDITIONS

Obesity adds time and decreases image quality. Cardiac and renal diseases limit contrast load and increase its complications. Patients with prohibitive risk for surgery may be better treated with endovascular intervention, even if the lesions are not particularly favorable for this approach.

Questions to Consider Before Arteriography

1. Can the patient be treated without arteriography?
2. What is the crucial information that arteriography will provide?
3. Is an aortogram necessary?
4. Is contralateral runoff needed?
5. How much contrast can the patient tolerate?
6. Could this be embolic disease?
7. Is selective catheterization required?
8. Is conversion to endovascular therapy likely?

Evaluation Before Angiography

Before performing arteriography the medical status of the patient must be evaluated. Potential puncture sites are checked to be certain that the skin is free of infection. Current medications are reviewed. Those taking Glucophage™ or Metformin™ should stop it two days prior to the procedure. Insulin dosage should be decreased appropriately for nothing per oral (NPO) status on the day of the arteriogram. Intravenous hydration is begun when the patient arrives. Coumadin™ should be held for five days before the arteriogram if the international ratio (INR) is expected to be fully normalized. If anticoagulation must be continued, the patient may be hospitalized and converted to intravenous heparin administration or an outpatient heparin window can be arranged using subcutaneous administration of Lovenox. A closure device may be used to manage the arteriotomy at the conclusion of the procedure. However, the plan to use a closure device may be changed or interrupted by findings or occurrences at the time of the procedure.

Allergies to medications should be clearly noted, as for any procedure. Patients with contrast allergies should be asked about what type of reaction occurred and what the circumstances were. An earlier anaphylactic reaction is a contraindication to contrast administration. Patients with dermatologic or other systemic reactions may be pretreated with prednisone and Benadryl. Management of contrast allergies and medication dosing is discussed in chapter 15.

Cardiac and pulmonary insufficiency may also present difficulties in performing arteriography. The patient must be able to lie in the supine position for a lengthy period of time. Breath holds are often required to obtain reasonable images of any part of the body cavities. Patients with severe congestive heart failure, poor cardiac output, diastolic dysfunction, or a history of flash pulmonary edema may not be able to tolerate the osmotic load presented by the contrast.

Renal insufficiency may be worsened by contrast administration, and precautionary maneuvers should be undertaken to minimize nephrotoxicity

Table 3 Preventing Contrast-Induced Renal Failure

Use alternative imaging methods	Use duplex or MRA
Minimize iodinated contrast during arteriography	Obtain imaging studies to complement and minimize extent of arteriogram (duplex, MRA)
	Use alternative contrast agents (CO_2)
Hydrate	Before, during, after procedure with normal saline
	Or consider bicarbonate infusion
Premedicate	Mucomyst, 600-mg po bid on day before procedure, 600-mg po on day of procedure

(Table 3). Alternative imaging methods, such as duplex, MRA, or CT angiography should be considered, either to replace the arteriogram or to minimize the amount of contrast required for a more limited arteriographic study. If an arteriogram is still required, iodinated contrast may be minimized or possibly eliminated by using alternative contrast agents, such as CO_2. When iodinated contrast is required, preprocedural hydration is performed, usually with normal saline. Patients should also be treated with mucomyst. Fenoldopam may also be considered. These medications are discussed in more detail in chapter 15.

Informed consent is best obtained in the office well before the arteriogram or intervention so that the patient has time to become educated about the procedure and family members may ask questions and be reassured.

Deciding Where to Puncture

Selecting a puncture site is similar to planning an incision. Puncture site choice is based upon where the operator believes the pathology is located. The person performing the procedure should understand the patient's problem well. The correct puncture site location decreases the likelihood of complications and shortens the length of the procedure. The essential data for choosing the best puncture site are derived from the physical examination and supplemented by noninvasive studies. Table 1 in chapter 3 includes a detailed list of which puncture sites are best for access to various anatomic segments. Puncture in an area of significant plaque formation, such as a bulky common femoral artery lesion, should be avoided when possible. Substantial femoral artery lesions may often be identified by palpation and further evaluated by duplex scanning.

When there is no overriding concern about approach, most operators choose to perform a retrograde femoral puncture on the side that is easiest to reach with forehand positioning because of ease of guidewire and catheter placement. If the femoral pulses are equal, a right-handed operator usually punctures the right common femoral artery. If femoral pulses are diminished, the least diseased side is punctured. If a renal stenting is likely, most operators begin with an approach from the femoral. If the arterial angle of origin is acute, the best approach may be through a proximal puncture site. This is a common finding with the visceral vessels.

Infrarenal occlusive disease is usually approached with a retrograde femoral artery puncture on the side contralateral to the worst disease (Fig. 1).

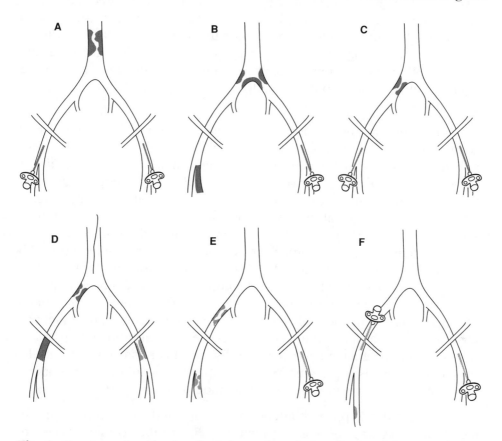

Fig. 1 Puncture site selection for infrarenal occlusive disease. (**A**) Aortic disease may be treated with access through either femoral artery. When the two sides are relatively equal, the operator usually goes to the side where the forehand approach is easier. The right-handed surgeon would likely go to the patient's right side. (**B**) When aortoiliac disease is similar bilaterally, the side with the least infrainguinal occlusive disease is punctured. This can usually be ascertained using physical examination, ankle-brachial indices, and/or other noninvasive studies. (**C**) A focal iliac artery stenosis can be evaluated through a puncture of either femoral artery. Usually the side contralateral to the disease is used as access for arteriography. If endovascular therapy is planned, an ipsilateral retrograde approach may also be used. (**D**) Severe common femoral artery occlusive disease is an indication for a proximal approach. (**E**) Infrarenal occlusive disease is usually approached with a retrograde femoral artery puncture on the side opposite the worst disease. (**F**) Isolated infrainguinal occlusive disease may be approached through an ipsilateral antegrade femoral puncture or a contralateral approach and up-and-over guidewire passage.

This location provides maximum flexibility if the procedure is converted to endovascular therapy and avoids a puncture site in an area of low flow. If a puncture contralateral to femoral artery approach with the worst disease is not possible, puncture on the same side as an iliac lesion may still be considered. In this setting, it is best if other imaging has been performed to be sure that it is not a distal external iliac artery lesion. A proximal approach, through the brachial arteries, may also be considered. Focal iliac artery lesions, identified by duplex scanning or MRA, which are likely to be reasonable candidates for endovascular therapy, can be reached with an initial ipsilateral retrograde femoral artery puncture and undergo immediate treatment. If an iliac lesion is located in the distal external iliac artery, a contralateral puncture should be performed, whether endoluminal therapy is planned or not.

When the presence of aortoiliac disease can be ruled out by physical examination and noninvasive studies, only femoral arteriography may be required. This can be performed through an ipsilateral antegrade or retrograde femoral puncture or a contralateral retrograde puncture and passage of the catheter over the aortic bifurcation. If noninvasive data demonstrate infrainguinal occlusive disease and endovascular treatment is reasonable, either an up-and-over approach from the other side or an antegrade femoral artery approach is appropriate. An antegrade approach is useful when the infrainguinal disease is very distal in location; this permits distal contrast delivery and if endovascular treatment is required, it provides better guidewire and catheter control. A contralateral femoral artery puncture with the catheter passed over the aortic bifurcation and into the superficial femoral artery (SFA) is the most appropriate approach to evaluation of infrainguinal occlusive disease.This approach is especially indicated if there is a proximal SFA lesion, which would render working room inadequate with an ipsilateral, antegrade puncture.

Since proximal approach arteries are smaller and more prone to spasm and thrombosis, and the risks of neurologic and other complications are higher, these are usually a second choice for routine access. Nevertheless, there are several situations in which proximal access is advised (Table 4). These indications include severe bilateral infrarenal or common femoral occlusive disease, hostile groins, a more favorable angle of approach to aortic branches through a proximal approach, and a retrograde approach to subclavian or axillary artery lesions.

ANGIO CONSULT: HOW CAN DUPLEX SCANNING HELP IN CHOOSING A PUNCTURE SITE?

1. The integration of hemodynamic information from duplex scanning into the planning of strategic arteriography and endovascular therapy permits better decision making on the patient's behalf. Choices

Table 4 When to Use a Proximal Puncture Site Access Through the Brachial Arteries

---

Severe infrarenal occlusive disease
Aortic occlusion
Bilateral critical/diffuse iliac occlusive disease
Bilateral common femoral artery disease
Common femoral artery occlusion
Severe common femoral artery stenosis
Femoral puncture contraindicated
Recent surgery
Infection
Aneurysm
Pseudoaneurysm
Angle of approach more favorable
Selective catheterization of or endovascular intervention in mesenteric arteries
Acute angle at origin of renal arteries
Retrograde approach to endovascular therapy
Subclavian lesions
Axillary lesions

---

   of puncture sites, approaches, and therapy can be focused and specific.

2. Use duplex scanning to rule out lesions in the common femoral artery that may contraindicate puncture of that vessel.

3. When duplex scanning shows an isolated, focal iliac artery stenosis and therapy is intended, consider an ipsilateral, retrograde femoral artery puncture for arteriography and angioplasty.

4. When duplex scanning shows extensive aortoiliac occlusive disease and it is unclear whether an endovascular or an open surgical technique will be required, consider a retrograde femoral artery puncture on the side with the least amount of inflow disease.

5. When duplex scanning shows severe common femoral artery disease, puncture the least diseased side or use a proximal puncture site.

6. When duplex scanning shows a tight, proximal superficial femoral artery stenosis, avoid puncture of the adjacent common femoral artery.

7. When the superficial femoral artery is occluded and duplex scanning shows a significant proximal stenosis of the deep femoral artery, avoid puncture of the adjacent common femoral artery.

8. When an antegrade femoral artery puncture is considered, use duplex scanning to ensure that there is no large femoral bifurcation plaque.

9. Identify a high origin of the deep femoral artery before performing an antegrade femoral artery puncture.

10. Evaluate an infrainguinal vein graft with duplex scanning to identify the proximal anastomotic site and its distance from a common femoral artery puncture site. This is one factor in deciding whether to use an ipsilateral antegrade or an alternative approach.

Catheter Placement

The technique of arterial puncture is described in chapter 3. After the optimal puncture site is selected, access is obtained and the guidewire is placed in the desired location. The usual initial guidewire choice for routine strategic arteriography is a floppy-tip, 0.035-in. diameter, and 145-cm length starting guidewire (see table 1 in chap. 5). The guidewire is advanced to a location where the floppy tip is several centimeters beyond the intended location of the catheter head. Aortography is usually performed with a pigtail or tennis racket catheter that has many side holes and is able to create a contrast blush in a short period of injection time. Catheter types and lengths are discussed in chapter 5. Some common catheter choices for flush aortography are listed in table 1 in chapter 5. Catheter placement for aortography is based upon fluoroscopically visible landmarks (Fig. 2). Arch aortography is performed with the catheter head in the ascending aorta, well distal to the coronary ostia but proximal to the innominate artery. Thoracic aortography is performed with the catheter head placed just distal to the left subclavian origin, usually at the location where the aorta begins to straighten to descend into the thorax. The paravisceral segment of the aorta is seen best when the catheter is placed at or just proximal to the level of the diaphragm. A lateral projection is required to evaluate the celiac and superior mesenteric arteries in profile. Aortorenal arteriography requires catheter head placement at or just below the level of the renal arteries, usually over the first lumbar vertebral body or at the junction of the first and second lumbar vertebral bodies (fig. 1 in chap. 7). More details about catheter head placement are provided in the later sections that describe different types of arteriograms.

Following removal of the guidewire, the flush catheter head takes its preformed shape. Play with the catheter for a moment to make sure that the catheter is free in the large aortic lumen and that the flush catheter tip has not engaged a branch orifice. Contrast may be puffed through the catheter to confirm the correct location. The catheter is flushed with heparin–saline solution. The catheter is permitted to backbleed momentarily while the sterile tubing of the automated power injector is purged. After the air bubbles are removed from the system, the catheter is connected to the sterile tubing. The catheter is again aspirated through the power injector to check the system for microbubbles.

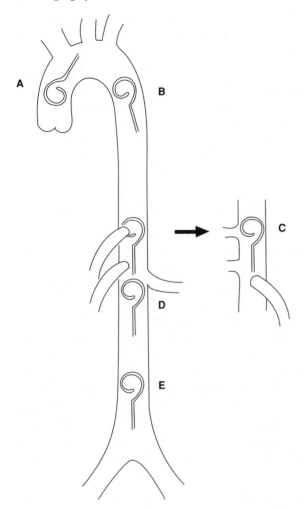

Fig. 2 Catheter position for aortography. (**A**) Arch aortography is performed with the catheter head in the mid-ascending aorta. (**B**) A thoracic aortogram is performed with the catheter head positioned in the proximal descending aorta. (**C**) The paravisceral aorta is evaluated in the lateral projection with the catheter head at the level of the celiac artery. (**D**) Catheter head placement at the level of the renal arteries provides reflux of contrast into the renal arteries and a flush of contrast into the infrarenal aorta. (**E**) When the side holes are placed just proximal to the aortic bifurcation, pelvic and bilateral lower extremity arteriographic runoff can be performed.

Contrast Administration and Image Acquisition

The power injector and its usage in arteriography are described in chapter 8. Power injection in the aorta causes contrast to reflux several centimeters against the direction of flow before the contrast bolus moves forward with the flow stream. During routine abdominal aortography, for example, contrast refluxes proximally the distance of approximately one vertebral body. If severe occlusive disease is present in the aorta or iliac arteries, contrast may reflux further and run off through the visceral arteries. Reflux during arch aortography is usually less since it is higher flow, there is more mixing with nonopacified blood, and juxtaposed occlusive disease is much less common. Because the flush catheter is placed into a curved position over the arch, there is often observed significant recoil of the catheter due to the high pressure exerted during contrast administration. The injection (volume and rate) and imaging of contrast depend on the size of the patient, the expected rate of blood flow, the type of filming selected (digital subtraction or cut film), and the area of arterial anatomy to be surveyed (trunk, neck, or extremity).

Digital subtraction arteriography (DSA) is often performed at one station (field of view) at a time. A mask is created for later subtraction, contrast is injected, and the image intensifier and the object are held in a constant position. Motion artifact is detrimental to digital images because the computer attempts to subtract the static image from the contrast column after the images have been acquired. DSA within a body cavity requires that the patient perform breath holding during image acquisition to minimize motion artifact. Digital images are acquired at rates of 1 to 30 per second, depending upon the type of arteriogram and the lesion being interrogated. Aortography is usually performed at 3 to 4 images per second. High-flow aortic branches such as carotid, subclavian, or renal arteries require at least three images (or "frames") per second for evaluation. Very slow pedal artery flow may be well evaluated with images acquired at 1 or 2 per second. A high-flow arteriovenous fistula may require up to 30 frames per second to capture the detail since the passage of contrast through the lesion may be brisk.

Bolus chase technology is available in many arteriographic systems for lower extremity runoff imaging. Contrast is administered and the table moves the patient as the image intensifier is maintained in a fixed position and images are acquired. After the run, the table returns to its starting position and the filming sequence and table movement are repeated without contrast administration to create a mask that is then subtracted from the initial contrast run to produce the final arteriogram.

Arteriography Sequences

Strategic arteriography requires specific contrast injection and filming or image acquisition sequences depending on the vasculature being studied (Table 5). The clinical and arteriographic pictures should be reconciled to determine when the study has yielded adequate information and may be concluded. A clear understanding of the patient's clinical problem prevents the continued accumulation of noncontributory views and filming runs. In

Table 5 Strategic Arteriography: Contrast Administration and Image Acquisition

Type of arteriogram	Catheter placement	Type		Contrast Administration				Image Acquisition	
		Flush	Selective	Volume (mL)	Time (sec)	Rate[a]	Delay (sec)	Sequence (images per sec/no. of sec)	
Brachiocephalic									
Arch aortogram	Ascending aorta	X		30	2	15 for 30	0	4 per sec for 4–6 sec	
Innominate arteriogram	Innominate artery		X	15	3–4	5 for 15	0	4 per sec for 4–8 sec	
Carotid arteriogram	Common carotid artery		X	6–12	2	4 for 8	0	4 per sec for 4–8 sec	
Subclavian arteriogram	Subclavian artery		X	6–15	2	5 for 10	0	4 per sec for 4–8 sec	
Axillary arteriogram	Axillary artery		X	6–10	3	3 for 9	0	4 per sec for 4–10 sec	
Thoracic									
Descending thoracic aortogram	Proximal descending aorta	X		30	2	15 for 30	0	4 per sec for 4–8 sec	
Visceral									
Paravisceral aortogram	Distal descending aorta	X		24	2	12 for 24	0	4 per sec for 4–8 sec	
Celiac/SMA arteriogram	Visceral artery		X	6–18	3	4 for 12	0	4 per sec for 4–10 sec	
Renal arteriogram	Renal artery		X	8	2	4 for 8	0	4 per sec for 4–10 sec	

(Continued)

Table 5 (*Continued*)

Type of arteriogram	Catheter placement	Type		Contrast Administration			Image Acquisition	
		Flush	Selective	Volume (mL)	Time (sec)	Rate[a]	Delay (sec)	Sequence (images per sec/no. of sec)
Aortoiliac								
Aortoiliac arteriogram	Pararenal aorta	X		18–24	3	8 for 24	0	4 per sec for 4–8 sec
Abdominal aortogram with runoff	Pararenal aorta	X		60–90	6–12	8 for 72	1 or 2	4 per sec for 6–12 sec
Infrainguinal								
Bilateral runoff	Infrarenal aorta	X		60–70	6–8	8 for 64	2–4	2–4 per second for 8–20 sec.
Femoral arteriogram	External iliac or femoral	X	X	10	2	5 for 10	0	2–4 per sec for 4–20 sec. (4 or 5) stations
Tibiopedal arteriogram	Femoral or popliteal	X	X	4–12	2–3	3 for 9	0–4	2 per sec for 4–20 sec.

[a]Commonly used injection rates are shown. They are described in terms of the amount of contrast administered per second and the total volume injected.

the discussion that follows, DSA techniques are described. Cut film arteriography was the method of choice for decades and is no longer used. Veterans of this method acquired a respect for the complexities of arteriography. Digital systems are simpler, faster, less labor intensive, and provide a better finished product.

Table 5 offers some guidelines for contrast administration and image acquisition. It is the operator's experience, knowledge of the patient's problem, and estimation of likely volume and blood flow rate to an interrogated organ that will determine the best sequences in a given situation. When contrast is administered, imaging must be initiated just prior to contrast reaching the field of view since the first digital image is used for subtraction purposes. Any preprogrammed delay between contrast administration and initiation of imaging is intended to avoid useless radiation usage and exposure. Once imaging has been initiated, all extraneous movement of the field of view must be prevented to avoid motion artifact. The contrast volume must be adjusted based on the operator's estimate of the amount and flow rate of nonopacified blood entering the field. An arch aortogram requires a larger contrast bolus than the single stage of a femoral arteriogram, for example. As discussed earlier, where there is high flow in a large caliber artery, a flush catheter is needed to create an adequate blush of contrast. In the smaller caliber branch arteries, a selective catheter is needed to enter the artery, and the single end hole of the catheter is adequate to deliver the appropriate amount of contrast. In higher resistance outflow beds, the contrast should be administered in smaller amounts per second over a slightly longer period of time. The rate of image acquisition or frame rate is increased in rapid flow situations and decreased when there is slow flow, such as diseased tibial or pedal bed. The key is to get an accurate representation of the anatomy, and some clues to the accompanying physiology, without gratuitous X-ray exposure.

Arteriography of the Brachiocephalic Arteries

Brachiocephalic arteriography differs from many other types of arteriography for two reasons: (1) it is fairly remote from femoral artery puncture sites and longer guidewires and catheters must be used than for many other types of arteriography (see tables 2 and 3 in chapter 5); and (2) there is a small but real risk of stroke, which may be caused by guidewire–catheter manipulation, microbubbles, or catheter thrombus.

ARCH AORTOGRAPHY

Sheath access is obtained with a standard 4- or 5-Fr femoral sheath. Heparin is administered. Carotid and cerebral arteriography is the only type of strategic arteriography where anticoagulation is used routinely, even though no treatment is planned at the time of catheterization. This is to minimize stroke risk. The guidewire is introduced and its floppy tip is placed in the ascending aorta. Care must be taken to avoid placing the guidewire in the left ventricle or into the coronary arteries and causing arrhythmias. A 90-cm pigtail catheter is placed over the guidewire and the catheter head is placed in the distal ascending aorta, just proximal to where the aorta begins to turn to the left to form the arch (Fig. 2). The image intensifier is positioned so that the aortic arch and the extracranial carotid and vertebral arteries are within the field of view. The catheter crossing the arch provides a marker for the inferior aspect of the field. The presence of the guidewire in the catheter helps to clearly visualize how much left anterior obliquity is needed from the image intensifier position. The guidewire is removed, and the catheter is flushed and then connected to the power injector. Care must be taken to avoid the injection of microbubbles. The catheter hook-up process is described in chapter 8 and in the earlier section on catheter placement. The patient is asked to hold breath and avoid swallowing during image acquisition. Contrast injection is usually 15 for 30, or 15 ml/sec for two consecutive seconds (Table 5). Image acquisition is variable, but a common sequence would be four images per second for six to eight seconds or until contrast washes out.

The left anterior oblique (LAO) projection is used to separate the arch branches during aortography. The LAO view of the arch establishes the landmarks required for selective catheterization of the aortic arch branches. Figure 1 in chapter 9 demonstrates the LAO projection.

CAROTID ARTERIOGRAPHY

The arch is inspected for evidence of occlusive disease at the origins of its branches and for evidence of disease within the arch that may cause embolization. If either of these are present, the risk of stroke from catheter manipulation is substantial and the operator may consider alternative methods of imaging.

Chapter 9 contains a discussion of selective catheterization of arch branches. The arch aortogram is used to assist in choosing a selective cerebral catheter. The steerable, hydrophilic guidewire (Glidewire or similar product) is placed through the pigtail catheter, and the pigtail catheter is removed. The selective cerebral catheter is introduced over the guidewire and advanced to a position beyond the arch branch intended for catheterization. The image intensifier is not moved after the arch aortogram and is maintained in its LAO position so that landmarks may be used to guide selective catheterization. The guidewire is withdrawn into the catheter to permit the catheter head to assume its intended shape (Fig. 3, see also figs. 3 to 5 in chap. 9). The catheter is slowly withdrawn until the branch is engaged. The catheter may

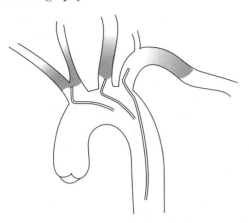

Fig. 3 Cerebral arteriography. A simple-curve selective cerebral catheter is advanced into each of the arch branches. The tip of the catheter must be a few centimeters or more into the artery to prevent the catheter from popping out of the artery and into the arch. There is some recoil of the catheter during contrast administration. See also Figures 3 to 7 in chapter 6 for more about selective arch branch catheterization.

be gently manipulated to permit the catheter tip to engage the branch orifice a little more securely. The steerable guidewire is slowly advanced into the artery for a few centimeters, with care to avoid advancing the guidewire into the carotid bifurcation. The arch aortogram, if it appropriately includes the field up to and including the mandible, usually demonstrates the location of the bifurcation that must be avoided with guidewire passage. The catheter is advanced over the guidewire while the guidewire is maintained in a stationary position. Because of the large caliber and curvature of the aorta, extra slack may be present along the length of the guidewire and care must be taken to avoid advancing the guidewire while the catheter is placed into the cerebral artery. After the catheter is a few centimeters within the origin of the intended artery, the guidewire is removed and the catheter is aspirated and gently flushed again. The shape of the guidewire, as it curves from the arch into the carotid artery, is observed as the catheter is advanced. If the guidewire becomes more tightly curved as the catheter is advanced, this is a sign that there may be too much torque and the catheter tip may drag the guidewire out of the arch branch and back into the arch.

Contrast is puffed into the artery to confirm correct positioning of the catheter tip. The catheter tip should not be placed into the sidewall of the artery or near a lesion. The selective catheters have an end hole but no side holes. Pressure injection should not be performed until the position of the catheter is confirmed within the lumen of the origin of the branch artery. Because there is only an end hole for contrast administration, there may be recoil of the catheter under pressure, so the catheter must be placed at least a few centimeters into the artery to prevent it from popping out. The catheter is aspirated, flushed with heparinized saline, and connected to the power injector tubing. The catheter is aspirated through the injector and the tubing is checked again for microbubbles.

Injection rates and filming sequences are summarized in Table 5. Injection of contrast into the innominate artery should be in the range of 4 to 8 ml/sec over three or four seconds. An example sequence is 5 for 15, or 5 ml/sec for three seconds. Image acquisition should be at four images per second. The pressure limit is usually decreased to 300 to 500 psi, and a 0.3 to 0.5 rate of pressure rise is programmed into the injector as a safety maneuver. A right anterior oblique (RAO) view of the innominate artery is usually required to open the bifurcation to evaluate the origins of the right subclavian and right common carotid arteries. Injection into the common carotid artery is usually performed with 3 to 5 ml/sec over two or three seconds. Example sequences include 4 for 8 (4 ml/sec for two seconds), 3 for 9 (3 ml/sec for three seconds), or 4 for 12 (4 ml/sec for three seconds).

The carotid bifurcation is usually evaluated in the antero-posterior (AP) and lateral projections. Since the bifurcation and proximal internal carotid artery disease is worst along the posterior wall, addition steep oblique views may be required to demonstrate the most significant segment of the stenosis in profile.During image acquisition, the patient is coached to hold breath, to drop the shoulders, and to lengthen the neck.

SUBCLAVIAN ARTERIOGRAPHY

The first step in transfemoral subclavian arteriography is an arch aortogram (figs. 6 and 7 in chap. 9). It is often possible to evaluate either subclavian artery with an arch injection. However, if the subclavian artery is significantly diseased, it may fill very slowly in comparison to the other arch branches. After arch studies are performed, the need for selective arteriography is assessed. The same steps are followed for selective subclavian arteriography as have been discussed in the earlier section on carotid arteriography. A selective catheter with either a simple curve or a complex curve is chosen and advanced into the origin of the subclavian artery using anatomic landmarks. Selective subclavian artery catheterization is discussed in detail in chapter 9. The selective catheter is positioned a few centimeters within the origin of the subclavian artery. The catheter is aspirated, checked for microbubbles, irrigated with heparinized saline, and connected to the automated power injector. Contrast administration is usually at 4 to 6 ml/sec for three or four seconds. An example sequence is 4 for 12, or 4 ml/sec for three seconds with image acquisition at four frames per second until contrast washes out. Injection within the subclavian artery should not be performed in proximity to the origin of the vertebral artery to avoid dissection and/or embolization. Most of the time, adequate information about the vertebral artery can be obtained with subclavian artery contrast injection. When detailed vertebral anatomy must be delineated, the vertebral artery may be selectively cannulated and a lower pressure injection may be performed. The vertebral artery is also prone to vasospasm. When subclavian steal is present, extended filming is required to demonstrate reversed flow in the vertebral artery ipsilateral to the lesion.

The subclavian artery may also be approached through an ipsilateral brachial puncture (chap. 3). The upper extremity approach may be useful for arteriography and interventions in a variety of situations (Table 4). Transbrachial catheterization of the subclavian and axillary arteries is described in chapter 9 (fig. 8 in chap. 9). After access is secured, and a straight catheter is placed, a hand-powered injection of 4 to 8 ml of contrast is usually adequate to obtain a subclavian arteriogram, especially if antegrade flow is reduced because of a proximal subclavian artery stenosis or occlusion. However, keep in mind that a brachial puncture ipsilateral to a significant lesion is more difficult to perform. In addition, there is a higher likelihood of thrombosis if the lesion is not treated to improve inflow.

Thoracic Aortography

A 90-cm pigtail catheter is introduced into the proximal thoracic aorta. When aortic arch or left subclavian artery anatomy is important, an arch aortogram may be performed initially and the location of the left subclavian artery may be identified. The catheter head is withdrawn and positioned at a level just distal to the origin of the left subclavian artery (Fig. 2). The catheter is connected to the sterile tubing for the power injector using the same routine. The patient is instructed to hold breath. Thoracic aortography requires 12 to 20 ml of contrast injection per second for two to three seconds. An example sequence is 15 for 30, or 15 ml/sec for two seconds, with filming at four frames per second. There is some debate about the safety and efficacy of selective arteriography of the spinal cord blood supply. This is beyond the scope of this text.

Arteriography of the Visceral and Renal Arteries

Arteriography of the visceral and renal arteries is characterized by factors that differentiate it from other types of arteriography. These include: (1) these arteries are more prone to spasm during manipulation, which may lead to end organ complication; (2) the anatomy of these arteries may be significantly altered by ventilatory motion and diaphragmatic movement; and (3) the angle of approach from the femoral artery to the visceral and renal arteries is usually fairly acute, and in some cases may be more favorable to approach from a proximal access site.

Arteriography of the Celiac and Superior Mesenteric Arteries

A starting guidewire is introduced through the femoral artery and a 65-cm length, 4- or 5-Fr pigtail or Omni-flush catheter is placed over it. The catheter head is placed at or just proximal to the level of the diaphragm (Fig. 2). Aortography of the paravisceral segment is performed using the power injector to administer 8 to 12 ml of contrast per second over three seconds. An AP aortogram is performed, the catheter head may be adjusted slightly, and a magnified lateral view is obtained. The lateral is performed with the patient's arms extended above the head. Chapter 9 details selective catheterization of the visceral arteries. The selective catheter must be placed 1 to 2 cm within the origin of the artery to avoid having the catheter pop out with diaphragmatic excursion or with pressure injection (Fig. 4). The catheter is connected to the power injector tubing after the system is irrigated and purged of microbubbles. Selective arteriography of either the celiac or superior mesenteric arteries may be performed with 4 to 6 ml of contrast injected per second over three seconds with image acquisition at four frames per second (Table 5). The origins of the celiac and superior mesenteric arteries are best visualized in the lateral position. The more distally located branches of each of these arteries are best evaluated in the AP position or at a slight oblique. Images are acquired for as long as it takes to get the desired information. Imaging at the origin of the visceral arteries takes only a few seconds but it may take many seconds for contrast to reach the small distal branches.

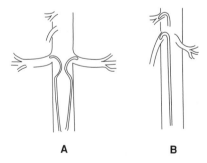

A   B

Fig. 4   Selective visceral and renal arteriography. (**A**) A C2 cobra catheter is used to cannulate the renal artery. Contrast may be puffed from the position shown. There is some catheter recoil with pressure injection, and the catheter tip must be inside the artery to perform detailed arteriography. (**B**) A hook-shaped catheter is used for selective arteriography of the celiac and superior mesenteric arteries.

If the catheter is in the artery for more than a few minutes, consider administering nitroglycerine to prevent spasm. If there is very slow flow due to a lesion at the origin of the artery, it is usually not advisable to cross it unless therapy is planned to follow immediately. In that case, consider systemic heparinization prior to crossing the lesion.

ARTERIOGRAPHY OF THE RENAL ARTERY

Renal arteriography begins with a pararenal aortogram if the patient can tolerate the contrast load. The catheter head is placed at or just below the renal arteries (Fig. 2). Reflux of contrast into the superior mesenteric artery is undesirable because its image frequently obscures the left renal artery orifice. The image acquisition is extended for several seconds so that bilateral nephrograms may be evaluated. The catheter head may be adjusted slightly, based upon the contrast flow pattern seen on the initial AP aortogram. If one renal artery origin is of particular interest, consider a repeat aortogram using a smaller field of view to provide a magnified arterial image. Since the renal artery origins are posterolateral, the orifice of the artery is often obscured by the aortic wall (Fig. 5). A 10-degree ipsilateral anterior oblique projection is performed. The images are inspected and selective catheterization is considered. Selective renal artery catheterization is detailed in chapter 9. The flush catheter is exchanged for a selective catheter, usually a 65-cm C2 cobra catheter (fig. 9 in chap. 9). The tip of the selective catheter is directed into the origin of the artery (Fig. 4). Selective renal arteriography may be performed with 3 to 6 ml/sec for two or three seconds (Table 5). If the catheter remains in the artery for more than a few minutes or therapy is planned, consider systemic heparin administration prior to entering the artery and local nitroglycerine administration after crossing the lesion.

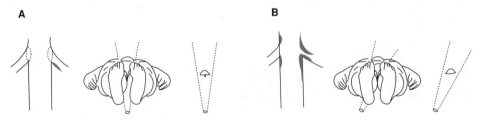

Fig. 5 Oblique projection for renal arteriography. Renal artery origins are posterolateral. (**A**) Origin lesions may be obscured by aortic plaque or contrast on the standard anteroposterior projection used for aortography. (**B**) An ipsilateral anterior oblique projection permits enhanced visualization of the renal artery origin.

Arteriography of the Infrarenal Arteries

Occlusive and aneurysmal diseases involving the infrarenal arteries comprise a significant proportion of contemporary vascular practice. Because there are many competing options available for treatment of lesions in these arteries, the operator's understanding of the patient's clinical problem has a direct impact upon the quality and appropriateness of the study. This is also a vascular bed where arteriography is likely to progress to endovascular therapy during the same intervention, so the arteriogram must be planned to dovetail with therapy.

Arteriography of the Abdominal Aorta and Iliac Arteries

Aortoiliac arteriography is usually performed with a 65-cm length, 4- or 5-Fr flush catheter, such as a pigtail, tennis racket, or Omni-flush catheter. The catheter head is placed at the level of the renal arteries (Fig. 2). When the patient is under consideration for any type of complex reconstruction involving multiple stents or a stent–graft, a calibrated catheter with 1-cm markers is used, and the first marker should be placed just below the renal arteries. The catheter is aspirated, flushed, and connected to the injector. The field of view should extend superiorly to the T12-L1 disc space. Laterally, the field should be wide enough to include both nephrograms. The patient is coached at breath holding. A DSA is obtained with 6 to 15 ml of contrast injected per second over two to three seconds (Table 5). A common sequence would be 8 for 24, or 8 ml/sec for three seconds. Image acquisition is at four frames per second until contrast washes out, usually requiring only a few seconds. Whether evaluating occlusive or aneurysmal disease, 30-degree anterior oblique projections may also be performed to provide additional anatomic detail. This provides a better view of the contralateral iliac artery bifurcation and the ipsilateral femoral bifurcation. The inferior aspect of the field of view for the obliques should include the common femoral arteries and their bifurcations so that these arteries may also be assessed.

Infrarenal Aortography with Lower-Extremity Runoff

An aortogram with lower-extremity runoff may be accomplished by placing the catheter at the level of the renal arteries and performing a sequence of films that covers the distance from the aorta to the feet. This is the "bolus chase" method.Another option is to perform an aortoiliac arteriogram, withdraw the catheter to the distal aorta, and follow with a filming sequence from the aortic bifurcation to the feet. A common method is to perform the runoff at one station, or field of view, at a time with a separate contrast injection at each level and to progress down the leg.

A digital aortogram with bilateral runoff using bolus chase is performed in the following manner. The locations of the patient's hips, knees, and feet are put into line using fluoroscopy and moving the angiographic table only cephalad and caudad, without side-to-side motion. The beginning and ending locations of the sequence are determined and locked into place. The contrast is administered. A hand-held table motion device is used by the operator to move the table to keep the contrast bolus within the field of view as it is followed toward the patient's feet. After the sequence is completed, the patient remains still and the sequence is repeated without contrast to obtain a mask. Contrast is usually administered at 7 to 10 ml/sec for 8 to 12 seconds.

The ability to perform an aortogram with bilateral runoff, using the bolus chase technique, provides the opportunity to cover a long distance within the arterial system by following a single large bolus injection. However, when the pattern of occlusive disease is significantly different from one leg to the other, the contrast may travel at different rates in each limb, making the resultant study suboptimal in one of the limbs. In this case, additional unilateral views will be required to supplement the study. Another disadvantage of this type of study is that in patients with multiple levels of disease, sufficient concentrations of contrast may not reach the feet to obtain adequate pedal arteriograms after an injection of contrast in the aorta. Subsequent study is then required, usually with contrast administered in a more distal location.

FEMORAL ARTERIOGRAPHY

Femoral arteriography may be performed with a catheter placed either up and over the aortic bifurcation or in a retrograde or antegrade direction through the common femoral artery ipsilateral to the lesion (Fig. 6). Femoral arteriography may be performed using a standard angiographic catheter or a dilator.

Using a contralateral approach, a straight or curved arteriographic catheter is placed over the aortic bifurcation for an injection at the level of the distal iliac artery or common femoral artery. An ipsilateral approach is performed using a short, straight catheter or dilator placed either retrograde or antegrade. Contrast is administered by hand or power injector. The simplest method for performing a DSA femoral arteriogram is to obtain one field of view at a time with a separate small injection of 6 to 10 ml of contrast at

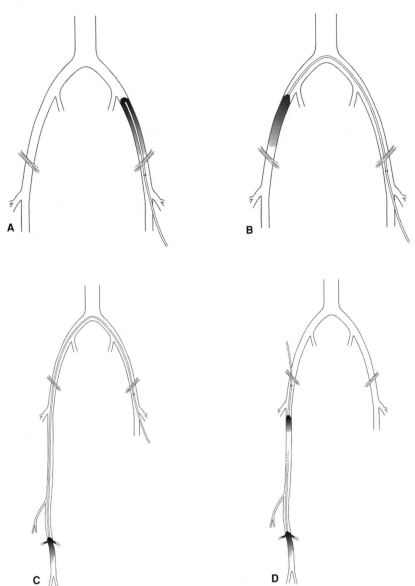

Fig. 6 Catheter placement for femoral arteriography. (**A**) An ipsilateral retrograde femoral puncture can be performed for femoral arteriography. A 4-Fr dilator can be used as the catheter. This approach is not well suited to endovascular therapy. (**B**) Contralateral access with catheter passage over the aortic bifurcation is a reasonable approach for arteriography, and it is easily converted to a therapeutic approach. (**C**) The catheter may be advanced further on the contralateral side to obtain more detailed arteriography of the lower extremity. (**D**) If aortoiliac disease has already been ruled out, an ipsilateral antegrade femoral puncture provides excellent control and pushability, especially if infrageniculate disease is the focus of the investigation.

each of several stations (usually four or five to the foot) while filming at two to four frames per second.

In patients with inflow to the knee but with severe tibial and/or pedal occlusive disease, as often occurs in diabetics, selective infrapopliteal arteriography may be required. The catheter is placed as distally as possible using an antegrade approach, either up and over the aortic bifurcation or as an ipsilateral antegrade femoral puncture (Fig. 6). A long, straight, multi-side-hole catheter is used, and 3 to 10 ml of contrast is administered directly into the popliteal artery.

The femoral bifurcation is best viewed with an ipsilateral anterior oblique projection. Oblique views of the SFA and popliteal arteries are sometimes useful to delineate back wall plaque. The trifurcation is opened up with an ipsilateral anterior oblique projection that permits the tibia and fibula to be more widely separated than in a standard AP view. A lateral view of the lower leg, ankle, and foot are helpful to separate the tibial arteries.

PEDAL ARTERIOGRAPHY

It is not usually possible to obtain detailed pedal arteriography with contrast administered through an arteriographic catheter placed in the aorta. Inadequate pedal arteriography may lead to the subsequent surprise of the "angiographically occult" outflow artery in the foot. When detail is required at the ankle and foot, such as target site identification, either selective catheterization with injection in the popliteal artery is required or an extended filming sequence must be performed after a femoral artery injection (Fig. 7).

Contrast displaces what little blood is flowing to an ischemic foot, so arteriography causes discomfort, which prompts movement. This movement diminishes film quality but also indicates the timing of the contrast flow to the foot. Once the transit time for contrast to flow from the injection site to the foot has been quantified, the delay between contrast administration and the initiation of imaging can be more readily predicted. Patients with very ischemic limbs may require a 20-second delay after administration of contrast into the femoral artery. The foot is padded and taped in the lateral position (hip externally rotated and knee flexed). The pain of contrast reaching an ischemic foot can be a memorable and upsetting experience for the patient, and sedation should be administered prior to selective pedal arteriography. Hand-powered injection of 5 to 10 ml of contrast over one or two seconds is performed with the catheter tip placed in the popliteal artery if possible. When there is an ipsilateral SFA occlusion, contrast is administered into the common femoral artery. A larger bolus of contrast may be required since there is more mixing of contrast with unopacified blood from collaterals prior to reaching the foot.

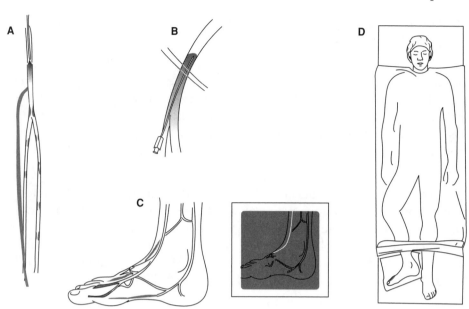

Fig. 7 Pedal arteriography. (**A**) Antegrade placement of the arteriographic catheter is optimal to evaluate infrageniculate occlusive disease. (**B**) When antegrade catheter placement is not possible, a straight 4- or 5-Fr dilator can be placed retrograde in the femoral artery and contrast administered. Delayed filming is performed. (**C**) The foot is imaged in the lateral position. The image intensifier is placed over the area of interest. Contrast may require 20 to 30 seconds to flow from the femoral segment to the foot. (**D**) The foot must be completely immobilized to prevent motion artifact.

EVALUATION OF A DIABETIC WITH AN ISCHEMIC FOOT LESION

Assess the patient for evidence of inflow disease by physical examination and duplex. Check renal function and estimate the ability of the patient to tolerate iodinated contrast. Perform a retrograde femoral puncture on the side opposite the ischemic foot lesion. Perform an aortoiliac arteriogram. If renal function is compromised, CO_2 may be used as a contrast agent to rule out lesions in the aortoiliac and femoral–popliteal segments. Place a catheter over the aortic bifurcation. Perform a lower-extremity arteriogram, including a pedal arteriogram. The catheter is advanced antegrade down the limb to the area where the significant disease is encountered, often below the knee. This permits better images with less contrast. Direct contrast administration into the arterial segment just proximal to the disease of interest permits better opacification. There is less nonopacified blood with which to mix and less chance that contrast-laden inflow will run off into collaterals. When the angiographic catheter is brought in proximity to the lesions, the contrast may be diluted with saline to lessen the contrast load. Inflow lesions are treated aggressively, whether in the aortoiliac or femoral–popliteal segments. If disease is limited to the infrageniculate segment, advance the catheter to the knee to obtain a quality arteriogram and measure the distances required to pass the sheath for treatment. If a contralateral retrograde femoral puncture is not possible, the choice is between an antegrade ipsilateral puncture and a brachial artery puncture. An antegrade puncture is only reasonable if inflow stenosis can be ruled out by duplex or some other noninvasive imaging. A brachial approach is feasible, but the distances are excessive. Angiography can be performed but infrageniculate intervention is not optimally performed through this route since it is about 100 cm just to get to the distal iliac level in a normal sized person. Pedal arteriography is discussed earlier but there are some caveats in diabetics with ischemic foot lesions. No complex salvage procedures should be performed without a good sense of the pedal arterial anatomy. A lateral and an AP view of the foot are very informative. Many diabetics have compartmentalization of flow with little crossover between the anterior and posterior pedal circulation. Salvage endovascular cases are almost doomed to failure if there is no named foot vessel that receives in-line flow as a result of the revascularization procedure.

ANGIO CONSULT: WHAT CAN I DO TO IDENTIFY ARTERIOGRAPHIC FAKEOUTS?

1. Posterior wall lesions. Obtain oblique or lateral views. Posterior wall plaque and bifurcation stenoses may appear insignificant in the anteroposterior projection, but sometimes a decrease in the density of the contrast column gives it away. Occlusive or embolizing lesions commonly occur along the posterior wall of the artery.
2. Juxtaposed aneurysmal and occlusive lesions. Filling an aneurysm with contrast can obscure the inflow and outflow arteries. Occlusive lesions are commonly present in these arteries and may be hidden.
3. Flow artifacts. These may occur at the leading edge of the contrast column. Flow artifacts usually result from incomplete mixing of blood and contrast and resolve on subsequent images.
4. Layering of contrast. If contrast is administered at inadequate pressure or volume, the contrast may layer within the artery and provide an image where the vessel is only partially opacified. This may create the impression that there is a filling defect. The contrast envelope is usually very smooth and contrast usually settles posteriorly.
5. Standing wave. Occasionally, contrast administration results in a standing wave. Although it represents only another mode of contrast flow, the artery may appear to be involved with fibromuscular disease because of a beaded appearance. This occurs in conduit arteries that travel at a regular rate over a distance of many centimeters without interruption by major branch points. The beads appear too regular and uniform to actually be lesions.
6. Parallax. This describes the differences in orientation and length measurement that may be expected when the image intensifier is

moved either toward or away from the patient. The radiographic image presents a three-dimensional subject in two dimensions. When bony landmarks are used to guide therapy, for example, movement of the image intensifier changes the relative relationship of the location of the arterial lesion and its bony landmarks. These landmarks must be rechecked before precise treatment may be undertaken.

7. Gas artifacts. If bowel gas mimics the appearance of an aortic or iliac lesion, obtain an additional view for clarification. Look for the same pattern on the mask to see if it was present and whether it was consistent with intestinal gas.

8. Catheter occlusion of the artery. If the residual lumen in a preocclusive stenosis is minimal enough that the guidewire or catheter occludes it, there may be no flow into the distal artery.

9. Spasm. If spasm occurs as a result of muscular reactivity to manipulation, administer vasodilators (e.g., nitroglycerin or papaverine) to reverse the effects. The infrapopliteal, renal, and upper-extremity arteries are most susceptible.

10. Filming error. If opacification of the vasculature is inadequate, there may have been a poor estimation of timing (flow), inadequate pressure or volume of contrast injection, or too much delay in filming. Determine that contrast was actually administered.

11. Patent "occlusion." If filling is very slow and filming is not extended adequately, patent arterial segments may appear to be occluded. This occurs commonly in the superficial femoral artery distal to an occlusion, especially when using cut film.

12. Viable foot/no outflow. If a foot is viable, but there is no outflow target vessel, pedal arteriography may have been inadequate.

13. Short-necked aneurysm. If the anteroposterior aortic view makes an aneurysm neck appear short (the aorta often turns anteriorly distal to the renal arteries), locate the neck on the video images as the place where the contrast column "stops." The contrast bolus dilutes with swirling blood in the aneurysmal sac. Obtain a cranial or caudal view with some degree of rotation to "unfold" the tortuous artery and provide additional detail.

14. Urinary contrast. Excreted contrast mixed with the fluid contents of the ureter are in motion and can be misinterpreted as arterial rupture, slow flow, dissection, or other abnormalities. Contrast in the bladder obscures the images of nearby structures, especially with oblique views of the pelvis.

15. Lesions difficult to characterize. Shelf-like lesions and those associated with severe calcification can be difficult to assess. Also, a lesion in a low-flow distal runoff bed can be difficult to illuminate, especially if there is a more proximal lesion that is reducing flow to the area.

Lesion Interrogation: Special Views

The aortic arch is demonstrated en face when a LAO projection is used (fig. 1 in chapter 9). This helps to separate the origins of the arch branches. If an area of expected critical stenosis appears only mildly diseased, additional interrogation, such as oblique views, should be considered. The degree of stenosis at the carotid bifurcation and proximal internal carotid artery is best evaluated with lateral or steep oblique views. During arch aortography, the patient should turn the head 20 degrees to 30 degrees to the right. This maneuver helps to separate the carotid and vertebral arteries. The innominate artery bifurcation into proximal right common carotid and right subclavian is best viewed in a RAO projection. The vertebral artery usually has its origin from the posterior wall of the subclavian artery. Therefore, to view the proximal vertebral artery, which often harbors orificial stenosis, the image intensifier is placed into a slight craniocaudal position, and may require some angulation as well.

The celiac artery, superior mesenteric artery, and paravisceral aorta require lateral views to evaluate branch artery orifice lesions and posterior wall aortic plaque or aneurysm (Figs. 2 and 4) The origins of the renal arteries are best evaluated with a slight ipsilateral anterior oblique (Fig. 5).

Disease at iliac and femoral bifurcations often requires visualization with oblique views (Fig. 8). The common iliac bifurcation and posterior wall external iliac disease are best delineated using a contralateral anterior oblique projection. The common femoral bifurcation and common femoral artery posterior wall are investigated using an ipsilateral anterior oblique projection. Occasionally, when there is a high take off of the profunda femoris artery, with a short common femoral artery, the profunda femoris artery exits from the common femoral artery in a straight lateral projection. This occurs more commonly in women and is best visualized in the AP projection. Popliteal and tibioperoneal occlusive disease is often diffuse, and an accurate assessment of severity sometimes requires oblique views of these arteries. The distal tibial and pedal arteries are evaluated with a lateral projection that separates the tibial and pedal arteries, as mentioned earlier.

CARBON DIOXIDE ARTERIOGRAPHY

Carbon dioxide can be administered into the vascular system, is absorbed, and is excreted from the body by exhalation. When renal function is severely diminished, CO_2 is the only contrast available that is not nephrotoxic. CO_2 has some very specific use issues that are discussed here. CO_2 may not be used in the brain or heart and many operators are only comfortable using it in the infrarenal aorta and more distally. In the brain and the heart, where there is a moment-to-moment dependence on perfusion, the passage of gas

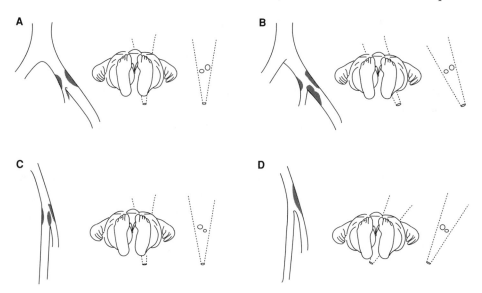

Fig. 8 Oblique projections of the iliac and femoral bifurcations. (**A**) Occlusive disease at the common iliac artery bifurcation is not clearly delineated with the standard anteroposterior projection used for aortoiliac arteriography. (**B**) A contralateral anterior oblique projection permits the iliac bifurcation to be viewed en face. (**C**) Occlusive disease at the femoral bifurcation is sometimes difficult to visualize because of overlap between the proximal superficial femoral artery and deep femoral artery. (**D**) An ipsilateral anterior oblique projection allows the femoral bifurcation to "open up" so that the proximal portions of the branches do not overlap.

through the arteriolar bed will temporarily diminish end-organ flow and cause ischemic events. In the intestinal arteries, the risk is that an air lock will form that becomes stationary and prevent forward flow. In the lower extremities, CO_2 is very well tolerated. Special settings at a high frame rate are required to image CO_2. This particular contrast forms a gas cloud in the vasculature. It rises against gravity and therefore the patient is placed in Trendelenburg when it is administered to decrease the likelihood that it could pass into the cerebral arteries.CO_2 must be medical grade, the tank must be appropriately maintained, and the CO_2 reservoir used during the endovascular procedure must not be contaminated with air. CO_2 is used to fill a sterile, airtight bag; the bag has a one-way valve so that air cannot be entrained. The tubing is purged several times before use. The tubing is connected to the angiographic catheter. A small amount of CO_2 is drawn into the syringe, about 5cc, and slowly administered into the catheter. This clears the catheter of fluid to avoid a sudden jet of gas-propelled saline that could cause injury to the artery during injection. An aortoiliac arteriogram can be performed with 20 cc of CO_2. When the CO_2 passes through normal arteries, the flow pattern of the gas is unpredictable. Therefore, in postprocessing, some type of longitudinal image stacking is usually required to form a reasonable arteriographic representation of the system being interrogated. When the CO_2 encounters significant disease, the gas begins to fragment into bubbles and this makes it very challenging to properly evaluate severely diseased segments. CO_2 is usually used in combination with dilute iodinated contrast in order to make a complete study. Between CO_2 administrations, wait about 2 minutes for the contrast to pass. Each time the angiographic catheter is connected to the CO_2 reservoir, the lines must be carefully purged of air and the catheter must be emptied of fluid prior to a CO_2 angiographic run.

Pressure Measurement

Pressure measurement is time-consuming and is usually performed selectively. However, it is the only quantitative physiologic data that may be yielded by the arteriographic study. Pressure measurements are required only when the results will influence the treatment plan. This situation arises most commonly with moderate degrees of stenosis where the decision about whether to treat depends on the hemodynamic significance of the lesion. Decisions about the treatment of either critical or mild degrees of stenosis can usually be made on the basis of the images alone.

Pressure may be measured through a selective catheter, a diagnostic catheter, or a sheath. The transducer is placed at the level of the right atrium. The shortest adequate extension tubing is flushed with heparin–saline solution, zeroed, and connected to the catheter hub. Blood does not come into contact with the pressure transducer.

Pressure measurements vary from one cardiac cycle to the next. The systolic or mean values are observed until stable and then averaged over five readings. The catheter head is moved to the other end of the lesion and the process is repeated. If the catheter has been placed through a sheath at least one French size larger than the catheter, the distal pressure can be measured through the sidearm of the sheath. During measurement, pressure may continue to fluctuate. If a small gradient is present (less than 10 mm & Hg systolic) or if the lesion in question is potentially physiologically important, papaverine (1 ampule, 30 mg) is administered through the catheter and into the limb or end organ. Diminished peripheral resistance exacerbates any gradient across the lesion and is revealed by immediately repeating the measurements. The converse is also true: if there is increased resistance in the outflow bed, for example very poor runoff, the pressure will tend to equalize in all the artery segments proximal to that and will underestimate the true gradient across a lesion. Pitfalls associated with pressure measurement across lesions are listed in Table 6. No one really knows how much of a gradient is significant. The catheter must be placed across the lesion to do the measurement. At that point, the added morbidity of going ahead with treatment is minimal.

Table 6 Pitfalls Associated with Pressure Measurements Across Occlusive Lesions

Systemic pressure fluctuation	Variations in systemic blood pressure during the few minutes it takes to measure pressure influence the results of pressure measurement proximal and distal to a lesion.
Pressure in end organ arteries	Measuring pressure in an end organ artery, such as the renal artery, presupposes that the lesion must be crossed. The catheter used to measure pressure must occupy a portion of the residual lumen. In a tight stenosis, this may falsely lower the distal pressure.
Poor outflow	If outflow distal to a lesion is poor, pressure tends to equalize proximal and distal to the lesion.
Pressure does not equal flow	Although pressure measurement provides hemodynamic quantitation, it does not provide what is really required, which is a quantitaive assessment of flow across a lesion.
Pressure is not measured under physiologic conditions	Occlusive lesions often become hemodynamically significant only with exercise. Although vasodilators may mimic this, it is usually not an accurate representation of physiologic conditions.

Arteriography of Aneurysms

Arteriography has some distinct advantages and disadvantages with respect to the assessment of aneurysms. Arteriography is not useful in determining the size of an aneurysm or the configuration of an aneurysmal segment. However, arteriography is a very good option for evaluating inflow and outflow arteries, flow surface contour, and associated aneurysm or occlusive disease in juxtaposed arteries. There is usually slow flow and substantial mixing of the contrast bolus with nonopacified blood. Larger contrast volumes administered over a longer period of time are often used. The proximal neck is the location where the contrast bolus seems to stop on the cine loop during DSA. Contrast is administered proximal to an aneurysm, since injecting within an aneurysm may cause thrombus disruption and embolization. Oblique views or special angles may be required to fully evaluate the proximal and distal necks of the aneurysm. Evaluation of runoff distal to an aneurysm may be difficult since the contrast bolus becomes so diluted. Additional contrast injections may be required distal to the aneurysm.

ANGIO CONSULT: HOW CAN I USE DUPLEX SCANNING TO LIMIT THE AMOUNT OF ARTERIOGRAPHY REQUIRED?

1. Unilateral lower-extremity ischemia and a normal femoral pulse. Obtain femoral waveform and femoral acceleration time and evaluate aortoiliac segments directly with duplex scanning. If these are normal, consider unilateral femoral arteriography without aortography.

2. Diabetic with gangrene and normal femoral artery and popliteal artery pulses. Evaluate aortoiliac and femoral segments with duplex scanning. If these are normal, consider an antegrade femoral artery approach and infrageniculate arteriography only.

3. Diminished femoral artery pulse and no tissue loss. Evaluate aortoiliac and femoral-popliteal segments with duplex scanning. If a focal iliac artery lesion is identified and the femoral–popliteal segment is without significant disease, consider proceeding to aortography and balloon angioplasty without performing arteriographic runoff.

4. Patient with an abdominal aortic aneurysm, indications for arteriography, and palpable pedal pulses. Evaluate popliteal arteries with duplex scanning if any enlargement is suggested by physical examination. If these are normal, consider aortoiliac arteriography only without runoff.

5. Recurrent lower-extremity symptoms after a previous reconstruction. Identify the flow-limiting lesion with duplex scanning. If a focal lesion is identified, consider either very limited arteriography for lesion anatomy or no arteriography at all.

6. Suspected occlusion in the aortoiliac segment that requires therapy. Assess the location and length of the lesion with duplex scanning to help determine whether an effort at recanalization is reasonable. If not, detailed arteriographic interrogation of occluded arteries is not necessary.

7. Superficial femoral artery occlusion that requires therapy. Identify the length of the occlusion and the location where flow reconstitutes with duplex scanning. If it is a short occlusion and not at the superficial femoral artery origin, consider an antegrade approach and recanalization. If it is a long occlusion with reconstitution above the knee, consider an above-knee femoral–popliteal bypass without arteriography.

8. Use noninvasive methods to evaluate the lower-extremity contralateral to the symptomatic limb to avoid performing bilateral runoff studies.

Selected Readings

AbuRahma AF, Robinson PA, Boland JP, et al. Complications of arteriography in a recent series of 707 cases: Factors affecting outcome. Ann Vasc Surg 1993; 7(2):122–129.

Anderson J. Techniques in diagnostic angiography. In: Criado FJ, ed. Endovascular Intervention: Basic Concepts and Techniques. Armonk, NY: Futura, 1999: 31–55.

Jacobs JJ. Diagnostic neuroangiography: Basic techniques. In: Osborne AG, ed. Diagnostic Cerebral Angiography. Philadelphia, PA: Lippincott Williams & Wilkins, 1999:421–446.

Jaff MR, Goldmakher GV, Lev MH, et al. Imaging of the carotid arteries: The role of duplex ultrasonography, magnetic resonance arteriography, and computerized tomographic arteriography. Vasc Med 2008; 13(4):281–292.

11

Setting Up the Therapeutic Maneuver: Crossing Lesions

There are only two reasons to cross an occlusive arterial lesion. The first is to set up a therapeutic intervention. The second reason to cross a lesion is because this may be the best option for evaluating that lesion (i.e., by measuring pressure) and the surrounding vasculature (e.g., no other reasonable route to perform an arteriogram). Guidewire advancement is performed deliberately but gently. The principles of guidewire handling are presented in chapter 5. In the present chapter, these principles are applied in concept and practice to the management of occlusive lesions. The ideally placed guidewire will "dance" across the lesion. Negotiating guidewire passage across a reluctant arterial segment leads to a rewarding sense of accomplishment.

In general, a comprehensive approach with a multistep plan has the highest chance of success. If treatment of the lesion is planned, place the guiding sheath early and use it as a platform to launch the chosen catheter and guidewire. Waiting until the lesion is crossed before placing the sheath is the hard way to do it. Access for intervention is covered in detail in chapter 14. Assess flow conditions proximal and distal to the lesion to avoid stagnant flow and the risk of thrombus formation. Choose the puncture site with the likely treatment in mind and estimate the distance between the access site and the target lesion to give yourself all the advantage possible before attempting to cross the lesion.

Three Types of Lesions

The challenge to any endovascular operator is posed by the lesions that are encountered. There are three general types of lesions facing every endovascular surgeon, including (1) lesions that the guidewire sails across easily; (2) lesions that require multiple tricks to get across; and (3) lesions that are impossible, almost no matter what is done (Fig. 1). Although this is an oversimplification, categorizing lesions as such may help to shorten the learning curve by focusing our attention on the difficult ones and what needs to be done to get across them. Lesions included in each of these categories may vary depending upon the place along the learning curve where each operator is working and how many tricks are at immediate disposal. As endovascular skills and new devices develop, the first category may not change much but the second category should get larger as the third category, comprised of impossible lesions, becomes smaller. It used to be in earlier years that occlusions were in this third category of impossible or nearly impossible lesions. Now we have many tools for crossing occlusions, such as subintimal angioplasty and reentry devices, and these are being used with increasing frequency.

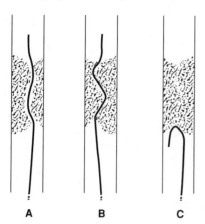

Fig. 1 Three kinds of lesions. (**A**) A guidewire may sail across a lesion, sometimes even one that looks complicated. (**B**) A lesion may require multiple guidewire–catheter tricks to traverse it. (**C**) Some lesions are impossible, or seemingly so. The farther along the learning curve an endovascular surgeon progresses, the smaller this third category becomes.

Crossing Stenoses

The stenotic lesion should be visualized with arteriography before one attempts to cross it. Oblique projections may be required for a full evaluation. Sometimes, the passageway through the lesion is only visible on a certain oblique and occasionally it cannot be identified. The guidewire is selected on the basis of the lesion's appearance. A steel body, floppy-tip starting guidewire is satisfactory for many routine cases with mild or moderate lesions. If the lesion is complex, a hydrophilic-coated guidewire is a good choice. When the lesion also contains a critical stenosis, a steerable tip may be used. Lesions near branch points are best managed with steerable guidewires. Don't lead with a stiff guidewire or a catheter tip. There is some advantage to the use of 0.014-in. guidewires when crossing long diseased segments, especially in small caliber vessels. The 0.014-in. guidewire may be supported with either a microcatheter or a 4- or 5-Fr angiographic catheter with a Tuohy-Borst adapter. Many of the 0.014-in. guidewires have tips that can be shaped and steered across the lesion. Since the 0.014-in. guidewire has less than one-half the caliber of a 0.035-in. guidewire, the ability to cross a tight lesion without stopping forward flow is much better. Smaller caliber treatment platforms are discussed in chapter 6.

Encounters between guidewires and lesions are observed using fluoroscopy. When a guidewire fails to cross, its behavior as it encounters the lesion may reveal information that will assist subsequent passage using an alternative technique. Using the shortest and most direct route between the entry site and the arterial segment of interest offers the operator the most

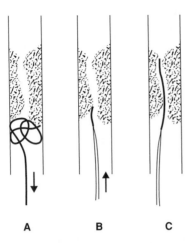

A   B   C

Fig. 2 Stiffen the guidewire by passing a catheter. A straight catheter passed over a guidewire gives additional stiffness and body to its shaft. (**A**) The guidewire is unable to traverse the lesion and the floppy-tip guidewire piles up proximal to the lesion. The guidewire is partially withdrawn. (**B**) A straight catheter is passed over the guidewire. The tip of the guidewire protrudes from the catheter and probes the lesion. (**C**) The guidewire is advanced through the lesion.

guidewire control at the site of the lesion. This approach assumes a minimum adequate working room, or distance, between the access site and the lesion (usually the length of a standard access sheath, 10–15 cm). When distance results in poor guidewire control once it has reached the lesion, passing a catheter over the guidewire improves support and a selective catheter improves directionality.

Direct incremental advancement of a floppy-tip guidewire results in passage across long distances of normal or mildly diseased conduit artery. If, for some reason, passage of the floppy-tip guidewire stalls or is unsuccessful, the guidewire should not be forced. If the guidewire tip buckles, the leading elbow of the guidewire loop may find the lumen and pass with the guidewire doubled over on itself (see fig. 1 in chap. 5). This is a useful maneuver but it is not advisable when crossing significant stenoses. In this case, the guidewire may enter a dissection plane and act as a loop stripper. If the guidewire begins to buckle, but continues to accumulate into several loops and piles up proximal to the lesion, withdraw the guidewire and change course to use one of several options that may facilitate guidewire passage.

A catheter passed over the guidewire gives additional support to the guidewire shaft and secures the access site (Fig. 2). The guidewire tip remains a few centimeters beyond the leading end of the catheter, and the guidewire is used to probe the lesion. Another option is to exchange the floppy-tip starting guidewire for a hydrophilic-coated guidewire, which may cross the lesion, even a preocclusive stenosis, on the first pass. Hydrophilic-coated guidewires may be obtained with either a straight or angled tip. The angled

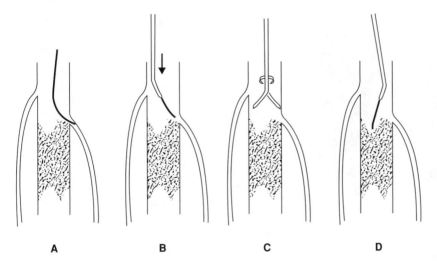

Fig. 3 Use a catheter to steer the guidewire. A Berenstein catheter (5 Fr) passed over a steerable or standard guidewire can help steer the guidewire tip into the desired location. (**A**) The guidewire enters a collateral proximal to the lesion intended for passage. (**B**) A bent-tip Berenstein catheter is passed over the guidewire. (**C**) The catheter is rotated to redirect the guidewire. (**D**) The guidewire is advanced into the lesion.

tip is steerable with a torque device and may be used to find the entrance to an eccentric lesion (see fig. 7 in chap. 5). Hydrophilic guidewires have been a tremendous advance in crossing lesions but are more challenging to use for treatment because of their handling difficulty. Road mapping facilitates this maneuver (see fig. 3 in chap. 8). A 5-Fr bent-tip catheter, such as a Berenstein or a Teg-T catheter, may help steer the guidewire into the desired location (Fig. 3). The catheter may be advanced as the guidewire makes forward progress, but the catheter should not be advanced into a lesion until the guidewire is across the lesion. A special exception to this is when the guidewire will not cross an occlusion and the lesion is crossed in the subintimal plane. This is performed by using the catheter at the plaque wall interface and advancing the guidewire into it. Otherwise, the catheter tip itself, without the guidewire protruding from it, should not encounter the lesion because it is too stiff and may disrupt plaque.

Contrast may be puffed through the tip of the catheter to ensure that its position is intraluminal (Fig. 4). If significant resistance occurs, the guidewire may have passed outside the course of the artery lumen. Most of the time, guidewire does not cause pain but if the patient develops discomfort, subintimal dissection should be suspected. Whenever a lesion is crossed, always confirm intraluminal position on the far side of the lesion before proceeding to treatment.

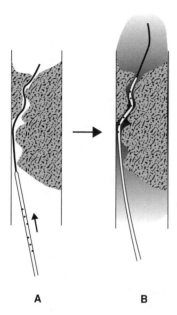

A   B

Fig. 4 Puff contrast into the lesion. (**A**) After a difficult guidewire passage, a multi-side-hole, straight, exchange catheter may be placed over the guidewire. The catheter maintains the position through the lesion. (**B**) Contrast is puffed through the catheter, and its side holes allow the lesion to fill with contrast. The guidewire may be withdrawn and contrast administered directly with the catheter tip through the lesion. Another option is to place a smaller caliber guidewire, such as a 0.018 in. or 0.025 in. and a Tuohy-Borst adapter.

Crossing lesions in well-collateralized arteries, such as the superficial femoral artery, presents an additional challenge. A large juxtaposed collateral just proximal to a critical stenosis may be the preferential course for a passing guidewire. The guidewire may be mistakenly advanced into a collateral that parallels the treatment artery (Fig. 5). Guidewire position must be confirmed before larger endovascular devices are passed over it. A steerable guidewire is useful for avoiding collaterals and maintaining position in the flow stream. A directional catheter may be used to point the guidewire away from the collaterals.

An oblique projection, as mentioned earlier, may be useful not only for evaluation of the lesion, but for opening up the entrance to the lesion and showing the way to cross it (Fig. 6). Occasionally, the steerable guidewire will require multiple manipulations to wind its way through a highly irregular stenosis (Fig. 7). When the approach artery is highly tortuous, it can be difficult to advance through a lesion after the guidewire has passed through several opposing curves. A 5-Fr catheter passed over the guidewire can lessen the curvature of some of the turns through which the guidewire must proceed. Sometimes it is necessary to place a sheath to give the advantage to the guidewire–catheter apparatus.

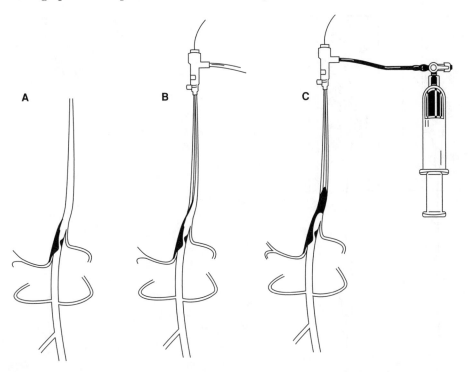

Fig. 5 Determine that the guidewire is really in the lumen. (**A**) Large perigenicular collaterals may be the preferential course for a guidewire attempting to cross a superficial femoral artery or popliteal artery lesion. (**B**) Under fluoroscopy, the guidewire appears to have crossed the proximal popliteal artery stenosis but is actually in a collateral that parallels the artery. (**C**) Arteriography performed by administering contrast through the sidearm of the sheath reveals the true course of the guidewire and that the lesion has not been traversed.

Occasionally, a critically stenotic segment cannot be crossed in the chosen direction, and a separate puncture and an approach from the opposite direction are required (Fig. 8). After guidewire passage, control of the guidewire should not be relinquished until after treatment is completed. When guidewire control is inadvertently lost, it may be exceedingly difficult to cross the lesion a second time. Inexplicably, the same guidewire using the same technique across the same lesion may not recross easily.

Lesions at the orifice of major branch arteries, such as occur in the subclavian or renal arteries, may also be a challenge to cross. Selective catheters and steerable guidewires are routinely used to cross these. The tip of the selective catheter must provide substantial support to the guidewire despite being perpendicular to the aortic flow stream. Selective catheters appropriate for these arteries are presented in chapter 9. The usual intent in crossing a lesion in one of these locations is intervention. Before the lesion is crossed, appropriate planning should be undertaken so that access for endovascular therapy with a guiding catheter or guiding sheath is prepared. Chapter 14

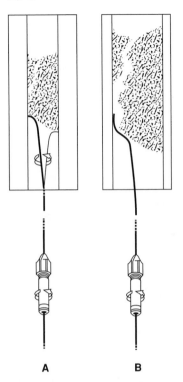

                    A   B

Fig. 6 Magnified oblique view. (**A**) A complex lesion is encountered by the probing guidewire. (**B**) The field is magnified and an oblique projection helps to open up the entrance to the lesion.

contains further discussion of appropriate access options for endovascular therapy. Once the branch artery lesion has been crossed, subsequent placement of a guiding sheath may pull the guidewire from its location and back into the aorta. Chapters 24 and 25 provide a step-by-step approach to the treatment of subclavian and renal lesions. After an orifice lesion has been crossed in one of these arteries, care must be taken to prevent dislodgment of the guidewire during other maneuvers. This is especially true in the renal artery, where the distance to the renal parenchyma is relatively short and the length of guidewire across the lesion is limited. This is combined with a sharp turn, often more than 90 degrees from the aorta into the branch artery.

After the guidewire is in place across the lesion, the chosen catheter is advanced (see chap. 5 for a detailed discussion of techniques for catheter placement). If there is a minimal lumen diameter at the site of the lesion, the guidewire–catheter combination may occlude it. Heparin should be administered to prevent thrombosis or the lesion should be dilated without delay so that flow resumes.

PLAN OF ATTACK: CROSSING A STENOSIS

1. Don't raise a dissection plane. This can be done easily by using excessive force, pushing a hydrophilic-coated guidewire, or

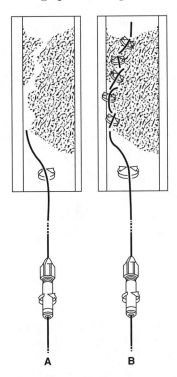

Fig. 7 Multiple maneuvers are sometimes required. (**A**) A steerable guidewire probes a complex lesion. (**B**) Multiple maneuvers are required to steer the guidewire across the lesion.

attempting to advance the catheter without the guidewire (see Angio Consult).

2. Buckle the guidewire to form a leading edge across a mild stenosis, a long segment of artery, or a previously placed stent. Don't force the elbow.

3. Use a catheter to confer directionality or stiffness to the guidewire (Fig. 2).

4. If a standard steel guidewire won't cross the lesion easily, use a hydrophilic-coated guidewire.

5. Exchange for a steerable guidewire (Fig. 7, see also fig. 7 in chap. 5).

6. Obtain oblique views of the lesion to get more information, especially if it is an eccentric or posterior wall lesion or located at a bifurcation or branch point (Fig. 6).

7. Road map the lesion to provide real-time guidance (see fig. 3 in chap. 8).

8. Use a selective catheter to provide additional directionality and to steer the guidewire (Fig. 3).

9. Once across the lesion, puff contrast to ensure that the guidewire did not pass through a dissection plane or into a collateral juxtaposed

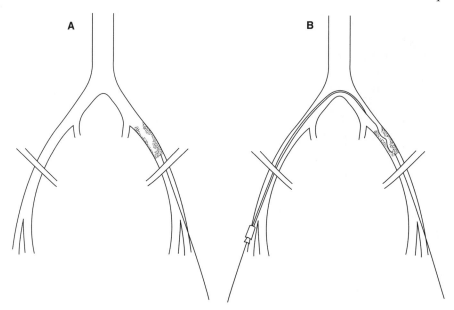

Fig. 8 Approach the lesion from the opposite direction. After attempting various maneuvers to cross a lesion, it is sometimes better to approach the lesion from the other end rather than force it and cause a complication. (**A**) Ipsilateral retrograde passage of a guidewire is unsuccessful at crossing an external iliac artery stenosis. (**B**) A second puncture is performed in the contralateral femoral artery, a catheter is passed over the aortic bifurcation, and the guidewire is advanced antegrade through the iliac stenosis.

to the lesion (Fig. 4). Make sure that the catheter is in the artery distal to the lesion.

10. If the guidewire impedes flow, administer heparin.
11. If endovascular therapy is planned, advance an exchange catheter and place a stiffer guidewire to maintain control of the lesion.
12. If the lesion still can't be traversed, approach from the opposite direction and repeat these maneuvers (e.g., if a retrograde approach to an iliac artery lesion is not successful, try an antegrade approach) (Fig. 8).

ANGIO CONSULT: AVOIDING SUBINTIMAL GUIDEWIRE DISSECTION, UNLESS OF COURSE YOU INTEND A SUBINTIMAL COURSE

1. Most stenoses can be crossed with the guidewire maintained in the true lumen, even long and challenging stenotic lesions with multiple preocclusive stenoses.
2. Staying in the true lumen when possible, obviates the need to reenter the true lumen. This would be the case when the subintimal plane is entered.

3. Crossing a lengthy and challenging stenosis with multiple critical areas is facilitated by the following maneuvers: place the tip of the sheath close to the lesion, use a 0.014-in. directional guidewire, and support the guidewire with a catheter, either a microcatheter or a 4-Fr directional, hydrophilic catheter with a Tuohy-Borst adapter.

4. Most guidewire-induced subintimal dissections occur at the leading edge of a lesion at the interface with the wall of the artery. Care must be taken during the initial encounter with the lesion. Occasionally, even innocuous-appearing lesions will dissect.

5. Puff contrast as often as is required to see where you are going. Make sure there is blood return before administering contrast.

6. "Dance" through the stenosis with a steerable-tip guidewire.

7. Use continuous fluoroscopy while the guidewire is in motion through a lesion.

8. Go fast with the guidewire until you get close to the lesion and then make small incremental and deliberate movements after that.

9. Be aware that a hydrophilic-coated guidewire may pass effortlessly along a dissection plane. If the guidewire tip catches on a lesion, don't keep pushing to form a loop unless you intend to go into the subintimal space. This is a good way to enter the subintimal space. This is described in greater detail in the next section and also in chapters 22, 26, and 27.

10. Anticipate where cleavage planes might be in the plaque, such as bifurcations and branch origins, and be extra careful around these areas, especially if they are also calcified and/or tortuous.

11. If a dissection plane placement is suspected, twirl the guidewire to be certain that it behaves as a free guidewire should in the vasculature distal to the lesion. When the guidewire encounters unexpected obstructions or appears constrained, it may be in the wall of the artery.

12. A suspected guidewire dissection may be evaluated by advancing a 4-Fr straight catheter over the guidewire and puffing a tiny amount of contrast. If it is subintimal, the contrast will be stationary in the arterial wall.

13. If a dissection occurs, remove the guidewire and start again, unless of course the procedure is intended to be performed in the subintimal space after that.

14. Subintimal angioplasty is often best for treating occlusions. This is discussed in next section and in chapters 22, 26, and 27.

Crossing Occlusions

Crossing occlusions is more challenging and less reproducible than crossing stenotic lesions. The only reason to cross an occlusion is in preparation for an attempt at recanalization. An ill-fated attempt at crossing and recanalizing an occlusion that results in distal embolization can be one of the most costly complications of endovascular intervention because of the potential that relatively stable chronic ischemia will be converted to acute ischemia. Acute ischemia due to embolization may also be untreatable if it is caused by plaque contents occluding the distal runoff of the organ system in question. Along the length of an occluded arterial segment, there is usually an underlying critical stenosis from a progressive atherosclerotic plaque that went finally on to thrombose and occlude. There is usually an accumulation of compacted chronic thrombus proximal and distal to the lesion that extends to the next substantial collateral. There are usually substantial collaterals just proximal and just distal to the occlusion that maintain flow to the distal reconstituted segment and also help to prevent the occlusion from propagating.

These collaterals come into play in several ways when managing occlusions. An approaching, probing guidewire usually passes preferentially into the large collateral immediately preceding the occlusion, rather than into the lesion itself. When the occlusion is crossed in the subintimal plane, an attempt is made distal to the occlusion to reenter the true lumen close to where it reconstitutes. This is in an effort to maintain the patency of the distal reconstituting collaterals. In addition, when reconstructing after subintimal passage and true lumen reentry, any stent or stent–graft should be placed such that the distal collateral is preserved. When the occluded artery is tortuous or the underlying atherosclerotic lesion is diffuse or heavily calcified, the likelihood of passing a guidewire along the true lumen is decreased and the risk of perforation is increased. The dual antegrade and retrograde approach to a lesion is more often required for occlusions than for stenoses.

When endovascular recanalization is considered, adequate arteriography includes delayed films to assess the length of the occlusion and its runoff (Fig. 9). For iliac artery occlusions, digital subtraction arteriography (DSA) with delayed pelvic filming is required. For superficial femoral artery occlusions, extended DSA is performed in the area where reconstitution is expected.

Occasionally, when crossing an occlusion, it is possible to keep the guidewire in the intraluminal space. If the occlusion can be crossed intraluminal, there is no reentry required and the shortest possible reconstruction can be performed. A straight tip hydrophilic guidewire or a hydrophilic catheter with a stiff tip (Quick-cross catheter, Spectranetics, Colorado, U.S.) can be used to enter an occlusion and push across it. The combination of the hydrophilic guidewire and the catheter with the stiff tip can be very effective as well (Fig. 10).

Most often, the guidewire finds its way into the subintimal plane regardless of what the operator does. Many specialists seek this out at the beginning of the case and don't worry about it, especially when treating a long

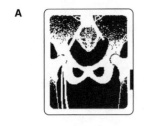

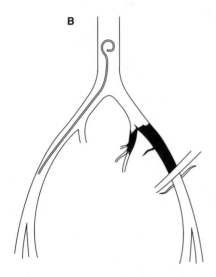

Fig. 9 Use delayed filming to show the true length of an occlusion. The length of an occluded segment can affect the decision as to whether recanalization should be attempted. (**A**) Cut film arteriography tends to overestimate the length of an occlusion. The late filling of contrast into the distal, underperfused segments is usually missed by a multistep filming sequence. (**B**) The length of an occlusion is best determined by placing the image intensifier over the area of interest, injecting contrast, and performing delayed filming as contrast slowly fills the segment immediately distal to the occlusion. This is most simply accomplished with DSA.

occlusion. The most common approach is to use a hydrophilic-coated guidewire in the shape of a loop and pass it in the subintimal plane. A relatively stiff, angled catheter is used to back up the guidewire. The catheter tip is pointed into the stump of the occluded artery. The hydrophilic guidewire is used to jab and probe until the tip catches and the guidewire forms a loop. The loop is advanced for a few centimeters. The catheter is advanced a few centimeters up to the beginning of the loop but the loop is not straightened out. Then the loop is advanced again, and the catheter is subsequently advanced in a step-by-step fashion. If the loop is advanced too far on its own, the loop will begin to spiral around the inside of the artery. Adjuncts that may be employed for crossing occlusions are listed in Table 1.

Once a dissection plane is raised in juxtaposition to an occluded arterial segment, it may be difficult to redirect the guidewire into the lumen. The

A   B   C

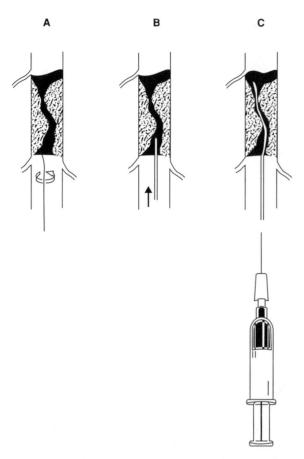

Fig. 10 Crossing an occlusion. (**A**) A Wholey guidewire approaches the occlusion. The guidewire tip enters the thrombus but advancement stops. (**B**) A straight catheter is passed over the guidewire. The guidewire is advanced while its tip is rotated. (**C**) The catheter is advanced gradually and intermittently over the guidewire. Occasionally the guidewire is removed and contrast is puffed through the catheter to check progress and position.

Table 1 Adjunctive Tools for Crossing Occlusions

Loop of hydrophilic guidewire pushed into subintimal space
Low profile, stiff hydrophilic catheters (Quick-cross, Spectranetics)
Entry catheters (Frontrunner, Cordis)
Reentry catheters (Outback, Cordis) and Pioneer (Medtronic)
Intravascular ultrasound (for identifying presence in true lumen)
Laser
Approach lesion from opposite direction

subintimal angioplasty procedure is more technically demanding because of the challenge of reentering the true lumen at the optimal location. Although subintimal balloon angioplasty is a second choice to angioplasty within the true lumen of the artery, it has gained increasing usage in the past few years.

In general, the shorter the occlusion and the less calcified, the easier it is to cross. Once the guidewire is through the most narrowed segment with the heaviest plaque formation, it usually slides through the compacted thrombus. If a short but difficult segment of the occlusion remains to be crossed or the entire lesion is short (2 cm or less) but heavily calcified, a straight catheter is advanced to the base of the J tip on the guidewire and the guidewire–catheter combination is advanced together. Longer occlusions may also be treated, especially in the superficial femoral arteries and iliac arteries with a variety of steps that are detailed in a later chapter. Endovascular treatment cannot be achieved unless the guidewire is completely across the occluded segment. Always be sure that the guidewire is in the true lumen distal to the occlusion before beginning the treatment.

PLAN OF ATTACK: CROSSING AN OCCLUSION

1. Assess proximal and distal patent arteries arteriographically to measure occluded distance and to ensure that the plaque load is small enough that a recanalized occlusion has a reasonable likelihood of continued patency. DSA is best for this task.
2. If there is the option that access could be obtained both proximal and distal to the lesion (such as an iliac artery occlusion), keep this in mind for planning so that this option can be maintained. This is a good back up plan if crossing of the lesion is not successful in the first go round.
3. Road map the lesion. An extended road-mapping run usually allows both ends of the occlusion to be visualized simultaneously (Fig. 9, see also fig. 3 in chap. 8).
4. Place the tip of the sheath close to the occlusion. This permits enhanced pushability and also allows interval arteriography with minimal contrast.
5. Advance a relatively stiff, angled-tip catheter through the sheath and into the stump of the occluded artery.
6. Probe, drill, and push a 0.035-in. angled-tip, hydrophilic guidewire into the stump of the occluded artery. The best place to point the catheter is toward the interface between the plaque and the artery wall that is opposite the largest collateral.
7. When the tip of the guidewire grabs and sticks in the plaque, the flexible guidewire right behind the tip will form a loop. The loop is then advanced.

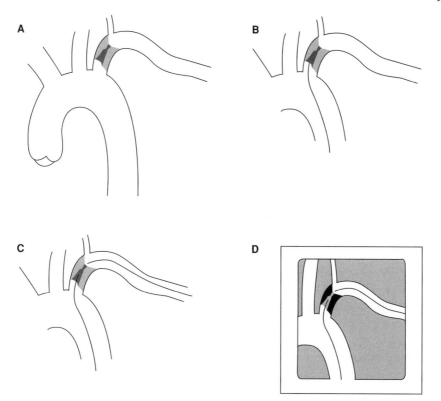

Fig. 11 Leave guidewire that won't cross occlusion as a marker. (**A**) A proximal subclavian artery occlusion can be approached either antegrade (transfemoral) or retrograde (transbrachial). (**B**) An unsuccessful antegrade approach results in the partial passage of a guidewire tip across the occluded segment. (**C**) The first guidewire is temporarily left in place and serves as a marker for an alternate retrograde approach to the same lesion. (**D**) Using fluoroscopic guidance, the distance between the tips of the two guidewires can be assessed.

8. Watch the trajectory of the loop and be sure that it is going along a pathway where the artery should be. Clues about this can often be obtained using plain fluoroscopy to look for calcification.
9. After the guidewire loop is a few centimeters along the subintimal plane, advance the catheter behind the guidewire. Alternate between pushing the looped guidewire and pushing the supporting guidewire.
10. Assess the course of the guidewire and the distance from the other end of the occlusion with oblique views or with continued use of a road map. If the sheath that supports the procedure is well placed, the administration of contrast into the sheath will opacify the collaterals that reconstitute the artery distal to the occlusion.

11. Push the loop of guidewire supported by the catheter until it reaches the location where the artery reconstitutes. Usually the loop will reenter the true lumen.
12. If the loop does not reenter, the options include using an angled catheter to attempt reentry, using a specially designed reentry catheter (discussed in chap. 27), or coming from the opposite direction.
13. If the guidewire won't cross the occlusion completely, leave it in place as a marker and approach the lesion from the opposite direction (Fig. 11).

ANGIO CONSULT: WHEN IS ROAD MAPPING USEFUL TO CROSS LESIONS?

1. Road mapping is a helpful adjunct for treating occlusions. Both ends of the occlusion may be visualized simultaneously. The progress of the guidewire across the occluded segment may be monitored in real time.
2. Road mapping may not be as useful for crossing stenoses. Most operators use other tricks before going to the effort to construct a road map.
3. Consider a road map for approaching complex lesions that could not be crossed after many different maneuvers have been attempted. The road map provides another option for attacking the lesion.
4. Road mapping simplifies the approach to lesions near the origins of branch arteries since it permits simultaneous visualization of the location of the branch that must be entered and the lesion that must be crossed.

Selected Readings

Kerlan RK. Angioplasty. In: LaBerge JM, Gordon RL, Kerlan RK, Wilson MW, eds. Interventional Radiology Essentials. Philadelphia, PA: Lippincott Williams & Wilkins, 2000:147–164.
Uflacker R. Angioplasty procedures. In: Uflacker R, ed. Endovascular Therapy. Philadelphia, PA: Lippincott Williams & Wilkins, 2002:1–60.

Part II

Endovascular Therapy

12

Strategy for Endovascular Therapy

Endovascular Skills

Endovascular therapy has prompted an ongoing reinvention of vascular care that has permanently changed the spectrum of vascular practice. As in so many other disciplines, a set of skills comprise the foundation upon which complex therapy is provided, thus making endovascular skills integral to vascular patient care. Part I (chaps. 1 through 11) provided an overview of basic endovascular skills. Part II presents techniques in endovascular therapy that build upon the basic skills. Endovascular therapy is performed with fairly simple tools, such as guidewires and catheters. However, guidewire–catheter skill development is a dynamic process. As techniques and devices are refined, the capability of the catheter and its attachments to render treatment will continue to expand.

Impact of Endovascular Therapy

Balloon angioplasty has offered an alternative to open surgery for several decades. This technique was initially complementary to bypass operations and was reserved primarily for lower-extremity revascularization in patients with focal occlusive disease in larger arteries. Since the widespread introduction of stents in the first half of the 1990s, endovascular therapy of both occlusive and aneurysm disease has advanced rapidly. Advances include the capability of treating more severe disease morphology, a broadening of endovascular therapy to include all vascular beds, and the development of stent–graft treatment of aneurysmal disease. Endovascular therapy has had a huge impact upon vascular practice. This impact will continue to increase as techniques and devices develop and more data becomes available to guide treatment. Table 1 offers a summary of one practitioner's view of the impact of endovascular therapy upon the management of vascular disease in various vascular beds. Endovascular intervention has traditionally provided an option for treatment in patients with mild forms of occlusive disease or those who are not surgical candidates. The scope of endovascular intervention has increased to replace surgery in some vascular beds and to be a more competitive adjunct in others. Endovascular intervention has become the treatment of choice in most patients with aortic, iliac, and renal artery occlusive disease and has become a prominent part of treatment for carotid, subclavian and infrainguinal occlusive disease, and aortoiliac aneurysm. The future of endovascular therapy is bright. The impact of carotid balloon angioplasty and stent placement remains to be seen but it is likely to play a major role in future carotid treatment.

Steps to Endovascular Therapy

Performing endovascular therapy is a multiple-step process (Table 2). The conduct of the intervention is important but is only one of the many steps

Table 1 Overall Impact of Endovascular Intervention in Various Noncoronary Vascular Beds Upon Vascular Therapy Practice

	Current		
	Provides treatment option for patients who are not surgical candidates	Replaces surgery for patients who were candidates for operation	Likely to be future treatment of choice
Carotid bifurcation	****	**	*→ *****[a]
Common carotid[b]	****	****	****
Innominate	***	***	***
Subclavian	****	***	***
Axillary	**	**	**
Brachial	O	O	O
Celiac/superior mesenteric artery	****	***	***
Renal	****	****	****
Infrarenal aorta	***	****	****
Iliac	***	****	****
Femoropopliteal	***	***	***
Tibial	***	**	**
Pedal	*	O	O

[a] Depends upon the results of prospective randomized trials of endarterectomy versus carotid stent.
[b] Isolated common carotid artery stenosis.
Abbreviations: O, no impact on vascular therapy; *, minimal impact; **, moderate impact; ***, substantial impact; ****, profound impact.

Table 2 Steps to Endovascular Therapy

Step	Physician responsible
Identify symptoms and signs of vascular disease	Primary physician; vascular specialist
History and physical examination of vascular system	Vascular specialist
Order appropriate laboratory and noninvasive tests	Vascular specialist
Interpret results of testing	Vascular specialist
Assess treatment options	Vascular specialist
Obtain nonvascular studies to assess medical risk of intervention	Vascular specialist, primary physician
Counsel patient and family with recommendations	Vascular specialist
Admit patient (if necessary) Endovascular operation	Vascular specialist
	Vascular specialist or nonclinical interventionist
Periprocedural management	Vascular specialist
Manage complications	Vascular specialist
Discharge patient, arrange follow-up, provide results	Vascular specialist
Manage postprocedure outpatient issues as they arise	Vascular specialist
Long-term clinical and noninvasive follow-up	Vascular specialist

required. Actually pulling the trigger of an endovascular device takes skill, but patient selection, management, and follow-up also require judgment and vigilance that require enthusiasm and years of effort to develop. Vascular therapy is ideally practiced as a continuum: a long-term commitment to prevent, diagnose, treat, and follow patients with vascular problems. The person performing the procedure is effective only if there is a clear understanding of where a given patient is along the treatment curve and what the other treatment options are. The operator must also be focused on short-term results and longer-term outcomes if continuous quality improvement is to be possible. When a piece of the care, such as pulling the trigger on an endovascular device, is farmed out to another specialist, the opportunity for discontinuity in care is profound.

A Loaded System

Open surgery for vascular problems is a "front loaded system." Open surgery is expensive and has an inescapable risk of morbidity. The short-term costs and complications have the potential to be substantial. However, open surgery also offers the best long-term results among the various treatment options for many vascular problems. Conversely, endovascular intervention has lower associated perioperative morbidity, but it is also a "pay as you go system." The additive costs are high, with greater surveillance required, and higher rates of failure, and repeat therapy. Since almost any lesion may now be treated with endovascular intervention, it is important to be readily aware of the long-term consequences of the chosen therapy. In this context, understanding when not to do a particular procedure will take on greater value as technology progresses.

The Future of Endovascular Surgery

Endovascular therapy is here to stay and the likelihood is high that it will assume an expanded role in the coming years. There are applications in every vascular bed for the management of both aneurysmal and occlusive disease. Although the durability of many procedures is not yet known, technology and innovation will likely lead to further improvements. There will be many patients requiring vascular care but it is not clear who will be delivering that care or what the constraints will be from a standpoint of resource expenditure. The vascular specialist is well advised to be able to justify needed procedures from a risk–benefit standpoint.

Choosing Treatment: The Endovascular Therapy Curve

Deciding who gets what can be a challenge. Wrong choices are revealed only after the damage is done. When intervention is indicated, the choice

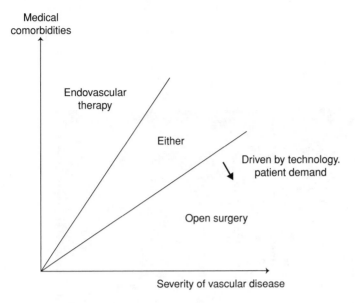

Fig. 1 Endovascular therapy curve.

of endovascular or open surgery is based upon the clinician's understanding of the balance in a given patient between medical comorbidities (perioperative risk) and lesion severity (likelihood of endovascular success). This is represented in a stylized graphical version in Figure 1. Endovascular therapy is most beneficial in patients with more severe medical comorbidities or with lesser forms of vascular disease. Open surgery is more successful when the medical risk is low and open surgery can usually be tailored to manage more severe disease morphology. When the extent of disease is severe enough that the results of open surgery are likely to be more durable in comparison to endovascular intervention, making the best decision in a given patient can be challenging. Demand for less invasive procedures is strong among patients, physician colleagues, and the heath-care system. There is an enlarging group of patients who could be considered for either type of treatment, open or endovascular. Nevertheless, advancing technology and demand for less invasive procedures is pushing the curve downward toward a decrease in open surgery and an increase in endovascular surgery.

Endovascular Decision Tree

Figure 2 shows an endovascular decision tree. This diagram helps to categorize the important decisions, which must be made to carry out therapy. The concept that multiple different specialists could be involved in this decision tree and each take responsibility for some small part of the process is an invitation to failure. Ideally, the physician who knows the patient and understands the problem is best suited to guide the patient through the decision-making process. When an approach is selected, the procedure

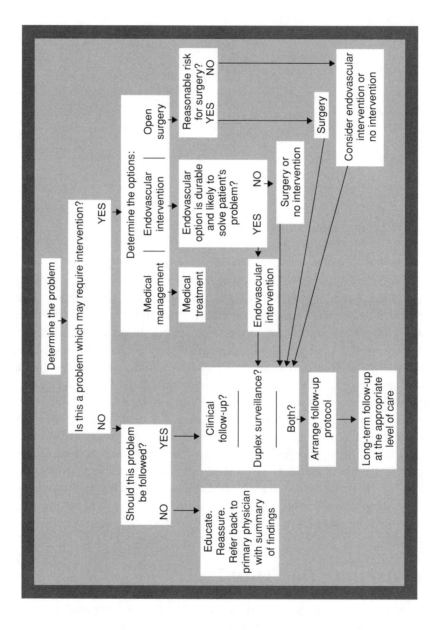

Fig. 2 Endovascular decision tree.

should be planned and controlled in the same way as an open operation. The case should be prepared in advance with a thorough understanding of the patient's desires and expectations, a careful physical examination, and noninvasive imaging to evaluate the location and severity of lesions. In that way, the scope of endovascular therapy can usually be determined ahead of time.

Converting a Strategic Arteriogram to Endovascular Treatment

Strategic arteriography should be planned so that when conversion to an endovascular operation is indicated, it can proceed with stepwise progression. Expectations generated by history, physical examination, and noninvasive studies as to the location and severity of disease determine not only the puncture site and arteriographic approach, but also the likelihood that the procedure may be converted to an endovascular operation. A contralateral or proximal approach for strategic arteriography permits maximal flexibility. Occasionally, a well-placed second puncture site in proximity to the area intended for therapy is a simple solution. Performing endovascular surgery from a very remote location increases catheter and procedure time, contrast load, and the number of exchanges necessary for longer guidewires and catheters.

13

Endovascular Workshop

Where We Work Determines What We Can do

Dramatic developments in endovascular intervention have prompted the common dilemma about where the modern vascular specialist should be working to get the best results: the operating room or the special procedures suite. In many institutions, endovascular operating rooms have been constructed to solve this problem and provide superior imaging in an operating room setting. Thoughtful and deliberate requests for expensive equipment and space are usually required to pave the way for this change in practice. The facility where the work is done can either promote or hamper success. Vascular specialists must be clear about what is required to provide high-quality care. Fixing vascular problems is already complicated without the case being placed at a disadvantage before the procedure starts. High-resolution imaging, endovascular inventory, and uniquely trained personnel are all required to deliver modern vascular care.

Operating Room vs. Special Procedures Suite

Operating rooms (ORs) are well suited to the sterile technique of open surgery, handling blood vessels, and implanting prosthetic material. Special procedures suites, such as angiographic suites and cardiac catheterization laboratories, are designed to support percutaneous interventions and generally have the best fluoroscopic imaging available. Table 1 compares these two environments. Special procedures suites were designed for what they are each named to do, either angiography in angio suites or cardiac catheterization in cath laboratories. The fact that these facilities usually have a high volume of foot traffic, poor lighting, poor airflow, marginal sterile technique, and excellent imaging makes sense.

Table 1 The Operating Room or the Special Procedures Suite

	Operating room	Special procedures suite
Advantages	Best sterile technique	Best imaging quality
	Handle blood vessels	Broader inventory of devices
	Manage bleeding	Personnel trained in interventions
	Implant prosthetic material	Personnel trained in imaging technique
	Better anesthetic capability	
Disadvantages	Lower imaging quality	Poor sterile technique
	Smaller endovascular inventory	Poor environment for open surgery
	Poor staff support for interventions	Inadequate equipment, lighting, and staff support
		Poor anesthetic capability

ORs were designed to meet the standards required to provide therapy: in terms of sterility, quality control, planning for contingencies, managing sick patients, and performing procedures efficiently. The primary advantage of special procedures suites over ORs, as they exist in most institutions, is radiographic imaging. There is a substantial trend toward recognition of high-resolution digital arteriography as an essential component of vascular procedures of all types, including open vascular operations. There is some validity to the concept that quality imaging is required in the OR, regardless of whether the majority of endovascular interventions are performed there. The unsatisfactory choice of multiple suboptimal facility options is being resolved in each institution. Eventually, most institutions that can support modern vascular care will develop an endovascular OR for this work to be done.

Stationary vs. Portable Imaging Systems

Table 2 compares stationary and portable fluoroscopic imaging equipment. Angiographic suites are constructed with stationary imaging equipment, including a ceiling- or floor-mounted C-arm configuration (Fig. 1).

In most surgical ORs, portable C-arm digital arteriographic imaging can be obtained when necessary (Fig. 2).

Stationary equipment offers high resolution and maximal C-arm mobility for multiple views. Portable, digital arteriographic units have been developed that produce adequate images for completing complex endovascular procedures. Available features include multiple frame rates, digital storage, road mapping, video playback, last image hold, postimage processing, and variable fields of view. The portable fluoroscopic unit lacks the convenience of a specially designed room. It is more cumbersome to position and use

Table 2 Stationary Versus Portable Fluoroscopic Imaging Equipment

	Stationary	Portable
Advantages	Better resolution	Less expensive
	Easy to use	Can be used in different locations
	Versatile positioning	Best units available simulate quality
	Bolus chase	of stationary equipment-resolution,
		road mapping, postimage
		processing, and storage
Disadvantages	More expensive	Inconvenient and cumbersome to
	Usage restricted to single location	move and position
	Some units difficult to adapt to	Resolution inferior to fixed unit
	use with open surgery	Impractical for survey arteriography
	Requires room renovation	Often no dedicated personnel

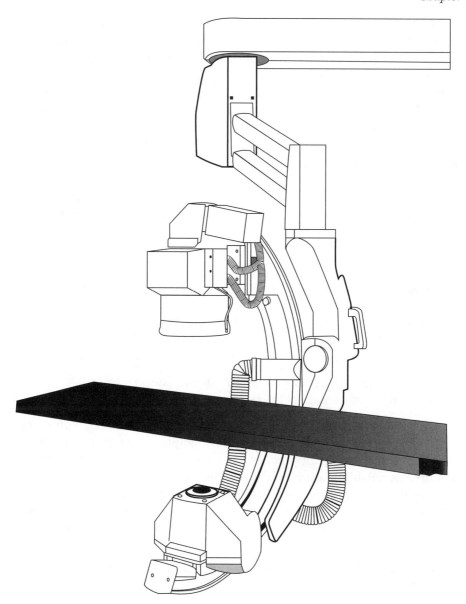

Fig. 1 Stationary imaging system. The C-arm may be either ceiling mounted, as in this example, or floor mounted. Monitors are usually ceiling mounted on booms. These systems usually have larger generators for better image quality. A floor-mounted table on a pillar provides imaging access to the entire body.

portable equipment and more setup time is required. The hard copy obtained with a portable imaging system is frequently not as good as the visual image on the monitor at the time of the arteriogram. However, portable units are cheaper and can be used (and therefore justified) by many different services in the same institution. The most complex procedures in endovascular

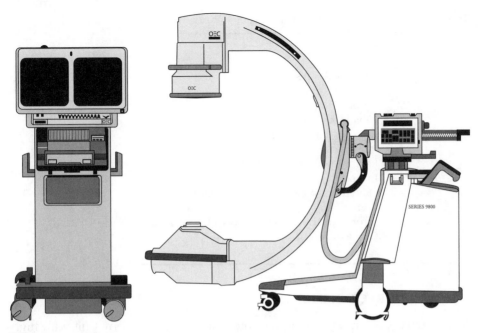

Fig. 2 The portable imaging system provides more flexibility and can be moved from room to room. It consists of a portable C-arm (image intensifier and X-ray tube) and a portable monitor. These generally have a smaller generator and lower heat capacity.

intervention, such as endovascular aortic grafts, have been performed in the OR with portable digital imaging systems, and with very acceptable results. Nevertheless, this approach is more challenging than it would be with improved imaging capabilities.

The Ideal Vascular Workshop

Important components that should be included in a vascular workshop are listed in Table 3. There are facility, equipment, and personnel requirements to consider.

FACILITY REQUIREMENTS

The facility should have a minimum of 750 ft^2. It will need lead-lined walls. The regulations that govern this vary from one state to another. The structure should be able to support the mounting of ceiling-based fluoroscopic and monitoring units. Further requirements that are standard for open surgery include the availability of anesthetic gases, adequate overhead lighting, appropriate airflow, and limited foot traffic.

Table 3 Components of the Ideal Vascular Workshop

Facility	Space
	Lighting
	Lead-lined walls
	Anesthetic gases
	Air flow
	Limit foot traffic
Equipment	High-resolution imaging
	Pressure injector
	Radiographic table
	Inventory
	Other Ultrasound Intravascular ultrasound
Personnel	X-ray technologist
	Scrub (both open and endovascular technique)
	Circulator
	Anesthesia

EQUIPMENT REQUIREMENTS

A stationary, preferably ceiling-mounted, digital fluoroscopy unit with high-resolution capability, road mapping, postimage processing, digital storage, last-image hold, variable frame rates, multiple fields of view, and versatile image intensifier positioning is desirable. A radiographic table that permits positioning for open surgical cases and the placement of self-retaining retractors is also important. A pressure injector is necessary.

PERSONNEL REQUIREMENTS

Scrub and circulating personnel must have expertise in both open and endovascular techniques and a familiarity with the inventory of supplies, devices, and instruments. X-ray technologists with an understanding of endovascular surgery are needed for help with positioning the image intensifier, enhancing imaging technique, and performing arteriographic sequences. Anesthetic personnel should be able to monitor the patient, perform conscious sedation, and perform other types of anesthesia when required. Support personnel must have a thorough knowledge of the inventory: where it is, what it does, how many of each there are, how it is prepared, and other features.

INVENTORY REQUIREMENTS

A broad inventory of endovascular supplies as well as surgical supplies and instruments are also required.

Converting an "OR" to a Vascular Workshop

Given the need for high-quality imaging in the OR and the challenges in performing open surgery in most special procedures suites, for many it makes the most sense to modify the operating room to provide the tools required to perform endovascular interventions. If modern vascular therapy is to be performed in an OR, it will need better imaging, a reasonable inventory, and trained personnel. Endovascular inventory and appropriate personnel are mobile and can be brought in. Better imaging capability, with a stationary unit, is expensive but is an important investment. Vascular therapy is not going to regress to the era of blind revascularizations.

Inventory

The inventory available must complement or exceed the ability of the endovascular surgeon. The availability of inventory to perform a challenging case is just as important as the technical know-how to do the case. Each operator must understand what is available in order to be effective. Look before the case starts. Be sure there is an extra one of the key items you need for the case. Pay attention to what you have and continuously update it. New products come out several times a year. The level of attention you pay to inventory depends upon the environment in which you work. The technicians and staff are often a resource and can facilitate inventory management. Gear the personal level of involvement with inventory to the type of environment in which the work is carried out. The less support is available, the more hands-on control the operator needs to keep track of the inventory.

Table 4 contains tips for inventory management. Use all the available resources to your advantage. See what others are using for various purposes and copy their inventory lists. When visiting colleagues, look through their closet and see if they have anything you can use. Focus your purchasing on two or three companies that are chosen on the basis of geography, price, and service. Most companies want to sell supplies to doctors of all different disciplines and the reps are caught in the middle. Don't take it out on the device reps. Get to know them. They have a tremendous wealth of knowledge and are a potential resource. They know what everyone else is doing and what the latest approaches are. They know what is selling. Get all the catalogues you can from companies that make endovascular supplies

Table 4 Tips for Inventory Management

Copy a colleague's inventory
Pick 2 or 3 companies: compare geography, price, and service
Check catalogues
Know your device reps
Read materials and methods
Use the case card approach
Put someone in charge of inventory
Review inventory every 3 mo

and have them available. When the endovascular journals come in, be sure to read the Materials and Methods section. Authors often share technique and inventory advice that can be put to good use. Each of the major cases should be summarized using case cards, the same as it would be for any surgical case. It must be clear who is in charge of the inventory and who is accountable for replenishing any item that is used. The inventory should be reviewed at every three months.

Selected Readings

Bell RS, Vo AH, Veznedaroglu E, et al. The endovascular operating room as an extension of the intensive care unit: Changing strategies in the management of neurovascular disease. Neurosurgery 2006; 59(5 Suppl 3):S56–S65.

Dietrich EB. Endovascular suite design. In: White RA, Fogarty TJ, eds. Peripheral Endovascular Interventions. St. Louis, MO: Mosby, 1996:129–139.

Mansour MA, Hodgson KJ. Preparing the endovascular operating room suite. In: Moore WS, Ann SS, eds. Endovascular Surgery. Philadelphia, PA: W. B. Saunders, 2001:3–13.

O'Brien-Irr MS, Harris LM, Dosluoglu HH, et al. Lower extremity endovascular interventions: Can we improve cost-efficiency? J Vasc Surg 2008; 47(5):982–987.

14

Access for Endovascular Therapy

Make Access as Simple as Possible

Endovascular therapy is performed using some type of delivery system: an access sheath, a guiding sheath, or a guiding catheter. Whichever one is used represents a "system" in the sense that the selected guidewire, balloon catheter, stent, therapeutic catheter, etc. must fit through the sheath and be able to travel over the chosen guidewire. Access for endovascular therapy has several goals: to secure the puncture site, maintain guidewire placement, deliver the therapeutic catheters, and maintain access for interval arteriography of the treatment site and its outflow bed. Selecting the best means of access is about anticipating the scope of the procedure and the sizing required. Choose the right access and you set yourself up for success. Problems with access are a common reason for a procedure to be prolonged, unnecessarily challenging, or complicated. Patience and planning are required to achieve safe and straightforward access.

There are some simple rules to follow in obtaining access for endovascular therapy (Table 1). Don't upsize to a larger sheath or use a specially designed guiding sheath or guiding catheter until it is certain that therapy will be performed. Otherwise, the arteriotomy has been enlarged without cause and the sheath wasted. Make sure you have the puncture site location you want before enlarging the arterial puncture. This rule comes into play when an arteriogram is converted to a therapeutic procedure. Occasionally, it is better to puncture at an alternative site, such as the contralateral femoral artery or an upper-extremity artery, rather than use the initial puncture site for therapy. This is sometimes the case with iliac, infrainguinal, or subclavian occlusive disease. When the artery chosen for entry is itself significantly diseased (e.g., a common femoral artery stenosis or aneurysm), it is usually best to pick another site and avoid the increased risk of puncture site thrombosis or hemorrhage. Use arterial dilators at the puncture site to gently and gradually enlarge the arteriotomy prior to placing the access sheath. A sheath is sized by its inside diameter (ID) (by what will fit through it). A dilator, like a catheter, is sized by the outside diameter (OD). A 6-Fr dilator has the same OD as a 5-Fr sheath and would therefore be used if full dilatation of the arteriotomy was desired before sheath placement. There is more about this in the next section. Check to see that the required guidewires

Table 1   Simple Rules of Access for Endovascular Therapy

Upsize the sheath when therapy is certain
Confirm that initial puncture site is the best one for therapy
Use dilators
Check availability of catheters and guidewires to go with sheath
Cross-check the size of the sheath with the therapeutic catheters
Anticipate the extent of the procedure and place the correct sheath initially
Determine whether a guiding sheath or guiding catheter is required

and catheters are available for the procedure you plan before you place the access sheath. Always cross-check the size of the sheath with the size of the balloon catheters and stent delivery catheters. The best way is to look for the ID of the sheath, which is in inches or millimeters or both, and compare it with the OD of the catheter intended for placement through it. These measured features are usually listed on the package. Anticipate the full extent of the procedure so that the best-sized sheath can be placed initially. This avoids stopping in the middle and placing a larger or differently shaped sheath. Mid-procedure sheath exchanges always seem to come at the wrong time, usually after it is clear that something important will not fit through it. Often the most useful stiffer guidewire for access placement has already been removed and a softer, more selective guidewire has been placed to perform therapy. If a mid-procedure sheath exchange is required, don't forget to give more local anesthetic at the access site. If the table and image intensifier position must be maintained, tamponading the arteriotomy and advancing a new sheath can be challenging and cumbersome. In some instances, sheath exchange may cause loss of guidewire position, which must be later regained after the correct sheath is in place. Part of planning the procedure is anticipating which guiding access device is likely to be the best one. This could be a longer straight sheath, a guiding sheath, or a guiding catheter. These devices are discussed in more detail later.

Sizing Considerations

Each endovascular device is measured and described in a different way (Table 2). Although the nomenclature can be confusing, mastering the language of endovascular intervention is essential to a successful practice.

GUIDEWIRES

Guidewires are described by diameter, which is measured in inches. A "035" is a guidewire that is 0.035 in. in diameter. A "014" guidewire has a diameter of 0.014 inches. Guidewires are described in detail in chapters 5 and 6. The most common guidewire thickness or diameter for general usage in the aorta and iliac arteries, for both occlusive and aneurysm disease, is 0.035 in. Branch arteries, such as carotid, renal, and tibial arteries, are increasingly treated with 0.014-in. guidewires. Other guidewire sizes used are 0.018, 0.025, and 0.038 in. in diameter, but these are only used in a limited manner. Each guidewire diameter has a catheter system sized appropriately for it.

DILATORS, FLUSH, AND SELECTIVE CATHETERS

Catheter sizes are described using the French system to signify the OD of the catheter. This is true for dilators, diagnostic catheters, and selective catheters.

Table 2 Sizing Considerations

| Accessory | Size measurement for endovascular accessories | |
	Measured feature	Units
Needles	Gauge	Inches[a]
Guidewires	Diameter	Inches[a]
Catheters	Outside diameter	French[b]
Dilator	Outside diameter	French
Access sheath	Inside diameter	French
Guide sheath	Inside diameter	French
Guiding catheter	Outside diameter	French
Balloon catheter	Outside diameter of shaft	French
	Diameter of balloon	Millimeters when inflated
	Length of balloon	Centimeters
Stent	Diameter	Millimeters
	Length	Millimeters

[a] Maximum guidewire diameter for 18-gauge needle is 0.038 in.; maximum guidewire diameter for 21-gauge needle is 0.018 in.
[b] French size ÷ 3.14 = diameter, mm.

Take the French size, divide by 3, and this provides the actual diameter. For example, a 5-Fr catheter has approximately a 1.6-mm OD. A 6-Fr catheter has about a 2-mm OD, and so on. When a catheter is placed percutaneously, it must always be exchanged for a catheter that is the same Fr size or larger so that the artery does not bleed around it. The most common flush and selective catheter sizes in practice are 4 and 5 Fr. Catheters are discussed in chapter 5.

ACCESS SHEATHS AND GUIDING SHEATHS

Access sheaths are also described using the French system, but the feature described is ID, not the OD. This explains how a standard 5-Fr diagnostic or selective catheter can fit through a 5-Fr access sheath. A sheath is purposely sized based upon what will be able to fit through it. However, the operator must be aware that a 5-Fr sheath makes a 6-Fr hole in the artery: it has a 5-Fr ID to accept the 5-Fr catheter but its OD is 6 Fr. Guiding sheaths are sized the same way as access sheaths. The main difference between an access sheath and a guiding sheath is that the former is short (usually 10–12 cm) and straight and the latter may be long (25–100 cm) and have a specially shaped tip for delivery of devices to a side branch (Fig. 1).

GUIDING CATHETERS

Guiding catheters are described by their OD using the French system, the same way that other catheters are described. A guiding catheter functions as

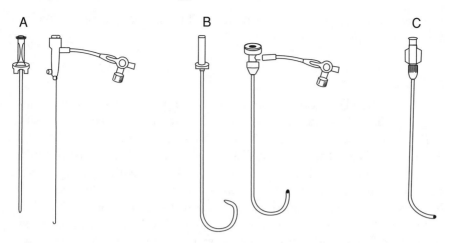

Fig. 1 Access for endovascular therapy. (**A**) A standard access sheath is 12 to 15 cm in length and has a hemostatic valve and a sidearm for administration of contrast and medication. The dilator is used during sheath placement to provide a smooth transition to the tip of the sheath and to provide shaft stiffness. (**B**) A guiding sheath has a dilator, hemostatic valve, and sidearm. It may be longer and it usually has a radiopaque band at the tip. Its tip also has a special shape that is functional for certain tasks. The guiding sheath in the example is used for passage over the aortic bifurcation. There are many different sizes and shapes available among guiding sheaths. (**C**) A guiding catheter is a large-bore catheter (larger than an arteriographic catheter) with a specially shaped tip. There is no dilator, sidearm, or hemostatic valve. The addition of a Tuohy-Borst adapter permits hemostasis since it has a hemostatic valve and an extra port for contrast administration.

access to side branches for delivery of endovascular therapy devices. Guiding catheters are usually introduced through standard hemostatic access sheaths. A 7-Fr guiding catheter requires a 7-Fr sheath (Fig. 1).

BALLOON CATHETERS

Balloon catheters are discussed in detail in chapter 16. The shaft of the balloon catheter is described, as any other catheter would be, by the French size of the OD. The balloon itself is described in terms of its diameter when inflated in millimeters and its length in centimeters with the diameter described first, followed by the length. A "5 by 4" balloon has a 5-mm diameter when inflated and a 4-cm length. An "8 by 2" has an 8-mm diameter and a 2-cm length, and so on. The balloon is tightly wrapped around the catheter when it comes out of the package. After angioplasty, the balloon material never quite folds down to the same profile, so the size of the device has increased slightly. This must be anticipated when choosing a sheath for angioplasty. A 6-mm diameter balloon and an 8-mm diameter balloon may be obtained on a 5-Fr shaft. The 6-mm balloon may be used through a 5-Fr sheath, but the 8-mm balloon should be used with a 6-Fr sheath. This is done to accommodate the balloon material during removal of the balloon catheter.

STENTS

Stents are described by width and length when expanded, usually in millimeters, with the diameter stated first. A "10 by 40" would be a 10-mm diameter and a 40-mm length. Stents generally come packaged with a description of the size of the access that is needed to deploy them. Stents are described in chapter 18. Balloon-expandable stents require a sheath large enough to accommodate the profile of the balloon, with about 1- to 2-Fr sizes added for the stent. Self-expanding stents are enclosed within a delivery catheter with a set sheath size described on the package. The usual minimum sheath size for both balloon and self-expanding stents using a 0.035-in. guidewire system is 6 or 7 Fr.

What Fits into What?

Taking this array of devices with varying size requirement and putting them together in a workable fashion permits endovascular interventions to proceed. Table 3 shows some examples of "what fits into what?" to make certain procedures possible. For example, a 6-Fr sheath can be used for a standard iliac artery balloon angioplasty up to about 8 mm. If an iliac artery stent is required, a 6-Fr sheath is usually adequate. If a larger balloon is required, a 7-Fr sheath is usually needed to accommodate balloon removal after the angioplasty.

General Principles of Sheath Placement During Therapy

Use the diagnostic catheter length to estimate the length of the sheath that will be needed to make it to the lesion or artery segment intended for treatment. When deciding where the sheath tip should be placed for treating the lesion, take into account the intended system for use, including monorail or coaxial, 014 or 035, and device choices. In general, the closer the tip of the sheath to the lesion, the better the control and the less contrast needed (Figs. 2 and 3). However, the sheath requires a stiff exchange guidewire for placement and the sheath itself can obstruct forward flow in some settings, and be difficult to remove if the pathway is highly tortuous. Choose a sheath that is large enough in caliber to accomplish the endovascular therapy, and keep in mind what will be required for a backup plan if the first plan does not work. In selecting a sheath size, also take into the account the tortuosity, calcification, and incidental atherosclerotic disease along the pathway to the

Table 3 Access for Endovascular Therapy: What Fits Into What?[a]

Sheath size (Fr)	Diameter of balloon (mm)	Balloon shaft (Fr)	Procedure	Stent
4	2–4	3	Small-vessel balloon angioplasty (0.014-in.guidewire system)	None
5	3–6	3 or 5	Infrainguinal balloon angioplasty	None
6	6–8	3 or 5	Balloon angioplasty—aortoiliac, carotid, renal, and subclavian	None
	5–7	5	Medium Palmaz stent placement—aortoiliac, renal, and subclavian with low-profile balloon	Balloon expandable
7	8–10	5	Balloon angioplasty—aortoiliac	None
	7–9	5	Medium Palmaz stent placement—aortoiliac	Balloon expandable
	5–10		Self-expanding stent placement (for 10-mm vessel, stent is 12 mm, oversized 2 mm to the artery)	Self-expanding
8	12	5.8	Balloon angioplasty—aorta	None
9	18	5.8	Balloon angioplasty—aorta	None
	8–12	5–5.8	Large Palmaz stent placement—aortoiliac	Balloon expandable
	12–14		Self-expanding stent placement—aorta	Self-expanding

[a] Modified from Schneider, 2001, p. 59.

lesion, all factors which are best managed by selecting the smallest caliber sheath that will do the job. Use a stiff enough guidewire for the size of the sheath and the tortuosity of the pathway. Don't cross the lesion intended for treatment with a stiff guidewire if it can be avoided. When advancing the sheath, keep an eye on landmarks so the sheath is not inadvertently placed across the lesion. If in placing the sheath, the advancement of the sheath is slow and difficult, it will also be difficult to remove. If the iliac arteries are tortuous proximal to a femoral access site, the iliac artery can sometimes be partially straightened by placing the nonsheath hand into the retroperitoneum and pushing on the iliac system.

When Do You Use a Guiding Sheath or a Guiding Catheter?

Whenever endovascular therapy is required to treat a side branch lesion, a guiding sheath or guiding catheter helps deliver the devices, maintains access, and permits interval arteriography. As more treatment is being rendered to major side branches, such as the subclavian, carotid, and renal

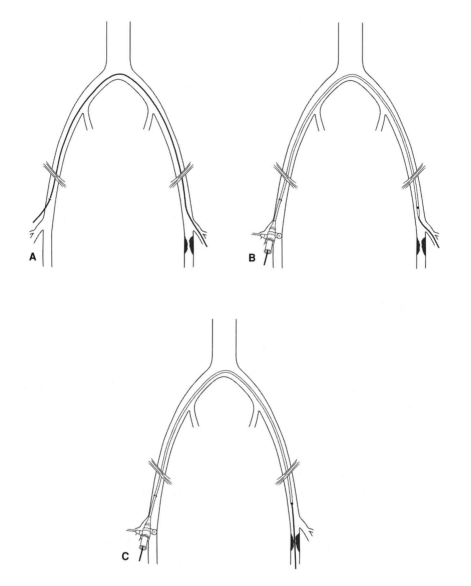

Fig. 2 Principles of sheath placement. (**A**) The stiff exchange guidewire is directed away from the lesion to be treated in the superficial femoral artery and into a safer branch artery nearby, namely the profunda femoris. (**B**) The sheath is advanced until its tip is in the common femoral artery. (**C**) The exchange guidewire and the dilator are removed and the treatment guidewire is advanced to cross the superficial femoral artery lesion.

arteries, guiding sheaths have advanced significantly and have become an important adjunct in treatment. A guiding sheath is designed for placement in a major branch vessel origin (Fig. 4). Like other sheaths, there is a dilator for use during placement, a sidearm port, and a hemostatic valve. The shape

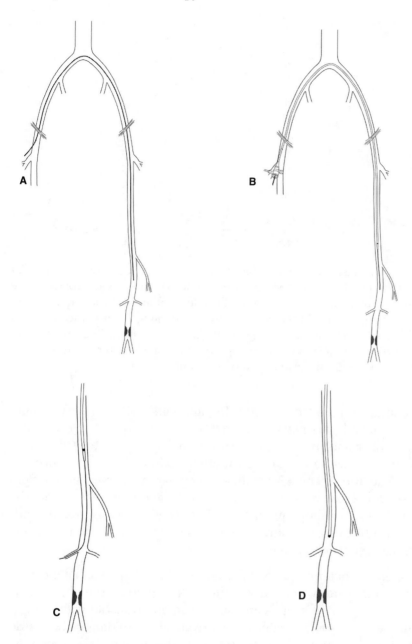

Fig. 3 Place the sheath tip as close to the target lesion as possible. (**A**) When treating infrageniculate lesions, getting the sheath tip in proper position can be challenging. The sheath will not advance near the lesion without adequate guidewire length and yet guidewire length past the lesion is not possible since it would add risk to try to cross the lesions with the stiffer wire. (**B**) The sheath is advanced as far as it will go. (**C**) The guidewire is redirected into a smaller branch or collateral to provide more guidewire length and the sheath is advanced. (**D**) When the exchange guidewire and the dilator are removed, the tip of the sheath is within a few centimeters of the target lesion.

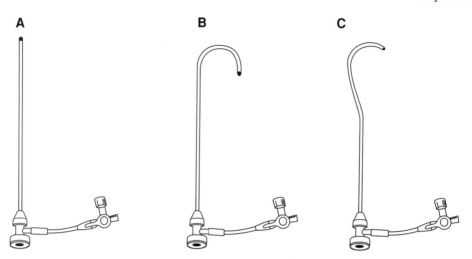

Fig. 4 Guiding sheaths. Guiding sheaths are the future of access for endovascular therapy. The special shapes and sizes have simplified access and provide more reliability. (**A**) A long straight sheath with a flexible shaft and a radiopaque tip can be used for brachiocephalic balloon angioplasty and stenting, such as the Shuttle or the Raabe sheaths (Cook, Inc., Bloomington, Indiana, U.S.A.). (**B**) The up-and-over guiding sheath has a long curve for passage over the aortic bifurcation. (**C**) The Ansel guiding sheath is used for renal artery interventions.

of the tip reflects its intended function. In Figure 4, a long (90 cm), straight sheath with a flexible tip may be used for brachiocephalic arteries. The 40-cm up-and-over sheath with the nearly semicircular curve of the tip is used to go up the iliac artery, over the aortic bifurcation, and down the contralateral iliac artery. The 45-cm sheath with various curved-tip configurations is used for renal artery balloon angioplasty and stent placement. The tip of the sheath has a radiopaque marker. The length of dilator that extends beyond the sheath is usually short to reflect its intended passage into a side branch that may contain a lesion.

The guiding catheter has a specially designed tip shape so that it can be used to enter a renal artery or a carotid artery like a guiding sheath. Guiding catheters offer many more shapes and sizes than are available with guiding sheaths, but there are some significant disadvantages. Guiding catheters do not have a dilator or obturator to facilitate smooth passage. To compensate for this, they are usually introduced through the soft tissue and into the artery through a standard, hemostatic access sheath. This generally means that the arteriotomy is slightly larger than would otherwise be necessary. After passage into the artery, they often require another device, such as a selective catheter, to act as an obturator for passage into the desired side-branch location. There is no end valve for hemostasis. A Tuohy-Borst adaptor must be used to make a guiding catheter hemostatic and to allow it to be flushed.

It is likely that when a broad array of guiding sheaths becomes available, guiding catheters will be used only rarely. Nevertheless, if a certain shape is required to guide passage and it is not available with a guiding sheath, a guiding catheter should be used.

In later chapters on balloon angioplasty and stent placement in various vascular beds, the placement of guiding sheaths is described when indicated. In general, placement of guiding sheaths is performed as follows. Flush aortography is performed. A selective catheter and steerable guidewire are used to cannulate the side branch of interest. The selective guidewire is removed and exchanged for an exchange guidewire. The arterial entry site is dilated and the selective sheath is advanced over the exchange guidewire. After the tip of the sheath is in the side branch, the dilator is removed, arteriography is performed, and therapy is initiated. An up-and-over sheath and a Raabe sheath (Cook, Inc., Bloomington, Indiana, U.S.A.) are good examples of frequently used guiding sheaths. These are useful for contralateral iliac or infrainguinal intervention. They maintain hemostatic access at the femoral artery, promote and maintain guidewire access across the lesion, permit interval arteriography, and enhance the ability to evaluate the runoff bed. The technique of placement of sheath over the aortic bifurcation is described in Figure 5.

TECHNIQUE: HOW TO PLACE AN UP-AND-OVER SHEATH

1. A starting guidewire is placed in the aorta through a retrograde femoral puncture. A hook-shaped catheter, such as an Omni-flush, is placed just above the aortic bifurcation, and a Glidewire is advanced antegrade into the contralateral iliac system. Selective catheterization of the aortic bifurcation is described in detail in chapter 9.
2. After the guidewire is advanced into the femoral artery, the hook-shaped catheter is advanced to the distal external iliac or proximal femoral artery.
3. A stiffer guidewire for exchange is placed, such as a Rosen (180-cm, 0.035-in., atraumatic J tip) or Amplatz super-stiff guidewire is required.
4. The catheter is removed and the entry site is enlarged with arterial dilators. The up-and-over sheath is advanced over the exchange guidewire. The radiopaque tip of the sheath can be followed with fluoroscopy to evaluate progress over the bifurcation. The sidearm of the sheath is oriented opposite the curvature in the sheath tip.
5. The sheath is advanced to its hub if it will go but if significant resistance occurs, the sheath tip can be parked anywhere in the contralateral iliac system.
6. The dilator is removed, and the sheath is aspirated and flushed.

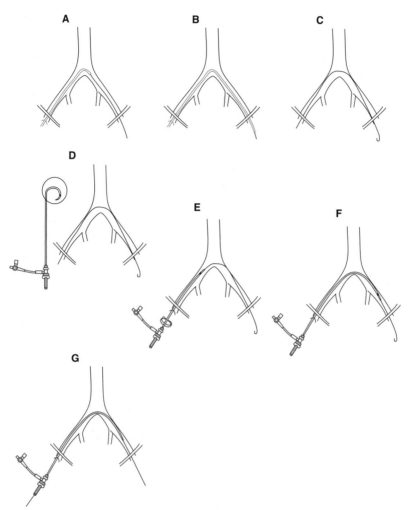

Fig. 5 Placement of up-and-over sheath. (**A**) A guidewire and catheter are passed over the aortic bifurcation (see fig. 10 of chap. 6). (**B**) The catheter is advanced into the contralateral femoral level. (**C**) An exchange guidewire, such as a J-tipped Rosen, is placed and the catheter is removed. (**D**) The arteriotomy is dilated, if this has not already been done. The up-and-over sheath is oriented with the tip directed toward the contralateral side and the sidearm of the sheath is directed toward the ipsilateral side. (**E**) The sheath is advanced over the guidewire. The dilator and the tip of the sheath are observed as they pass over the aortic bifurcation. A slight back-and-forth rotating motion along the shaft of the sheath is sometimes helpful during passage. (**F**) The sheath is advanced to its hub if it will go without significant resistance. If resistance is met, check to see that the guidewire is advanced far enough so that there is plenty of stiff guidewire to support the advancing sheath. The tip of the sheath may be placed anywhere from the mid-iliac to the proximal femoral level to be functional. If the sheath is not advanced to its hub and some length of it is left outside the access site, the extra length must be taken into account when guidewire and catheter length is considered. (**G**) The dilator is removed and the sheath is ready for use.

PLAN OF ATTACK: MANAGING A BRACHIAL ACCESS SITE

1. Consider using ultrasound guidance and a micropuncture needle for entry.
2. Because the brachial artery tends to spasm, consider placing the full-size sheath needed for treatment early in the course of the procedure.
3. Administer systemic heparin early in the case.
4. Monitor pulse at wrist and appearance of hand to have ongoing assessment of upper extremity perfusion distal to the puncture site.
5. Keep hand wrapped or covered to prevent distal vasospasm.
6. Use small doses of nitroglycerine (50–100 μg) into the brachial artery prior to sheath placement for distal vasodilatation.
7. Flush with heparinized saline in between all catheter exchanges.
8. Use dilators when establishing access.
9. A 7-Fr sheath can usually be accommodated with a percutaneous approach.
10. Distance to the arch is 40 to 55 cm and catheter lengths must take that into account.
11. If the subclavian and axillary arteries are redundant, these can be stretched out a bit and the path made smoother, by bringing the hand closer to the patient's side, instead of having it fully abducted.

Sheath Placement in Remote Branch Arteries

Sheath access is possible and can be done safely in any vascular bed in the body. However, for remote branch arteries such as the carotid or tibial arteries, multiple well-planned steps are required to avoid injury. Some of these steps are reviewed in the example in Figure 6 of a carotid access sheath placement. Many of the fundamentals reviewed in earlier chapters of this book come in handy in such an endeavor. Skill at handling guidewires and catheters and ability to do complex selective catheterization is required to get into the carotid artery. Emboli and microbubbles must be avoided with meticulous technique. Knowledge of carotid anatomy and imaging permits the bifurcation to be opened up so that the external carotid artery can be safely accessed. A stiff exchange guidewire is placed in a safe location, based on the operator's clinical sense of what the anatomy can handle, depending on configuration, tortuosity, calcification, and ectopic atherosclerotic disease present along the pathway. The sheath is selected with the reconstruction in mind and placed at the appropriate location to create a platform for a smooth procedure.

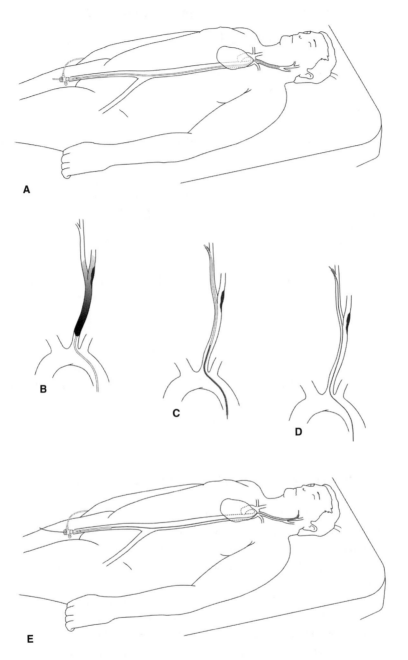

Fig. 6 Placement of a carotid sheath. (**A**) A standard femoral access sheath is placed. A selective catheter is used to catheterize the left common carotid artery. (**B**) The image intensifier is rotated to provide the best view that shows the bifurcation and the external carotid artery is road mapped. (**C**) The steerable guidewire is advanced into the external carotid artery and the selective catheter is advanced over it. The exchange guidewire is placed. (**D**) The catheter is removed leaving the exchange guidewire. (**E**) The sheath is advanced over the exchange guidewire.

Selected Readings

Andros G. Arterial access. In: Moore WS, Ahn SS, eds. Endovascular Surgery. Philadelphia, PA: W. B. Saunders, 2001:37–47.

Lee WA, Brown MP, Nelson PR, et al. Midterm outcomes of femoral arteries after percutaneous endovascular aortic repair using the Preclose technique. J Vasc Surg 2008; 47(5):919–923.

Schneider PA. Balloon angioplasty catheters. In: Moore WS, Ahn SS, eds. Endovascular Surgery. Philadelphia, PA: W. B. Saunders, 2001:55–63.

Silva MB, Haser PB, Coogan SM. Guidewires, catheters and sheaths. In: Moore WS, Ahn SS, eds. Endovascular Surgery Philadelphia, PA: W. B. Saunders, 2001: 48–53.

Wu CJ, Cheng CI, Hung WC, et al. Feasibility and safety of transbrachial approach for patients with severe carotid artery stenosis undergoing stenting. Catheter Cardiovasc Interv 2006; 67(6):967–971.

15

Medications for Endovascular Therapy

Sedation and Analgesia

Using low-osmolality contrast and thorough local anesthesia and performing an expeditious procedure help to limit the depth of sedation and pain relief required. Conscious sedation is required because the patients' cooperation is necessary to control ventilatory and other types of motion. Conscious sedation is usually performed using a combination of a narcotic and a sedative.

Opiate narcotics cause drowsiness and decrease the perception of pain. Fentanyl lasts 30 to 60 minutes and can be titrated with small, incremental intravenous doses. It is more potent than morphine and can be reversed with naloxone.

Midazolam (Versed™) relieves anxiety and causes amnesia. Intravenous midazolam is titrated in small doses of 1 or 2 mg and can be reversed with Romazicon.

Local Anesthetic

Plain lidocaine 1% is an excellent local anesthetic. It lasts up to two hours, which will cover most percutaneous procedures. The maximum dose of lidocaine is 5 to 7 mg/kg. Since 1% lidocaine contains 10 mg/ml, a 70-kg patient can be treated with 35 to 50 ml. Prior to using an access closure device at the conclusion of a case, consider adding more local anesthetic to the access site.

Prophylaxis with Antibiotics

Most strategic arteriography does not require antibiotic administration. However, patients with vascular prostheses in place or who will undergo placement of a stent or other foreign body should be treated with antibiotics. A first-generation cephalosporin such as cephazolin 1g is administered within one hour prior to the procedure. If a patient has ongoing evidence of bacteremia or localized infection, appropriate antibiotic coverage should be initiated prior to entry into the arterial system.

Anticoagulants

Heparin is routinely used in the saline flush solution during all arteriographic and endovascular therapy cases. Systemic heparinization is not usually required for strategic arteriography but is administered during carotid arteriography or when an arteriographic catheter is passed across a critical lesion. Intravenous boluses of heparin, ranging from 50 to 100 U/kg, are often used in conjunction with percutaneous interventions (table 4 in chap. 16). The half-life of heparin is one to one and a half hours and is prolonged in patients with renal or hepatic dysfunction. An activated clotting time (ACT; normal is 150 to 170 seconds) can be used to assess residual heparinization prior to sheath removal. Complex, small vessel endovascular cases, such as carotid or tibial cases, should be managed with an ACT of more than 250 seconds.

Vasodilators

Papaverine is a smooth-muscle relaxant and can be administered as a bolus (15 to 30 mg) or as an infusion at 1 to 3 mg/min. Papaverine is most commonly used to produce extremity vasodilatation in an effort to elicit evidence of the hemodynamic significance of a lesion. Papaverine will precipitate with heparin. Nitroglycerine (20 to 100 µg) is administered to prevent or treat vasospasm that may occur during endovascular therapy. Keep in mind that nitroglycerine administered into the cerebral circulation can cause headache. Vasodilators may also cause hypotension, but this is unusual at the small doses required for administration locally into an arterial segment.

Treatment of Contrast Reactions

Reactions to contrast media vary in severity and include a broad spectrum of potential symptoms. Nausea, vomiting, urticaria, pruritus, bronchospasm, upper respiratory congestion, facial edema, laryngospasm, glottic edema, respiratory distress, hypotension, and cardiac collapse represent some of these.

Four doses of prednisone (20 mg) are prescribed for the 18 hours leading up to the procedure in patients with an earlier history of contrast reaction. When a contrast reaction occurs, administer Benadryl™ (25 to 50 mg intravenous, intramuscular, or per oral), which blocks histamine receptors and treats contrast-induced urticaria. Provide oxygen, give inhaled albuterol treatment, and infuse epinephrine (1 to 3 ml of 1:10,000 IV). Administer fluid and elevate the legs for hypotension due to a vasodilation. Lasix is given to patients in pulmonary edema.

16

Balloon Angioplasty: Minimally Invasive Autologous Revascularization

Balloon Dilatation Causes Dissection

Some of the force exerted by the angioplasty balloon causes compression of the plaque and some causes plaque fracture. The radial force of the angioplasty balloon causes plaque fracture at areas of fixed stenosis, especially where the heterogeneous plaque forms a calcified circumferential ring (Fig. 1). There is often evidence of dissection on completion images immediately following the angioplasty, and the more thorough the investigation, the more that can be found. Contrast fills cracks in the plaque, most of which are longitudinal. Experience with balloon angioplasty before the development of stents indicates that most of these dissections, even dissections with seemingly terrible angiographic results, heal without treatment. The availability of stents has made it possible to treat most dissections safely and quickly. This has prompted the current dilemma. How aggressively should mild-to-moderate postangioplasty dissections be stented? This will gradually be solved in each vascular bed.

About Balloon Catheters

The coaxial balloon angioplasty catheter has two lumens. One lumen fills the balloon and the other lumen is used for placement over a guidewire (Fig. 2). The balloon is not preinflated because after inflation it assumes a higher profile and may be difficult to advance into the lesion. The catheter is irrigated and wiped with heparin–saline solution. Balloon catheters with inflated diameters of 3 to 12 mm may be obtained on 5-Fr shafts and can be placed over 0.035-in. guidewires. Balloon lengths of 2 and 4 cm are most commonly used, but lengths of up to 12 cm are available. Bursting pressure specifications usually range from 8 to 12 atm, but thicker polymer balloons have a bursting pressure of up to 30 atm. Radiopaque markers on the catheter at each end of the balloon are observed by using fluoroscopy to place the balloon in the correct location.

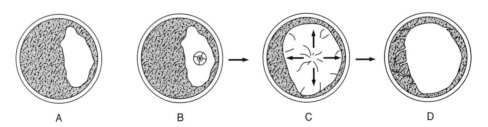

A   B   C   D

Fig. 1 Balloon dilatation causes plaque fracture. (**A**) A cross-sectional view of an atherosclerotic lesion. (**B**) A balloon catheter is placed in the lesion. (**C**) The radial force generated by dilatation is applied to the lesion. (**D**) Plaque fracture causes dissection, which is often observed during completion studies.

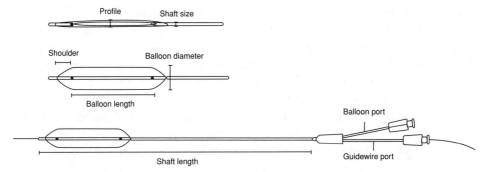

Fig. 2 Balloon angioplasty catheter. The width of the folded balloon over the catheter is the profile. The shaft size depends on the size and type of the balloon. A wide range of balloon diameters is available on a 5-Fr shaft. The shoulder is the distance from the radiopaque marker, where the balloon is filled out to its specified diameter, to the actual end of the balloon. The balloon diameter is the fully inflated diameter of the balloon. The length is the distance between the radiopaque markers. The shaft length provides working distance between the operator and the angioplasty site. The balloon port is used to inflate the balloon, and the guidewire or distal port extends the length of the catheter and is used for passage over the guidewire.

Desirable features for angioplasty balloon material are strength (rupture resistant), low compliance (maintains correct shape at high pressure), and low profile (enhances trackability and crossability). Most angioplasty is currently performed with balloons constructed of polyethylene terephthalate or a similar, low-compliance plastic polymer.

Reinforced high-pressure polymer balloons exert very high pressures (e.g., Blue Max, Boston Scientific Corp., Medi-Tech Division, Natick, Massachusetts, U.S.A. or Dorado, Cook, Inc, Bloomington, Indiana, U.S.A.) and are useful for residual, recurrent, calcified, or intimal hyperplastic lesions. These are mounted on slightly larger shafts of and assume a higher profile due to thicker balloon material. Larger balloons (from 14 to 28 mm inflated diameter) are available for use in endovascular aortic graft placement, large-vessel work, and cardiac valvuloplasty. These are on shafts that range from 5.8 to 7 Fr, and the redundancy of the balloon material requires that substantially larger sheaths be used.

Smaller platform balloons for branch vessel treatment, such as carotid or tibial angioplasty are available on a 3-Fr shaft that travels over a 0.014-in. guidewire. See chapter 6 for a discussion of monorail balloon catheters. The monorail system has several advantages for managing small-vessel angioplasty and stenting.

The Angioplasty Procedure

Percutaneous balloon angioplasty is similar to other surgical procedures. After patient selection and preparation, the next most important factor in success is a stepwise game plan that proceeds methodically, with contingencies available for managing any untoward events that may occur. The general steps include (1) identifying the lesion and confirming that it is a reasonable lesion for endovascular treatment (arteriography), (2) securing percutaneous access (sheath placement), (3) gaining control of the lesion (by passing a guidewire across the lesion), (4) selecting and preparing the balloon catheter, (5) placing the balloon, (6) dilating the lesion, and (7) confirming an acceptable result (completion arteriography). Steps 1 through 3 were covered in earlier chapters. Steps 4 through 7 are detailed in this chapter.

Balloon Selection

Choosing the balloon diameter is more art than science. It is unlikely that immediate trouble will be caused by selecting a balloon with a diameter that is a little too small. Underdilatation in the short term is an extra step, since the smaller-diameter balloon must be exchanged for a larger size to finish the procedure. If underdilatation is not recognized, it may result in a residual lesion that requires treatment at some later date. Conversely, significant overdilatation can cause immediate problems such as rupture or dissection.

Balloon selection was much simpler when cut film arteriography was the standard. The appropriate balloon diameter was selected by actually, physically measuring the diameter of the "normal" artery on the cut film just proximal or distal to the lesion and using that size balloon.

Digital subtraction arteriography is used exclusively in most institutions. In this case, there are two choices for balloon diameter sizing, the eyeball method and digital measurement:

1. After performing arteriography, choose a static image for analysis. (Table 1.) Assess the likely diameter of the "normal" artery proximal or distal to the lesion. Sizing the balloon to a segment of poststenotic dilatation will result in choosing a balloon diameter that is too large.

    Choose a slightly smaller than anticipated balloon diameter and dilate the artery without moving the image intensifier. When the balloon diameter is selected conservatively, the likelihood of significant overdilatation is low. The real-time image of the inflated balloon is juxtaposed to the image of the artery. Another method of doing the same thing is to perform a road map of the artery and inflate the balloon superimposed on the road map and look for the appropriateness of the size match. The operator will have a sense for whether the balloon appears appropriate for that artery (the "eyeball" method). If it appears that the balloon is too small, it may be exchanged for a larger one. If it appears to be appropriate in size, the operator proceeds to evaluate the treated artery for evidence of

Table 1 Balloon Sizing for Angioplasty[a]

Angioplasty site	Balloon diameter (mm)
Abdominal aorta	8–18
Aortic bifurcation[b]	6–10
Common iliac artery	6–10
External iliac artery	6–8
Superficial femoral artery	4–7
Popliteal artery	3–6
Tibial artery	1.5–4
Renal artery	4–7
Subclavian artery	5–8
Dialysis graft	4–6
Infrainguinal graft	2–5

[a] Each arterial segment has a general range of appropriate balloon sizes from which to choose.
[b] When kissing balloons are used at the aortic bifurcation, the diameters of the 2 balloons are additive. Kissing 10-mm balloons should be used only if the distal aorta can tolerate dilatation to 20 mm.

residual stenosis. Steps for assessing the adequacy of angioplasty are detailed later in this chapter.

2. Another option is to perform arteriography with a catheter that has graduated radiopaque centimeter markers and to use this known length to calculate vessel diameter. This method is not without the potential for error. If the catheter is traveling in the anteroposterior plane, the marked centimeter may appear shorter than it really is and cause an overestimation of vessel size. This method is also cumbersome since it requires the use of an extra catheter and the performance of real math. A variation of this method is available in some angio suite cockpits that have the software to estimate vessel diameter using a known standard for comparison, such as a 5-Fr catheter. This also takes enough time that it interrupts the procedure and there are major potential sources of error based upon where the cursor is placed to measure the walls of the catheter.

Most operators who have been doing angioplasty for a while just use the "eyeball" method described earlier. Dissection or rupture can result if the balloon is too large so, when in doubt, start small.

The balloon should be long enough to dilate the lesion and allow a short overhang on either end. Balloon length choices have increased significantly over the past few years. If a balloon is available that can be used to dilate the entire lesion at once, it is faster and probably a little less likely to cause as much dissection as when multiple overlapping inflations with a short balloon are performed. If the balloon used is too short to cover the whole diseased segment, additional inflations are required. Longer balloons have

Table 2 Angioplasty Balloon Catheter Length

Location of balloon angioplasty	Entry site	Length (cm)
Carotid	Femoral	110–130
Subclavian	Femoral	110–120
	Brachial	75
Visceral	Femoral	75–90
Renal	Femoral	75–90
	Brachial	90–110
Aorta	Femoral	65–75
Iliac	Ipsilateral femoral	40–75
	Contralateral femoral	75
Femoropopliteal	Ipsilateral femoral	75
	Contralateral femoral	75–110
Infrapopliteal	Ipsilateral femoral	75–90
	Contralateral femoral	90–150

been developed, especially for lesions of the superficial femoral and tibial arteries. The profile of the unexpanded balloon is important to ease passage through the sheath and across the lesion and should be minimized as much as possible. Other balloon types may be chosen for certain lesions. Reinforced polymer (high-pressure) balloons are used for recalcitrant lesions. Puncture-resistant balloons are used for placement of balloon expandable stents. The shaft length must be adequate to reach the lesion from the entry site. Shaft size should be as small as possible. Most angioplasty is performed with either 3- or 5-Fr balloon catheters. The hemostatic access sheath should be selected in anticipation of the balloon to be used. If a stent is likely to be required to treat the lesion, the operator will choose the sheath with the balloon–stent combination in mind. There is more information about sheaths in chapter 14.

The length of the balloon catheter itself must also be considered. There is more information about this in the individual chapters about intervention in specific vascular beds. Table 2 provides some guidelines. Balloon catheter lengths vary from 40 to 150 cm. A full complement of medium-length balloon catheters (75 or 80 cm) should be maintained in active inventory since these can be used for a wide range of balloon angioplasty procedures. Longer catheters, ranging from 90 to 120 cm, are also useful for angioplasty using remote access.

ANGIO CONSULT: HOW DO I CHOOSE THE RIGHT BALLOON FOR THE JOB?

1. Balloon diameter. Start small. Use guidelines based upon which artery is being dilated (Table 1).
2. Balloon length. Aim to cover the lesion and a little beyond.
3. Balloon type. Choose material based on the type of lesion.

4. Shaft length. Must reach the lesion from the entry site (range from 75 to 150 cm). Table 2 provides guidelines for choosing balloon catheter lengths. Additional information is available in the sections on angioplasty at specific sites.
5. Shaft size. Use as small as possible (usually 3 or 5 Fr).
6. Shoulder length. The length of the shoulder is important if the lesion is near an area that should not be dilated. The shoulder of the balloon is the end that extends beyond the radiopaque marker. If the shoulder extends into an adjacent branch vessel that is not intended for treatment, overdilatation may result.
7. Balloon profile. Lower is better but the profile varies with balloon type and somewhat from one manufacturer to another.

When to Use a Monorail System

Most larger platform devices (0.035 and 0.038-in. compatible) are designed for use in coaxial systems. Smaller platform systems (those designed for use with 0.014-in. guidewires) may be either coaxial or more commonly monorail systems. Some procedures are substantially facilitated by low profile, monorail systems. These include carotid stenting, tibial interventions, and other small artery procedures. The residual lumen of a critical or even pre-occlusive stenosis much more readily accepts a lower-profile guidewire. At the same time, the remote nature of the puncture site from the treatment site makes better control of the guidewire highly desirable and this is available with monorail systems. There are several situations where either a monorail or a coaxial system is satisfactory. These include superficial femoral artery interventions and renal and subclavian stenting. Many operators are using the monorail system with increasing frequency in these vascular beds, especially since a stent can often be placed through the lesion without predilatation when using the smaller platform systems. There are also some situations where the overall strength and profile of the 014 system are not adequate for the procedure, including aortic stent–graft cases.

Supplies For Percutaneous Balloon Angioplasty

Table 3 includes a list of items that should be available to initiate a balloon angioplasty procedure. The "arteriography pack" of basic supplies is included in table 1 of chapter 10. An inventory of disposable endovascular supplies, such as guidewires, catheters, sheaths, angioplasty balloons, and stents, must be maintained and continuously updated. In later chapters that cover intervention in different vascular beds, there is more specific information about which supplies should be available for balloon angioplasty.

Table 3   Supplies for Balloon Angioplasty

Starting guidewire	Balloon angioplasty catheter
Selective guidewire	Inflation device
Exchange guidewire	Balloon-expandable stent
Dilator	Self-expanding stent
Flush catheter	Arteriography pack
Selective catheter	Heparinized saline
Exchange catheter	Contrast
Access sheath	Protective gear (e.g., leaded apron)
Guide sheath	

Sheath Selection and Placement

Sheaths have been introduced and discussed in chapter 14. Sheath access to the arterial system is part of the standard approach to percutaneous balloon angioplasty.

The access sheath maintains control of the access site, provides hemostasis, and functions as a conduit for simple placement of balloon catheters and angiographic catheters. In general, the sheath is selected on the basis of the Fr sizing of its caliber and its length. General-access sheaths are straight and are available with radiopaque tips if desired. Special sheath configurations may be required for some types of angioplasty where a high degree of selectivity is required. These guiding sheaths are discussed in chapter 14.

The size of the sheath is selected to fit the endovascular device. In the case of balloon angioplasty, the sheath must accommodate the balloon after it has been inflated and aspirated and it is time to withdraw it from the patient. See the section in chapter 14, "What Fits Into What?" (table 3 of chap. 14). As a general rule, a 5-Fr sheath will accommodate balloons up to 6 mm. A 6-Fr sheath will permit balloons up to 8 mm to pass, especially if low-profile balloons are used. A 7-Fr sheath will accommodate a balloon up to 10 mm, as long as it is mounted on a 5-Fr shaft. Larger balloons may come on 5-Fr shafts or larger and generally require 8- to 10-Fr sheaths.

If stent placement is anticipated, the sheath size must be increased accordingly. Palmaz stents are placed through 7- or 9-Fr sheaths. Premounted Palmaz-type stents of 7 mm or less may be placed through 6-Fr sheaths. Self-expanding nitinol and other metal stents require 6- to 9-Fr sheaths, depending on the diameter of the stent. Vessel diameters up to 12 mm can be treated with self-expanding stents using 6-Fr sheaths. There is more information about sheath sizing requirements for stent placement in chapter 18.

The standard sheath length of 12 to 15 cm is often adequate for most ipsilateral iliac angioplasty. If the catheter must be guided over a bifurcation or into a specific branch vessel, such as the carotid or renal arteries, a longer sheath from 40 to 90 cm may be selected, often with a special curve to help smooth out the turns that must be negotiated.

The sheath is placed over the guidewire, usually in exchange for whichever angiographic catheter has been used to evaluate the lesion. Pressure is held at the arterial puncture site as the angiographic catheter and/or initial access sheath are removed. Preparation and management of the sheath are detailed in chapter 14. The sheath is advanced into the artery and the dilator is removed. Turn the sheath appropriately so that the sidearm is oriented toward the operator for ease of use. The sheath may be turned back and forth slightly to help make the advancement easier. As the tip of the sheath enters the skin entry site, the sheath is gripped by the operator along its shaft, close to its leading edge. Be sure to watch it so that the dilator does not pop backward. If the lesion is in proximity to the arterial entry site, care should be taken to avoid advancing the sheath across the lesion and unintentionally dottering the intended balloon angioplasty site. The sheath is generally advanced to its hub, unless it is too close to the lesion. The dilator is removed. The sheath is flushed with heparinized saline. Arteriographic projections are obtained prior to endovascular treatment. Placement of an external marker, such as radiopaque marking tape, is performed at this point if desired and a contrast run is performed with the marker in place.

Balloon Preparation and Placement

The balloon catheter is taken from its sterile package. The protective plastic cover that is placed over the balloon for shipping is removed. This is saved on the field so that it can be used to help refold the balloon wings later if the catheter is going to be used again during the same procedure. Balloons of widely varying diameters appear similar in the nondilated state. The operator must ensure that the correct size of balloon is being placed, by checking the size inscribed on the balloon catheter, prior to insertion. The catheter and balloon are wiped with a heparin–saline soaked gauze sponge. The distal or guidewire port is irrigated with heparin–saline. The balloon should not be preinflated; this raises the profile of the balloon and makes the operator look silly. The companies are responsible for quality control and do a remarkable job, in general. The balloon catheter is placed on the guidewire and advanced toward the entry site until guidewire is available to be grasped on the other end of the catheter. Do not insert the balloon catheter unless manual guidewire control has been achieved.

Monorail balloons are prepped by wiping the catheter. There is usually a throwaway metal wire or trocar in the short guidewire port to keep the treatment end of the balloon catheter straight and protected. This is removed. The balloon catheter usually comes with a small-gauge needle that is used

Table 4 Heparin Administration During Percutaneous Balloon
Angioplasty

Procedure	Systemic heparin administration (u/kg)	Other considerations
Brachiocephalic	100	IIb/IIIa inhibitors
Renal	50–75	Nitroglycerin for spasm
Aortoiliac		
Simple	25–50	
Complex	50–75	
Femoropopliteal		
Simple	25–75	
Complex	50–100	
Tibial	75–100	

with a 3-ml syringe to flush air out of the guidewire port. Don't kink the shaft
of the catheter, after that it will be difficult to pass the guidewire through it.
The balloon inflation port is not flushed but is aspirated to remove air and
replace it as much as possible with fluid.

Heparin is administered if indicated by the type of procedure being
performed (Table 4). When heparin administration is required, this should
occur at least three minutes prior to balloon inflation. In general, the more
distally the lesion is located or the more complex the planned reconstruction, the more likely the patient will be to benefit from heparin administration. As with open vascular surgery, there is a high degree of variability
between different vascular specialists as to appropriated heparin indications
and dosages. Table 4 is one operator's method and is intended for use as a
general guideline. Before placing the balloon catheter, confirm appropriate
heparin administration and prepare the inflation device so that angioplasty is
permitted to proceed as soon as the balloon is in place. The balloon catheter
is advanced through the sheath (Fig. 3) The location of the lesion is marked
after arteriography using bony landmarks or an external radiopaque marker
or road mapping. The catheter is advanced using fluoroscopic guidance, and
the radiopaque markers on the balloon are placed across the location of the
lesion. The shoulder of the balloon must not extend into an area where
angioplasty is not desired. The balloon is centered in the lesion so that the
most stenotic segment is dilated by the central portion of the balloon.

Balloon Inflation

Balloons can be inflated with anywhere from 2 to 12 ml of contrast and saline
solution, depending upon the diameter and length of the balloon. The inflation devices usually hold 10 to 15 ml. A 30% to 50% contrast solution allows
the outline of the balloon to be visualized fluoroscopically. Full-strength

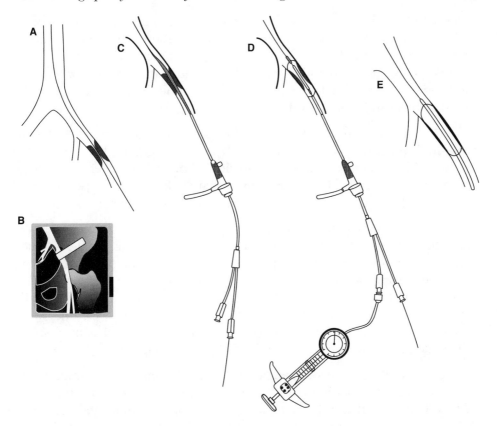

Fig. 3   Balloon angioplasty. (**A**) The guidewire is placed across an iliac artery stenosis. (**B**) The diameter of the balloon is selected based on the diameter of the uninvolved, juxtaposed iliac artery as measured on the cut film arteriogram. (**C**) The balloon catheter is passed over the guidewire, through the hemostatic sheath, and into position across the stenosis. (**D**) The balloon is inflated using an inflation device. Pressure within the angioplasty balloon can be monitored as the waist of atherosclerotic material resolves. (**E**) The lesion is fully dilated and the cylindric shape of the balloon is confirmed using fluoroscopy.

contrast is more viscous and therefore prolongs inflation and deflation. Air should be removed from the inflation device. Sizable air bubbles inside the balloon may make it difficult to tell whether or not the balloon is fully expanded. If the balloon breaks, the patient will receive an intra-arterial bolus of air. Balloon inflation is usually but not always performed with an inflation device. The plunger on the inflation device is compressed until a few atmospheres of pressure register on the pressure gauge. The plunger is locked in compression mode. At this point, the outline of the partially inflated balloon is visible on the fluoroscopic monitor. The inflation is completed by turning the screw handle to gradually increase pressure in the balloon while the fluoroscopic image is monitored for complete balloon dilatation. An inflation device permits pressure within the balloon to be measured during inflation to avoid exceeding the balloon's bursting pressure. Observation of balloon expansion can be compared with the pressure data to gain a better understanding of the lesion. Higher pressures required to dilate recalcitrant lesions can be sustained and monitored with an inflation device. When kissing balloons are required, as with aortic bifurcation lesions, pressure in the two balloons can be equalized.

The balloon may also be inflated by hand. A 10-ml syringe is filled to the 8-ml level and used to expand the balloon directly by hand-generated pressure. This is most effective with smaller balloons. Use a luer lock syringe when dilating by hand. In practice, this is simple, fast, and inexpensive, and it works well for most garden-variety atherosclerotic lesions.

Angioplasty is performed without delay after the balloon is placed, since the presence of the catheter alone in the remaining patent lumen can decrease flow and enhance thrombus formation. Angioplasty is always performed using fluoroscopic guidance. Atherosclerotic narrowing makes itself apparent on the outline of the balloon as it is being inflated under fluoroscopy (i.e., by the atherosclerotic waist). The atherosclerotic waist, which is present at the most stenotic part of the lesion, usually resolves when adequate pressure is applied by the balloon (Fig. 4).

There are many recommendations to guide inflation parameters but almost no data to support them—the amount of pressure to apply, the length of time balloon inflation is maintained, the number of times the balloon is expanded at the same location, and the length of time between inflations. A common approach is to dilate a lesion to a slightly higher pressure than that required for full balloon expansion as observed under fluoroscopy. A slow inflation is thought to decrease the rate of severe dissection. Inflation is maintained for a minimum 60 seconds. The balloon is deflated so that flow resumes, and then reinflated for another 60 seconds. A third inflation to higher pressure is recommended if a waist is still present at the lesion. Additional dilatations may be performed as needed. In practice, however, it is usually acceptable to dilate the lesion with a single-balloon inflation until the waist expands. Longer inflation times at higher pressures are required for intimal hyperplasia, recurrent lesions, residual lesions, and occasionally heavily calcified lesions. Most lesions are fully dilated with less than 8 atm of pressure. Intimal hyperplasia is a notable exception and may require 20 or 30 atm. Resolution of the waist is an important factor in assessing the adequacy of dilatation. If the balloon will not maintain pressure, this may be due to rupture of the balloon. Sometimes contrast can be seen leaking from the balloon on the fluoroscopic image. Aspiration of the balloon may reveal blood in the inflation mixture. Usually, the balloon must be exchanged in this case. Deflate the balloon as well as possible. Remove the balloon under fluoroscopic guidance to be certain that the irregular, torn balloon wings are not caught on the lesion.

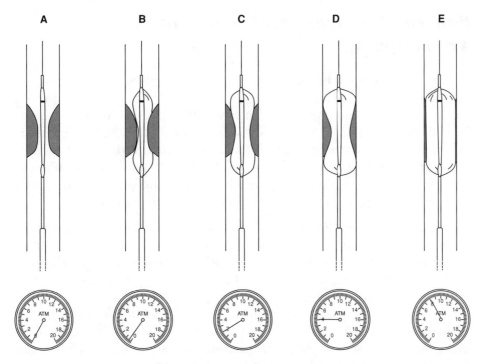

Fig. 4 Dilating the atherosclerotic waist. (**A**) The balloon catheter is placed within the lesion. The radiopaque markers straddle the stenosis. (**B**) The balloon begins to take shape at low pressure. (**C**) At 2 atm of pressure, the waist begins to become evident. A waist of atherosclerotic material represents the area of heaviest plaque formation and is usually the last area to be fully dilated. (**D**) At 4 atm of pressure exerted by the balloon, a substantial residual, unresolved stenosis is apparent. (**E**) When the pressure is doubled to 8 atm, the waist of atherosclerosis has been completely dilated.

The small caliber, lower profile, monorail system balloons are often compliant in order to adjust to small changes in the sizes of smaller arteries. In this case, the higher the administered pressure, the larger the resulting balloon diameter. Each compliant balloon comes with a specification sheet that correlates the number of atmospheres with the diameter of the balloon when inflated.

A common finding in the awake patient is a complaint of pain at the angioplasty site during balloon inflation. This generally is a sign that balloon pressure has reached its reasonable maximum. The pain should resolve when the balloon is deflated. Continued pain maybe a sign of dissection or rupture and should be evaluated with immediate repeat angiography.

After angioplasty, the balloon is completely deflated. The balloon port is aspirated vigorously using an empty 20-ml syringe. The balloon is not moved until it is visualized using fluoroscopy to ensure complete deflation.

Balloon Removal and Completion Arteriography

Withdraw the balloon but keep the guidewire in place. Occasionally, the balloon material catches on some irregular or sharp part of the dilated lesion, usually when there is significant calcification. If the balloon is caught, deflate the balloon again with constant negative pressure. Rotate the balloon on the guidewire. Advance the catheter a centimeter and then withdraw. Remember to hold the sheath so that it does not pull out when the balloon catheter is removed. When the balloon wings reach the tip of the sheath, there is some resistance as the redundant material is forced into the sheath.

There are several methods of assessing the results of balloon angioplasty (Table 5). Some combination of these methods is usually performed. Completion arteriography is the most widely applicable method. The quality of completion arteriography may be improved by magnified views of the angioplasty site, oblique views, and a qualitative assessment of contrast flow through the angioplasty site during digital subtraction arteriography. In general, a residual stenosis of less than 30% is acceptable, even if the angioplasty site has a somewhat irregular surface. Although completion arteriography is the most widely used and readily accessible method of assessing the results of balloon angioplasty, after the dissection planes are raised by angioplasty the degree of stenosis may be very difficult to assess. Pressure may be measured proximally and distally to the lesion. This is relatively simple to do by measuring pressure through an angiographic catheter placed over the guidewire that crosses the angioplasty site and measuring through the sidearm of the sheath that is on the other side of the angioplasty site. Any gradient following angioplasty is probably significant since it takes more than a 30% stenosis to cause a gradient. Remember that when outflow occlusion is present, the pressure will tend to equalize proximally and distally to

Table 5 How Do You Assess the Results of a Balloon Angioplasty?[a]

Method	Comment
Completion arteriogram	Performed in all cases; usually the only method required
Magnified view	Enhanced detail at angioplasty site
Oblique projection	Assesses residual stenosis or dissection flap
Measure pressure	Quantitative hemodynamic assessment
Intravascular ultrasound	Useful for evaluating residual stenosis. Adds cost to the case

Clinical evaluation
  Hemodynamic stability
  Pulse/color of extremity
  Flank pain
	Helpful in identifying complications

[a] Modified from Schneider, 2001, p. 61.

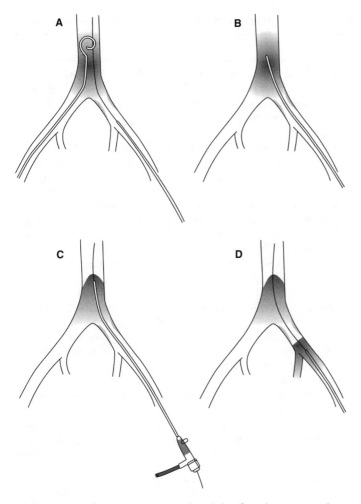

Fig. 5 Completion arteriography. (**A**) After iliac angioplasty, the balloon catheter is withdrawn from the angioplasty site. Completion arteriography can be performed through a proximal catheter placed in the aorta through the contralateral femoral artery. This is a reasonable approach if an arteriographic catheter had been originally placed to perform strategic aortography prior to the angioplasty procedure. (**B**) The balloon catheter can be removed completely and exchanged for an arteriographic catheter. Intraluminal position across the angioplasty site is maintained by the catheter itself. (**C**) If a long sheath has been used for the procedure, it may be most expedient to insert the dilator and advance the sheath through the lesion. Contrast administration through the sidearm of the sheath permits completion arteriography. (**D**) Retrograde arteriography can also be performed if the contrast can be delivered through a large-bore device such as a sheath. Power injection into a fresh angioplasty site should be avoided.

Table 6 Options for Completion Arteriography After Endovascular Intervention

General options	Technique
Proximal flush catheter	Place flush catheter over guidewire used for balloon angioplasty. Place catheter head proximal to balloon angioplasty site and administer contrast. Use flush catheter to maintain control at intervention site. This technique is most common in aortoiliac intervention.
Access sheath	Maintain guidewire control with original guidewire. Administer contrast through sidearm of access sheath. Tip of sheath must be proximal to lesion (e.g., in SFA balloon angioplasty) or just distal to the lesion (e.g., retrograde femoral approach to iliac lesion).
Straight catheter	Place multi-side-hole straight catheter through the lesion and remove the guidewire. The straight catheter may extend slightly beyond the lesion and is used to maintain control of the lesion. Contrast fills the angioplasty site by passing through the side holes on the catheter. This technique is useful for side branch balloon angioplasty, which is done without a guiding sheath (e.g., renal, subclavian).
Separate catheter	Administer contrast through a separately placed catheter. When arteriography is performed through one puncture site and intervention performed through an alternate site, the original access site can be used for the completion arteriogram. An example of this is a transfemoral arch aortogram, followed by transbrachial, retrograde subclavian intervention. The completion arteriogram is performed through a transfemoral catheter.
Guiding sheath	Long access sheaths with shaped tips are used for branch vessel balloon angioplasty (e.g., carotid, renal). After angioplasty, contrast is administered through the sheath and directly into the vessel origin.

the lesion or the angioplasty site. Intravascular ultrasound may also be used in this setting and is probably most accurate for assessing the precise degree of stenosis after angioplasty.

Figure 5 gives methods for performing completion arteriography after aortoiliac angioplasty. If the sheath tip is in proximity to the treatment site, contrast can usually be administered through the sheath and illuminate the results of balloon angioplasty. Completion arteriography may also be performed using a catheter placed through the sheath and over the access guidewire after the balloon catheter is removed. If a previous contralateral puncture has been performed, a separate catheter may be placed through this access site to obtain a completion study. Sometimes completion arteriography is performed simply by injecting contrast through the sidearm of the sheath with the tip either proximal or slightly distal to the angioplasty site. High-pressure contrast injection should not be performed directly into the fresh angioplasty site because it may extend a local dissection plane caused by the balloon injury. General options and techniques for completion arteriography at various sites are presented in Table 6. Further examples of completion arteriography are provided in the chapters on angioplasty in different vascular beds.

The guidewire is maintained in its position across the lesion until the completion arteriogram has been deemed satisfactory. If for some reason the guidewire is no longer across the lesion and more endovascular intervention is required, the lesion is recrossed with a J-tip guidewire to avoid entering a newly created dissection plane.

A balloon can be reused during the same angioplasty procedure. The balloon arrives in the package with a funnel-shaped plastic cover that protects the balloon during shipping. With a firm negative-pressure aspiration on the balloon port, the balloon material can be folded and reshaped by hand and advanced into the funnel to lower its profile for repeat use.

Selected Readings

Bosiers M, Deloose K, Verbist J, et al. Present and future of endovascular SFA treatment: Stents, stent-grafts, drug coated balloons and drug coated stents. J Cardiovasc Surg (Torino) 2008; 49(2):159–165.

Dick P, Sabeti S, Mlekusch W, et al. Conventional balloon angioplasty versus peripheral cutting balloon angioplasty for treatment of femoropopliteal artery in-stent restenosis: Initial experience. Radiology 2008; 248(1):297–302.

Schneider PA. Balloon angioplasty catheters. In: Moore WS, Ahn SS, eds. Endovascular Surgery. Philadelphia, PA: W. B. Saunders, 2001:55–63.

Schneider PA, Rutherford RB. Endovascular interventions in the management of chronic lower extremity ischemia. In: Rutherford RB, ed. Vascular Surgery. Philadelphia, PA: W. B. Saunders, 2000:1035–1069.

Werk M, Langner S, Reinkensmeier B, et al. Inhibition of restenosis in femoropopliteal arteries: Paclitaxel-coated versus uncoated balloon: Femoral paclitaxel randomized pilot trial. Circulation 2008; 118(13):1358–1365.

17

More About Balloon Angioplasty: Keeping Out of Trouble

Keeping Out of Trouble Is Simpler Than Getting Out of Trouble

There are numerous ways to get into trouble during the course of a balloon angioplasty procedure. Appropriate patient selection and lesion selection remain the two most important factors in preventing problems. However, premature loss of guidewire access, overdilatation of a lesion, thrombus generation caused by inadequate flushing or lengthy catheter times, and many other avoidable problems may occur. The best way to ensure success is to treat endovascular operations with the same selectivity, preparation, and methodical approach that is required for open operations. Balloon angioplasty may also help prevent or manage problems. It serves as a valuable adjunct to mechanical and laser atherectomy and also in the use of stents.

What's the Strategy for Managing Multiple Lesions?

When contemplating angioplasty for multiple sequential lesions, it is important to remember that the long-term success rate of the procedure decreases with each additional angioplasty site. This is especially true when there are several lesions in a series in the same conduit, such as a single iliac artery or superficial femoral artery.

When multiple sequential lesions require dilatation, angioplasty usually proceeds from proximal to distal, even if the proximal lesion is less stenotic (Fig. 1). Dilatation of a distal critical lesion is most likely to remain uncomplicated if there is adequate inflow to the area when the balloon is deflated. It is usually safest to dilate each lesion separately and to avoid angioplasty where it is not required between lesions.

Sequential ipsilateral lesions that occur in different arteries (e.g., the ipsilateral iliac artery and superficial femoral artery) are managed with angioplasty of the inflow artery first. Success rates after dilatation of the proximal (larger) artery are superior to that of the distal artery in most settings. The best approach is to assess the results of iliac angioplasty first and proceed with further angioplasty after the proximal lesion has been adequately treated.

When multiple sequential significant stenoses occur in the same conduit artery (e.g., the superficial femoral artery) without any significant branches between the stenoses, all the lesions should undergo angioplasty if any dilatation is performed. Angioplasty of only some of the lesions changes the anatomy but yields no hemodynamic improvement, and the lone angioplasty site(s) may thrombose because of continued low flow after dilatation. One possible exception to this is when a critical lesion is located in the middle

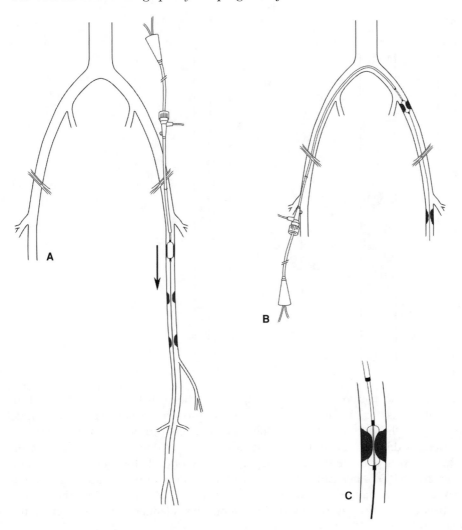

Fig. 1 Strategy for angioplasty of multiple lesions. The approach to angioplasty of multiple lesions is from proximal to distal, regardless of which lesion is most stenotic. (**A**) When multiple lesions are in the same conduit artery, and any requires dilatation, all the lesions are treated. (**B**) When sequential lesions are in different arteries, the proximal lesion is dilated first. (**C**) When a diffusely diseased artery requires treatment, consider dilating only the critical areas of stenosis.

of an arterial segment that is diffusely diseased but that is composed of only mild stenoses (Fig. 1). In this case, it may be better to dilate the single critical area only and then assess the results. The guidewire should be placed across the entire arterial segment in case extensive dissection occurs. An exception to the proximal to distal approach is when a distal lesion is so tight that the balloon is placed in that one first, since the balloon has the lowest profile prior to its first inflation. In other words, once the balloon is inflated to treat

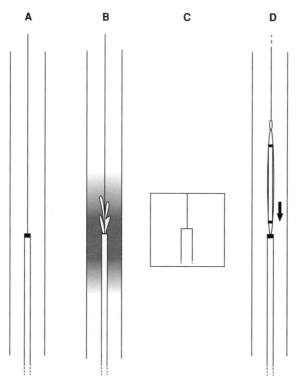

Fig. 2 How do you know where the tip of the sheath is located? Losing track of the sheath tip is a common mistake that leads to problems. (**A**) Use of a radiopaque sheath tip is the best way to keep track of the sheath location. (**B**) Contrast can be placed within the sheath to make it easier to see. Contrast puffed from the tip of the sheath is also useful. (**C**) A magnified view often helps identify the outline of the sheath. (**D**) After balloon angioplasty, the balloon on the end of the angio-plasty catheter usually is met with some resistance as it is pulled into the sheath. The balloon location as observed fluoroscopically identifies the location of the sheath tip.

another lesion, the profile of the balloon may be such that it will not cross the very tight lesion after that.

Complications are avoided if lesions dilated on the basis of clinical problem solving rather than the appearance of the lesions.

TECHNIQUE: KEEPING TRACK OF THE TIP OF THE SHEATH

During the angioplasty procedure, a common concern is keeping track of the location of the tip of the sheath (Fig. 2). Placement of the sheath too far within the artery may unintentionally dotter the lesion. Balloon inflation within the sheath tip may damage the sheath tip causing it to require exchange and risking damage to the artery when it is removed. The location of the sheath tip should be confirmed prior to inflation.

1. When working room between the sheath tip and the lesion is minimal, the sheath must occasionally be withdrawn partially to make way for the inflated balloon.
2. Many different types of sheaths are currently available with a radiopaque marker in the tip. This adds a little cost, but also simplifies the procedure and makes it more efficient. Some operators use these routinely.
3. A magnified view of the area of the sheath may also detect the end of the sheath along the guidewire where the profile of the guidewire changes.
4. Filling the sheath with contrast through its sidearm may also be helpful.
5. If the balloon catheter fits snugly within the sheath, the operator can usually sense when the balloon portion of the catheter is passing through the tip of the sheath because of the change in the friction applied to the catheter at this point. This location can be identified using fluoroscopy.

Which Lesions Should be Predilated?

When balloon angioplasty was performed in the past using cut film as a guide without the availability of stents, predilatation was only rarely required. There was not much benefit to this extra step: film development between steps took longer and balloon sizing based upon cut film was a little more life sized. The conversion of imaging to digital angiography has provided nearly immediate feedback on the results of angioplasty but has also introduced some additional uncertainty as to the optimal diameter of angioplasty at a given site. In addition, the ready availability but high cost of stents has created a situation where dilating first, assessing the results, then placing a stent or performing further dilatation is common practice. If a preocclusive stenosis cannot be crossed with an appropriately sized balloon because of the high profile of the catheter, a lower-profile balloon is required to pass through a residual lumen. The balloon catheter should not be kept in the lumen for longer than necessary since the potential for thrombosis at the angioplasty site is high. If a stent is required, but the minimal remaining lumen prevents passage of the appropriate sheath or stent delivery catheter, predilatation is required. It is sometimes useful to perform predilatation of heavily calcified but critically stenotic arteries to assess how the lesion will respond to angioplasty. When the correct balloon size is not clear based on arteriography, predilatation with a smaller balloon is reasonable to assess more accurately the correct sizing of the artery diameter.

Which Lesions are Most Likely to Embolize?

Embolization of clinical importance is not common after angioplasty but can be devastating. The incidence of embolization is minimized with appropriate anticoagulation, cautious passage of endovascular devices, and minimal manipulation of the lesion prior to definitive therapy. Some lesions pose a higher risk of embolization, including those that present with embolization, occlusions, lesions that are highly irregular or ulcerated, lesions that have fresh thrombus associated with them, lesions that are aneurysmal, and complex lesions located in the infrarenal abdominal aorta or the innominate artery. If the risk of embolization is high and endovascular treatment of the lesion is most appropriate, open arterial access and distal control of the outflow vessels should be considered. Another option more recently available is the potential of using a distal protection device. Primary stent placement or even placement of a covered stent may also be considered. Use very complete systemic anticoagulation when treating a potentially embologenic lesion. Also, the outflow bed may be evaluated angiographically prior to removing the guidewire and sheath. If the lower extremities are the outflow bed, simple clinical evaluation may be useful.

Which Lesions are Most Likely to Dissect?

Balloon angioplasty causes dissection. Thorough arteriographic inspection of a balloon angioplasty site usually reveals some evidence of dissection. Intravascular ultrasound will identify it more readily. Significant dissections may occur after balloon angioplasty of any artery. However, dissections tend to occur at branch points, in juxtaposition to very bulky or circumferential plaques, and in arteries with diffuse longitudinal plaque formation without natural cleavage planes, especially if the plaque is heavily calcified. The external iliac artery, especially near its origin, and the superficial femoral artery, especially at its origin and in the adductor canal, tend to dissect (Fig. 3). The aortic bifurcation, the common carotid artery, and the subclavian artery also share this propensity for dissection, although primary stent placement during treatment of these arteries is more common. Dissection may also occur as a result of inadvertent overdilatation of any artery.

Although dissection has been one of the feared complications of angioplasty in the past, the development of intravascular stents has made it possible to successfully treat postangioplasty dissection when it is recognized on the angiographic table. Nevertheless, it adds cost and needless excitement

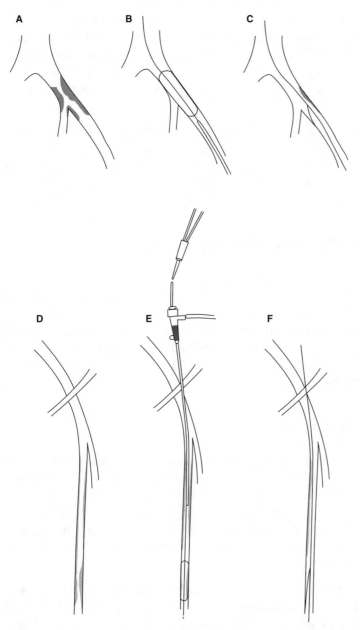

Fig. 3 Arterial dissection after balloon angioplasty. (**A**) A common iliac artery lesion extends into the proximal external iliac artery. (**B**) Balloon dilatation is performed across the iliac bifurcation. The balloon may be oversized for the proximal external iliac artery, especially if the location of the bifurcation is not completely clear or if the size differential between the common and external iliac arteries is not appreciated. A contralateral anterior oblique projection should be used for angioplasty of this segment. (**C**) A proximal external iliac artery flap is raised and it dissects distally. (**D**) A superficial femoral artery stenosis is identified in the adductor canal. (**E**) Balloon angioplasty is performed through an ipsilateral antegrade femoral artery approach. (**F**) A significant dissection occurs at the angioplasty site.

and, if dissection is not recognized or occurs at a later interval, it may cause acute failure of the procedure. Another benefit of stent availability is that a broader array of complex lesions may be considered for angioplasty, since a treatment option is available if the lesion is not adequately treated or is even worse after balloon angioplasty alone. This is discussed in greater detail in the next chapter.

A dissection may be recognized after balloon angioplasty by the appearance of parallel, wavy lines in the flow stream. These are elevated sheets of plaque. Contrast that remains trapped in the wall after the main bolus of contrast has passed is a sign of severe dissection. Flow in the artery may stop if the flap is pressed up against and opposing wall by oncoming inflow.

Pain During Balloon Angioplasty

Discomfort is common at the angioplasty site during balloon inflation. This usually indicates stretching of the adventitia. When pain occurs, do not push the pressure in the balloon higher. Deflation of the balloon should be followed by an immediate resolution of discomfort. If pain continues, it could represent rupture or dissection. These possibilities should be immediately ruled out with a completion arteriogram. The management of arterial rupture is discussed later in this chapter.

What About Spasm?

Spasm is not a frequent clinical problem. However, a small minority of patients seems to be prone to spasm. Patients with atherosclerosis are less likely to develop spasm since arterial wall thickening and plaque formation tend to prevent it. Younger patients with nonatherosclerotic conditions are more likely to develop spasm. When one considers how often and aggressively endoluminal arterial manipulation is performed, it is amazing that spasm does not occur more often.

Spasm is not much of a clinical issue at the balloon angioplasty site. More commonly, it may be considered as a possibility in the outflow bed for an angioplasty site or in a neighboring segment of the same artery being treated. If the operator is unable to visualize the end artery or outflow vessels, it may be poor technique, low flow, thrombosis, embolization, dissection, or spasm. Be sure that an adequate bolus of contrast was delivered and that the concentration was appropriate. Check to see if there are reasons for a low-flow state. The usual setting where this comes up is in the course of an endovascular intervention when an area of the outflow can no longer be visualized or appears substantially different than the preintervention arteriogram. When this occurs immediately after balloon angioplasty and it involves the angioplasty site, it is probably dissection. Usually there is some evidence of trapped contrast in the few centimeters distal to the angio-plasty site. If this occurs immediately after balloon angioplasty and involves a distant outflow bed, it is probably embolization and/or thrombus, espe-cially if the angioplasty site looks technically well treated but flow remains slow. Spasm may be initiated by endovascular manipulation, even by just a guidewire, ischemia, or contrast administration. The arteries most prone to spasm include the distal internal carotid, axillary, renal, and tibial arteries. Balloon angioplasty in these vascular beds often includes administration of a vasodilator, such as nitroglycerine. If spasm occurs, leave a guidewire across, but take off everything else you can, such as sheaths and catheters. Adminis-ter additional heparin intravenously and nitroglycerine into the treated artery.

PLAN OF ATTACK: OPTIONS FOR TREATING RESIDUAL STENOSIS AFTER BALLOON ANGIOPLASTY

Some residual stenoses do not require treatment. The degree of residual stenosis that may be acceptable is dictated by the clinical situation (Fig. 4). For example, a mild-to-moderate residual iliac artery stenosis may be acceptable after angioplasty of a critical lesion in a patient with rest pain and high surgical risk but not in a patient who also needs a femoral–tibial bypass for extensive pedal gangrene.

1. If the significance of a mild-to-moderate residual stenosis is not clear, measure pressure across the lesion. Proceed with other steps listed in table 5 in chapter 16 on assessing the results of balloon angioplasty.
2. If the atherosclerotic waist fails to resolve, repeat dilatation (up to several times) with the same-diameter balloon but to a higher pressure and with a longer expansion time.
3. If the initial balloon choice is unable to withstand higher pressures and it ruptures, use a high-pressure polymer balloon.
4. Place a stent and perform poststent placement balloon angioplasty, especially if the residual stenosis exceeds 30%. Stent placement is now fast, reliable, and durable and it may be more efficacious to proceed to stent placement early, rather than struggle with a difficult residual stenosis and risk arterial rupture from overdilatation (see chap. 18).

Preventing Puncture Site Thrombosis

Thrombosis at the access site is rare after arteriography since catheters are small in caliber and the indwelling times are short. However, this prob-lem is more common after endovascular therapy than after arteriography. When endovascular manipulation proceeds from strategic to therapeutic,

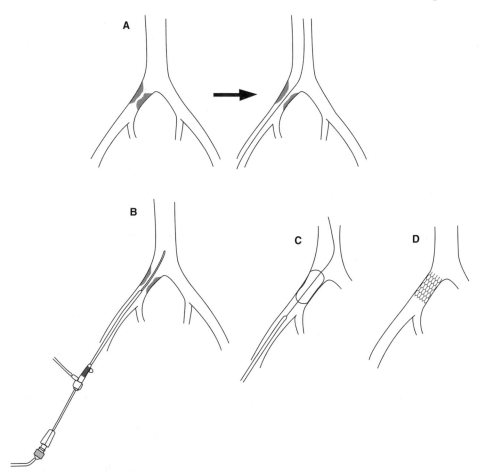

Fig. 4 Management of residual stenosis after angioplasty. (**A**) A residual common iliac artery stenosis remains after balloon angioplasty. (**B**) If the significance of the lesion is not clear, arterial pressure is measured proximally and distally to the lesion. The distal pressure is measured either through the straight catheter pulled down through the lesion or through the sidearm of the hemostatic sheath. (**C**) Repeat dilatation is performed to a higher pressure using longer expansion times. (**D**) A stent is placed at the site to treat the residual lesion.

the devices become larger, the length of time they are in the artery is longer, blood flow through the artery at the puncture site area may be altered by upstream endovascular intervention, and postprocedure hemostasis is more difficult after use of larger caliber sheaths. Avoiding puncture site thrombosis of the access artery during the angioplasty procedure relies upon skills learned in planning arterial access and in strategy for performing interventions (Table 1). Keep in mind how the sheath itself may alter flow. For example, if the puncture site is near a lesion, the presence of the sheath within a moderate lesion may cause a significant alteration in flow. If outflow is poor and inflow is improved and the puncture site is in between the two, hemostasis will be more challenging.

Table 1 Preventing Puncture Site Thrombosis After Endovascular Intervention

---

Palpate anatomy prior to puncture
Duplex scan the artery if uncertain
Do not puncture an aneurysm
Do not puncture a heavily calcified or critically stenotic artery
Do not puncture the femoral bifurcation
Use small-caliber catheters and sheaths whenever possible
Do not upsize the catheter or sheath if there is a critical lesion very near the puncture
When pressure is held, do not stop flow through the artery
Hold pressure carefully between all catheter or sheath exchanges to prevent the
    accumulation of blood under the skin around the puncture site
Treat the arterial access site gently; use dilators when the artery is diseased

---

Feel the artery. If it feels calcified or aneurysmal, perform a duplex evaluation. Access through a heavily calcified or critically stenotic common femoral artery is not advised. Do not puncture an aneurysm. Careful attention to anatomy and landmarks will assist the operator in avoiding a low puncture at the femoral bifurcation.

Access that is adequate for arteriography may not be satisfactory for endovascular therapy. If arteriography shows a critical lesion just distal to the location where the catheter goes into the artery, do not enlarge the arteriotomy with a sheath. Obtaining hemostasis later will be difficult without stopping flow altogether and risking thrombosis. Consider performing balloon angioplasty through an alternate access site.

After obtaining access, use the smallest-caliber catheters and sheaths that are adequate for the job. Arteriography can often be accomplished with 4-Fr catheters. Balloon angioplasty may be performed up to a diameter of 8 mm with a sheath of 6 Fr or smaller. Angioplasty of larger arteries or placement of stents usually requires 7- to 9-Fr sheaths. Upsizing of sheaths is done after consideration since it also increases the risk of puncture site problems.

After sheath removal, when manual pressure is held to achieve hemostasis, flow through the access artery should be permitted to continue so that platelets deposit at the puncture site. If pressure is held too aggressively and flow is stopped, a puncture site thrombosis is more likely to occur. When closure devices are used, obtain a femoral arteriogram first and follow the instructions for use for each specific device since they all have limitations.

Balloon Angioplasty Troubleshooting

Assessment of working room or distance between the arterial access site and the balloon angioplasty site is performed on every case. Long distances require that appropriate length guidewires and catheters are available (tables 2 and 3 in chap. 5). This is also discussed in greater detail in later chapters about angioplasty in specific arterial beds. Occasionally, working room is inadequate. Adequate working room requires that a standard 12-cm access sheath be able to fit between the puncture site and the lesion. If the tip of the sheath extends to the lesion, working room will not be satisfactory to pass catheters and perform interventions. Options include a percutaneous approach at an alternative location, an arterial cutdown at another location if percutaneous access is not possible, or proceeding with the same access site with the sheath partially withdrawn and well secured (Fig. 5).

Balloon rupture within the specified inflation pressure is possible when an attempt is made to dilate a sharp or heavily calcified lesion (Fig. 6). Occasionally, even after balloon rupture, a partial or complete dilatation of the lesion can be accomplished by exerting high pressure on the balloon. This allows the balloon to fill to the extent possible by overwhelming the leak. Usually, however, it is necessary to switch to a thicker and more puncture-resistant polymer balloon. The shoulder portion of the balloon often successfully dilates this type of lesion without rupture. The balloon is advanced in small increments and several inflations are required to dilate the entire lesion with the shoulder of the balloon. If the balloon ruptures again, placing a stent and dilating the lesion through the stent should be considered.

Occasionally, the nearly fully expanded balloon herniates past the resistant lesion, either proximally or distally, during an attempt to dilate (Fig. 7). This occurs more commonly during dilatation of intimal hyperplasia. Balloon herniation is observed using fluoroscopy. The balloon seems to pop out of the lesion just before it reaches its full, rounded profile. To minimize the likelihood of herniation, place the center of the balloon just beyond the center of the lesion, partially inflate the balloon to secure it, and then hold traction on the catheter shaft as inflation is completed. The balloon is held in place even though it tries to pop forward. Another option to prevent herniation is to use a longer balloon.

Dilating a lesion that is located adjacent to a large ulcer or an aneurysmal segment may be contraindicated by the increase in risk of embolization or rupture. If angioplasty is required in this setting, consider covering the entire segment with a stent or a covered stent. Open access for outflow control may also be a reasonable adjunct to prevent distal embolization.

Dilatation with a large (more than 10 mm) or compliant balloon is sometimes followed by an inability to empty contrast from the balloon in a timely manner because of an air lock. The balloon port should be aspirated with a large empty syringe (20 ml or larger) for a few seconds and the catheter and hub flicked with the finger to disrupt and mobilize any air bubbles. If the air lock remains, constant, high negative pressure is applied by withdrawing the plunger on the syringe and locking it in place with the plunger fully withdrawn and the syringe forming a vacuum. If negative pressure must be maintained during balloon catheter removal, a two-way stopcock may be

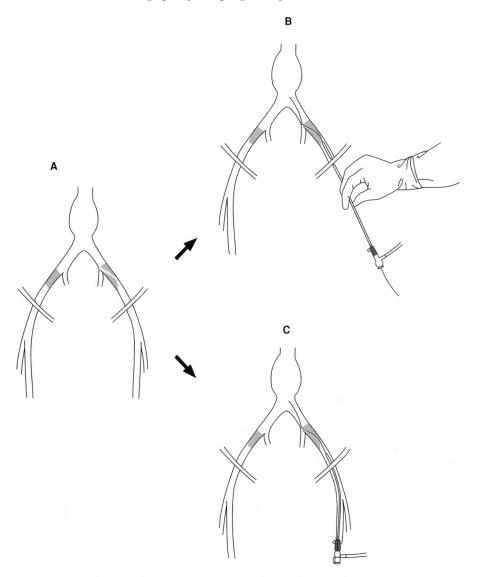

Fig. 5 Options for when working room is inadequate. (**A**) In this example, working room between femoral access sites and the iliac lesions is inadequate. A proximal, transbrachial approach is an option but is suboptimal because it must be performed across an aortic aneurysm. (**B**) Another option is to proceed with femoral access but to have the sheath only a few centimeters into the artery. If that option is chosen, the sheath must be secured so that it does not pop out at an inopportune time. One way to do this is to have an assistant to secure the sheath. (**C**) Another option is to create more working room by placing the sheath in the proximal superficial femoral artery, either percutaneously or through a cutdown.

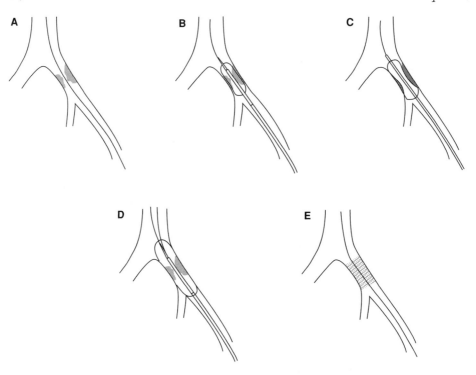

Fig. 6 Management when balloon ruptures on a calcified plaque. **(A)** A guidewire is placed across a common iliac artery stenosis. **(B)** The appropriately sized balloon is advanced into position but ruptures during inflation. Using fluoroscopy, contrast is seen extravasating from the balloon. Aspiration of the balloon port of the angioplasty catheter reveals bloody return fluid. **(C)** A more puncture-resistant, polymer balloon is used to dilate the lesion, which may require a larger sheath to accommodate the shaft size. **(D)** The lesion can also be dilated incrementally using the shoulder of the balloon, avoiding the sharpest part of the lesion until last. **(E)** A stent can also be placed to dilate the calcified lesion. Occasionally, a sharp lesion perforates the balloon through the struts during placement of a balloon-expandable stent.

placed on the syringe and closed with the syringe on full aspiration so that there is constant negative pressure (Fig. 8). These maneuvers maintain a vacuum by preventing the plunger from sliding back into the body of the syringe.

TECHNIQUE: SOLVING ANGIOPLASTY PROBLEMS

1. Balloon catheter won't track along the guidewire. Exchange for a stiffer guidewire and/or insert a long sheath (see fig. 4 in chap. 7).
2. Balloon won't advance through lesion. Determine that the guidewire is intraluminal, predilate by placing a 5- or 6-Fr catheter or dilate with a low-profile (smaller-diameter) balloon. Do not force.

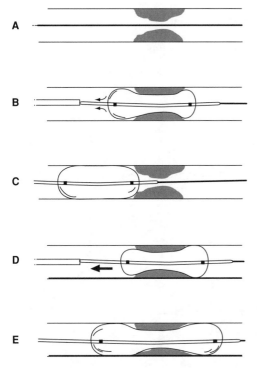

Fig. 7 Management when balloon herniates past the lesion during inflation. (**A**) A guidewire is passed through a stenosis. (**B**) As the balloon takes its shape, it begins to migrate out of the lesion. (**C**) The expanded balloon pops out of the angioplasty site. (**D**) The balloon catheter is deflated and advanced so that one radiopaque marker is well beyond the lesion. The balloon is reinflated while traction is applied to the catheter. As the balloon attempts to pop out of the lesion, it is held in place with manual traction. (**E**) The catheter can also be exchanged for a catheter with a longer balloon.

3. Balloon is unable to dilate residual atherosclerotic waist. Follow plan of attack outlined for residual stenosis after angioplasty (Fig. 4).
4. Balloon ruptures on calcified lesion. Use a thicker polymer balloon, dilate calcified portion with the shoulder of the balloon, or place stent and dilate (Fig. 6).
5. Balloon herniates past lesion during inflation. Apply traction to the catheter during inflation or use a longer balloon (Fig. 7).
6. Balloon won't empty after inflation (air lock). Apply continuous negative pressure with a large (20 ml or larger) syringe (Fig. 8).
7. Balloon can't be withdrawn into sheath. Rotate to fold wings and aspirate while applying steady traction.

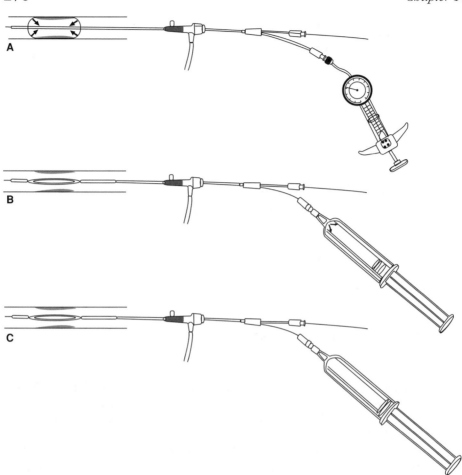

Fig. 8 Management when balloon will not empty or empties slowly. (**A**) Aspiration of a large balloon may produce minimal emptying. (**B**) A big, empty syringe generates more negative pressure. It is used to aspirate the balloon. (**C**) Continuous aspiration can be achieved by drawing the plunger back to the rubber seal of the syringe and locking it in place.

Management of Arterial Rupture

Acute, sharp, or unremitting pain may indicate arterial rupture, and an immediate arteriogram should be performed. If arterial rupture has occurred, the best maneuver is to advance the balloon back into the location of the rupture site and inflate it completely (Fig. 9). This tamponades bleeding until emergency repair can be performed with either an open surgery or a covered stent. If the patient is systemically anticoagulated, consider reversal.

If the patient is heavily sedated, however, or if the procedure is being performed concomitantly with another operation and the patient is under anesthesia, pain may not serve as a warning sign. Following angioplasty,

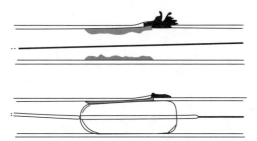

Fig. 9 Management of arterial rupture at the angioplasty site. (**A**) A rupture occurs at the interface between hard, calcified plaque and the adjacent soft artery after angioplasty. (**B**) The angioplasty balloon is reinserted and reinflated to tamponade the bleeding site.

several minutes may pass before completion arteriography is performed. Sudden hemodynamic instability in this setting should be considered a rupture until proved otherwise.

Any extravasation of contrast or vessel wall staining on completion arteriography is significant. Visualization of contrast extravasating through the arterial defect means that a high-flow rupture has occurred and that shock is only moments away. Contrast that has leaked beyond the confines of the vessel wall but appears to be stable may represent a contained rupture. A rupture after balloon angioplasty should not be stented because the stent is likely to reopen the incidental arteriotomy. This situation must be carefully distinguished from an acute local dissection, which is much more common and for which a stent is often indicated.

Rupture of the superficial femoral artery, popliteal artery, or tibial artery is much less likely to cause life-threatening hemorrhage and more often results in acute occlusion. Some localized ruptures heal or form chronic pseudoaneurysms. If a rupture occurs in the infrainguinal arteries, wait several minutes and repeat an arteriogram. If the artery remains patent and the extramural hematoma is not expanding, surgery may not be required.

The most common cause of postangioplasty arterial rupture is overdilatation. Rupture is rare if simple guidelines are followed:

Carefully consider the diameter of the chosen balloon prior to usage.
Double-check that the correct balloon is being advanced, especially if multiple different-sized catheters have been opened for the case.
Accept a decent result; don't be greedy about obtaining a cosmetically perfect completion image.
Know when to quit (or when to convert to surgery) if the limit of endovascular capability has been reached.

Conditions treated with balloon angioplasty are rarely, if ever, life threatening but arterial rupture is one complication that may result in death.

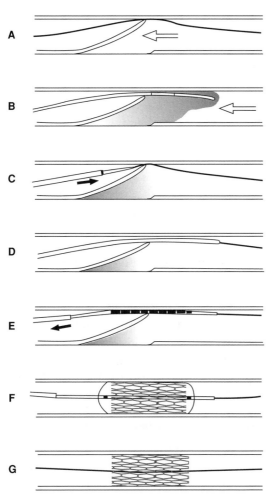

Fig. 10 Management of acute occlusion at the angioplasty site. The most common cause of acute occlusion after angioplasty is dissection. (**A**) A dissection flap is raised at the angioplasty site that occludes flow. (**B**) A catheter is passed over the guidewire and limited arteriography is performed. (**C**) A sheath and dilator are passed over the guidewire. (**D**) The dilator is removed. (**E**) An angioplasty balloon with a Palmaz stent is passed through the sheath and the sheath is withdrawn. (**F**) The balloon is inflated to deploy the stent at the site of the dissection. (**G**) The dissection flap is tacked down by the stent.

Ruptured arterial segments should not be treated with stents, but covered stents may obviate the need for emergency surgery in some cases.

Management of Embolization

In general, prior to balloon angioplasty, it is best to evaluate the runoff served by the artery to be treated and have a sense for the quality of the runoff. This

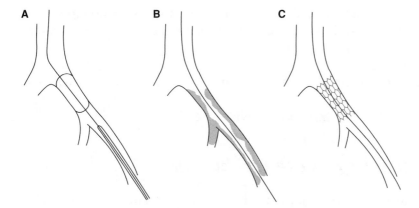

Fig. 11 Stent placement after dissection. (**A**) Balloon angioplasty of a focal, mid-common iliac artery lesion causes a dissection. (**B**) The dissection is identified by the appearance of contrast retained in the arterial wall, flow streaming effects through the lumen, and extension of abnormality well beyond the original lesion. Guidewire access is carefully maintained. (**C**) Stent placement at the original angioplasty site usually closes the false channels.

is helpful later if there is any question about whether embolization occurred. If the patient has a lesion which has previously embolized or looks like it might, use a distal protection device, use extra anticoagulation, consider IIb/IIIa receptor inhibitors, and consider primary coverage with a stent or a stent–graft. Clinically significant postangioplasty embolization is unusual but may result in organ or limb loss. In some angioplasty cases, the patient starts off with one problem (the lesion) and ends up with two problems (a partially treated, possibly unstable, upstream lesion and an ischemic or occluded outflow bed). Embolization may present as filling defects at some location distal to the angioplasty site or as pain experienced by the patient in the outflow vascular bed. If this occurs, the following steps should be taken.

1. Administer a fully anticoagulating dose of heparin.
2. Maintain any guidewire that is in the distal affected vascular bed.
3. Inspect sheaths that are already in place. Aspirate and flush.
4. Initiate intra-arterial heparin drip through the sheath.
5. Administer vasodilators.
6. Consider the cause. Is the embolus from the angioplasty site or the access site or is it due to thrombus formation from low flow?
7. Stabilize the angioplasty site as soon as possible. This usually means stent placement.
8. Place a multi-side-hole catheter distally into the affected outflow bed and perform a local arteriogram. Administer tissue plasminogen activator, 1 mg as a pulse spray over 10 min. Consider IIb/IIIa receptor inhibitors.

9. Use an aspiration catheter, such as an Export® (Medtronic) or Pronto® (Vascular Solutions) and aspirate the runoff bed as much as possible.
10. Repeat arteriogram.
11. If continued filling defects, continue tissue plasminogen activator at 1 mg/hr.
12. Use mechanical thrombolysis with AngioJet™.

Management of Acute Occlusion

An acute occlusion at the angioplasty site that occurs immediately after balloon angioplasty and is apparent on the completion arteriogram is usually caused by dissection (Figs. 10 and 11). The guidewire, left in place during completion arteriography, is exchanged for a stiff guidewire. A stent is placed at the same site where the balloon angioplasty was performed to tack down the dissection flap that has been elevated and propagated from the angioplasty site. After the placement of a single stent, arteriography usually demonstrates patency. If necessary, additional stents are placed distally and proximally to the first stent until patency is achieved.

18

Stents: Minimally Invasive Relining

Impact of Stents

Vascular stents have made it possible to reline a diseased artery. Stents have had a major impact on the development of endovascular surgery that is manifested in four ways.

1. The complications of balloon angioplasty, such as dissection and residual stenosis, may be immediately treated.
2. Lesions that otherwise would have required open surgery, such as occlusions or long lesions or recurrent stenoses, may be treated with endovascular surgery. This is particularly appropriate when it provides an additional option for the treatment of patients who are at high risk for open surgery.
3. The overall spectrum of arterial lesions that can be approached with endovascular techniques has broadened dramatically. Whether or not a particular lesion ultimately requires stent placement, the availability of stents has permanently altered the general approach and the consideration of options.
4. Combining stents with graft material to create stent–grafts has permitted the endovascular treatment of aneurysm disease.

Each stent application has its own cost and complication risks. The sheath must usually be upsized, a foreign body is implanted, the procedure time is often extended somewhat, and stents have their own unique complications. In addition, the cost of a single stent substantially increases the cost of an endovascular intervention. The placing of stents may be motivated by the wish to extend the short- or long-term success of balloon angioplasty, to avoid surgery, or to avoid repeat balloon angioplasty, but should be considered in each case. Stents have improved to the point where they can be easily and smoothly incorporated into a procedure, even if a stent was not necessarily intended from the start of the case. Future applications of stents may include further miniaturization and the ability to release antithrombotic agents, emit irradiation, or prevent intimal hyperplasia through bioengineering design changes.

Stent Choices

Stents are either balloon-expandable or self-expanding (Fig. 1). The main characteristics of these two types of stents are listed in Table 1.

The Palmaz stent (Cordis, a Johnson & Johnson Co., Miami, Florida, U.S.A.) was the original balloon-expandable stent design. This is a straight, metal, rigid, and balloon-expandable cylinder. The stent is crimped onto a standard angioplasty balloon and is deployed when the balloon is inflated. Initially, the stent had to be hand crimped on to the balloon catheter. Now the stents are premounted on the balloon catheters when ordered. The rigid

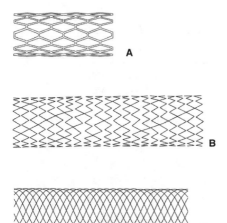

Fig. 1 Stent choices. (**A**) Balloon-expandable stents are rigid. The stent is crimped onto an angioplasty balloon and deployed by balloon inflation. (**B**) Self-expanding stents made of Nitinol, a nickel-titanium alloy, are flexible and may be delivered on low profile catheters. (**C**) The self-expanding, wire mesh stents may be made of either Nitinol or Elgiloy.

balloon-expandable stent has excellent hoop strength but can be crimped by external forces. These stents perform best when placed in locations that have no mobility, such as the aortic bifurcation. Balloon-expanding stents perform best when they are relatively short in length since they are rigid. These stents also shorten slightly as they expand in diameter. Most renal artery stents are between 1 and 2 cm, and most iliac stents are 3 to 4 cm. These are the places where balloon-expandable stents are most useful. The medium Palmaz stent can be expanded from a diameter of 4.0 to 9.0 mm and the large stent can be expanded from 8.0 to 12.0 mm. An aortic stent is also available that can be expanded to more than 2 cm in diameter.

The Wallstent (Medi-Tech, Natick, Massachusetts, U.S.A.) is a flexible, self-expanding, wire mesh tube that is deployed by retracting a covering sheath. This was the originally available self-expanding stent. Self-expanding stents are now more commonly constructed of Nitinol, a nickel-titanium alloy

Table 1 Stent Characteristics

Balloon-expandable stent	Self-expanding stent
Slotted-tube design	Wire mesh or slotted tube
High radial force	Low radial force (oversize for vessel)
Rigid	Flexible
Most functional at short lengths	Longer lengths very functional
Premounted, or mount onto balloon of choice	Delivery catheter with covering sheath
Some shortening with expansion	Variable shortening; some do not shorten
Steel or stainless steel	Nitinol or light metal alloy
Moderate radiopacity	Poor radiopacity (some have markers)

Table 2 Some Stents on the Market[a]

Type	Stent	Manufacturer
Balloon-expandable	Bridge Stent, extra support	Medtronic AVE
	Bridge stent, flexible	Medtronic AVE
	Herculink	Abbott
	Megalink	Abbott
	Palmaz[b]	Cordis
	Palmaz-Corinthian	Cordis
	Perflex	Cordis
Self-expanding	Luminex	Bard
	Memotherm	Bard
	SMART[b]	Cordis
	Symphony	Boston Scientific
	Wallstent[b]	Boston Scientific
	Zilver	Cook
	Precise	Cordis

[a] Many other stents are available that are not included here.
[b] Approved by the FDA for limited use in the noncoronary vasculature.

that has thermal memory and a high degree of contourability. Self-expanding stents are packaged on their own delivery catheters. Self-expanding stents are intentionally oversized at the time of deployment in the artery, usually by 2 to 3 mm, and they maintain continual outward radial force after deployment. They are not as susceptible to damage from external forces since they are more flexible, but they have much less hoop strength. Self-expanding stents cover more distance but they are more difficult to place with great accuracy.

Self-expanding and balloon-expandable stents tend to play complementary roles. Deciding which type of stent to use may be somewhat subjective from one practice to another, but endovascular specialists must become facile with the use of each of these two general stent types. In addition, there are numerous stents, both balloon- and self-expanding, that are available (Table 2). These compete with one another and have continued to improve over the past few years. The balloon-expandable stents have become lower profile and easier to deliver, continue to have excellent hoop strength, but are made of less metal then once was required. The self-expanding stents have a variety of designs, adding to flexibility. Delivery has improved and tends to be more accurate than previously. Visibility is also improved as many have radiopaque markers.

Indications for Stents: Primary or Selective Stent Placement

The key difference between primary and selective stent placement is that with primary placement the operator knows ahead of time that a stent will be placed versus the selective approach where the operator must decide during the procedure. The concept of primary stent placement presupposes that the patient is better off with a stent, regardless of the results of treatment of the lesion with balloon angioplasty alone. The operator places a stent at each site of intervention, without first performing a balloon angioplasty to see if this would be adequate treatment. This approach appears to work best for some lesions that were treated with balloon angioplasty alone in the past with marginal to mediocre results, including recurrent lesions, occlusions, orifice lesions, and others. Primary stent placement has made endovascular intervention a very reasonable option in some areas of treatment, such as for renal artery origin lesions. This approach has also been advocated for carotid bifurcation and aortoiliac occlusive disease. The idea behind primary stent placement is that the short- and/or long-term results are generally improved with stent placement to the point where it justifies the up-front increase in risk and cost. Taken to its fullest extent, however, every lesion in every patient would receive a stent, and this would be expensive and unnecessary.

Selective stent placement assumes that the cost and risk of stent placement are not justified in every case and that not every patient requires a stent to have acceptable treatment results. Balloon angioplasty was widely practiced for more than 15 years before stents became available. This experience yielded reasonable long-term results with balloon angioplasty for many aortoiliac, infrainguinal, nonorifice renal lesions, and some upper extremity lesions. Balloon angioplasty is performed. The results are assessed. If the results are not acceptable, stent placement is performed. Indications for selective stent placement after balloon angioplasty include residual stenosis, a persistent pressure gradient, and significant dissection.

The indications for stents have expanded steadily since they became available. Endovascular specialists have become more adept at placing stents, and the development of new stents and simpler ways of placing them have assisted in this process. Each stent added to the mix in a given case brings the entire process closer to a point of diminishing returns. The temptation with stents is to continue to lay them in place until the entire arterial tree appears to be perfect. The "stack o' stents" phenomenon should be avoided.

Which Lesions Should Be Stented?

Although each specialist must decide what the appropriate level of stent placement aggressiveness is, there are specific situations where stents are useful.

POSTANGIOPLASTY DISSECTION

Stent placement should be considered for any significant dissection after angioplasty, even if there is no gradient. Because plaque fracture is the

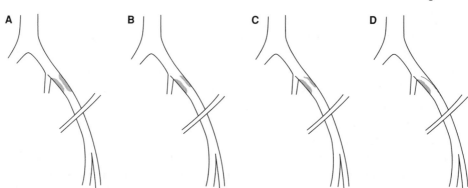

Fig. 2 Degrees of dissection after angioplasty. (**A**) An external iliac artery stenosis is treated with balloon angioplasty. (**B**) Angioplasty creates separations between the intima and media that are demonstrated by completion arteriography as small dissection flaps. (**C**) A more prominent dissection flap may not impede flow but does protrude into the lumen. Stent placement should be considered. (**D**) Dissections that impede flow, lengthen during the procedure, or extend into an adjacent nondiseased segment of artery should be stented.

mechanism of angioplasty, some degree of dissection is common. Unfortunately, there is no good method of assessing the severity of dissection or predicting its behavior (Fig. 2). As a result, many postangioplasty dissections that would have healed spontaneously in the past are currently not being given that opportunity and are stented immediately after balloon angioplasty. Stents should be placed for any false channel or for any intimal flaps that impede flow, increase in size during the procedure, or extend into a previously uninvolved segment of artery.

RESIDUAL STENOSIS AFTER ANGIOPLASTY

Residual stenosis can usually be resolved with stent placement. The concept of preventing recurrence by eliminating residual stenosis makes empiric sense. A 30% postangioplasty stenosis is used as a general threshold for continued intervention, although there is no convincing justification for using this particular degree of stenosis.

PRESSURE GRADIENT

A pressure gradient (more than 10 mm Hg systolic) after angioplasty usually indicates a residual stenosis or dissection that requires treatment. Again the threshold for treatment is somewhat arbitrary.

RECURRENT STENOSIS AFTER ANGIOPLASTY

Treating recurrence with stent placement after previous angioplasty is an empiric approach with reasonable results.

Table 3 Which Lesions Should Be Stented?

Indication	Rationale	Reality
Postangioplasty dissection	Prevents acute occlusion	Makes angioplasty safer because dissection can be managed without emergency open surgery. More complex lesions can be treated with angioplasty. Which dissections need stents is unknown. Most dissections healed without stents in the past.
Residual stenosis after angioplasty (> 30%)	Causes early failures and late recurrence	Makes empiric sense but there is little proof. Mild residual stenosis may not cause harm. Moderate residual stenosis (>50%) can almost always be resolved with stent placement.
Occlusion	Poor results with angioplasty alone	Better short- and long-term results with stents. Avoids open surgery in most patients with iliac occlusion.
Recurrence	Limited success of primary angioplasty	Repeat angioplasty alone has reasonable results in iliac artery. Makes empiric sense but there is no proof.
Long lesion	Not sure	More likely to dissect after angioplasty. Looks better with stents.
Embolizing lesion	Cages and compacts the embolic material	Makes sense and there are reports of success. Be certain it is not an aneurysm. Control outflow during procedure.
All lesions (primary stent placement)	Extends long-term results	Looks great. Provides excellent opportunity to practice stent placement. Unclear if long-term results justify the upfront cost and complications.

OCCLUSION

Balloon angioplasty alone for occlusions has only fair results and these may be improved with stent placement. Stent placement may make the procedure safer by stabilizing residual thrombus that could embolize from the lesion site. Stent placement in the treatment of iliac and superficial femoral artery occlusions is widely accepted.

EMBOLIZING LESION

Stent placement at the site of an embolizing lesion is thought to trap the embologenic plaque and prevent further embolization during intervention. Because embolizing lesions are often soft, care must be taken during guidewire and catheter crossing. The lesion must also be evaluated to be certain that it is not an aneurysm.

As experience is gained with stents, indications for their placement have been continuously modified (Table 3). Other relative indications include a significant ulceration, a long lesion, or a highly irregular, calcified plaque.

The location of the intended angioplasty site affects the likelihood of stent placement. Since most atherosclerotic renal artery lesions are aortic plaque that has spilled over into the renal artery, stent placement is usually necessary to resolve these stenoses. Stent placement appears to be safer than angioplasty alone at the carotid bifurcation, possibly because these are primarily embolizing lesions. Aortoiliac angioplasty is fairly durable without stents, and stents can be used selectively with reasonable results. Infrainguinal angioplasty is not as durable and stent placement offers little improvement in long-term results.

Placement Technique for Balloon-Expandable Stent

The selection of diameter is an important decision in the placement of balloon-expandable stents. The stent size is selected based on the anticipated diameter of the reconstructed artery. If the selected stent is too small in diameter, it may not adhere to the vessel wall after deployment and could migrate, even before it is more completely expanded. The balloon must be rapidly exchanged for a larger one, which is used to expand the stent further. If the stent is too large, it will overstretch the artery and may cause rupture, and it is not retrievable once it is deployed. If selective stent placement is performed, the inflated balloon profile from the initial angioplasty may be used to size the artery. When primary stent placement is performed, sometimes it is necessary to dilate the lesion with the balloon alone to size the lesion and to create enough space for the stent delivery catheter to be placed across the lesion. Balloon-expandable stents can be dilated a few millimeters larger than the intended specifications, but as the diameter increases, the length decreases. The shortest stent that covers the lesion (usually 1–4 cm) is placed. Longer balloon-expandable stents are available (up to almost 8 cm) but there are disadvantages to the rigidity of these stents over longer distances. They do not conform to any tortuosity or any change in vessel diameter along the length of the stent.

Prior to placing a stent, the lesion length is assessed as well as the tortuosity and tapering effect present at the segment, that intended for stenting. Balloon-expandable stents are usually premounted in the factory. However, if hand crimping is to be performed, the balloon chosen for deployment must be of either the same length or longer than the stent. If it is of the same length, mount the stent directly between the radiopaque markers. If the balloon is longer than the stent, it should not be more than a centimeter longer. The stent should be mounted so that the end of the stent is on either the proximal or distal radiopaque marker on the balloon, so that the stent's location is known when it is time for deployment. Vigorous crimping with the thumb and forefinger secures the stent without bending it. The stent should not be able to slide on the balloon unless firm traction is applied. Test the adherence of the stent to the balloon, but do not slide the stent back and forth on the balloon because the sharp end of the stent can pierce the balloon. Mounting of the stent on the balloon is best performed prior to advancing the sheath across the lesion so that the stent is ready for deployment. When advancing the catheter that has the stent mounted on it, support the stent at its training end as it is pushed through the head of the sheath so that the stent is not loosened on the balloon shaft. Each of the major endovascular companies makes a puncture-resistant balloon that is designed for stent delivery. A medium Palmaz or Palmaz style stent requires a 7-Fr sheath. Premounted knock off versions can be placed using a 6-Fr sheath. Larger vessel stents, such as that used for large iliacs up to 12 mm are placed through a 9-Fr sheath. An even larger, 5 cm length balloon-expandable stent is available for the infrarenal aorta and this stent has been used often in bailout of Type I endoleaks during stent–graft repair of aortic aneurysms.

For many years, the general approach to balloon-expandable stent placement has been to pass the appropriate sheath and dilator combination through the lesion and proceed to stent placement (Fig. 3). If the lesion has a residual lumen of less than the diameter of the sheath (for a 6 Fr sheath it is approximately 2.0 mm and for a 7 Fr sheath it is about 2.3 mm), the lesion should be predilated or the sheath and dilator will dotter the lesion. The sheath must be of adequate length to pass from the skin entry site to near the lesion. A radiopaque tip on the sheath is useful so that it is always clear where the sheath tip is located relative to the lesion. The dilator is removed and the sheath is flushed. The sheath may stop or impede blood flow, since it occupies the remaining lumen at the site of the lesion. If there is any question about the exact location for stent placement, a repeat arteriogram should be performed prior to sheath placement. The balloon catheter, with the stent crimped into place, is passed over the guidewire and into the sheath. A customized metal cannula may be used to temporarily open the hemostatic valve on the sheath. This cannula comes in the package with the stent. However, the stent may also be passed through the hemostatic valve by hand. Grab the balloon–stent with a pincer grasp at the end of the stent that is farthest from the valve and push the balloon and stent through the valve. Using fluoroscopy, the balloon and stent are passed into the appropriate location. Check the balloon while it is still in the sheath using a magnified field of view to visualize the stent on the balloon and ensure it is still located where it was crimped on the balloon. The sheath is withdrawn, exposing the balloon and stent. A sheath with a marker at the tip is very useful in this circumstance. Before deployment, it is important to make sure that the stent is still in the correct place on the balloon and that it is well positioned to cover the lesion. The balloon is then inflated to expand the stent. The stent should be slightly overdilated to embed its metal struts into the plaque.

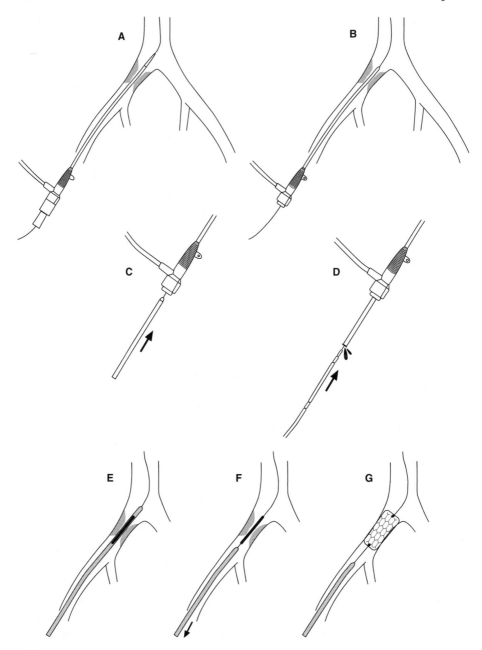

Fig. 3 Placement technique for balloon-expandable stent. (**A**) The dilator and sheath are advanced through the lesion. (**B**) The dilator is removed, leaving the sheath across the stenosis. (**C**) A metal introducer with a beveled end opens the hemostatic valve on the head of the sheath. (**D**) The stent is mounted on the balloon and crimped into place between the radiopaque markers. The balloon and stent are advanced through the metal introducer and into the sheath. (**E**) Using fluoroscopy, the stent is placed at the desired location within the lesion. (**F**) The sheath is withdrawn to expose the stent. (**G**) The balloon is inflated to deploy the stent.

Another option for access and one that is more commonly used at present is to pass the tip of the sheath toward the lesion but not through it. Be careful if you are passing it close to the lesion to avoid inadvertently passing the unmarked dilator across the lesion. The sheath tip is used as a platform for pushing, for easy arteriography, for stabilizing the back end of the stent after the stent is deployed, and for helping to gather up the balloon after it has expanded the stent. Lower-profile, well-secured, and premounted balloon-expandable stents have made it much less necessary to pass the sheath across the lesion to deliver the stent.

Palmaz stents expand initially to an hourglass shape with the proximal and distal ends flaring first and the middle portion of the stent filling out at the completion of the balloon inflation. The proximal or distal end of the stent is often only partially dilated into an oval shape, which is not always apparent on completion arteriography. The balloon is deflated after the stent has been fully deployed. The balloon is advanced slightly and reinflated so that the proximal end of the stent is fully dilated. This maneuver is repeated on the distal end of the stent.

If there is a sense that the stent is loose in the lesion, either because it is underdilated or because it migrated during deployment to an area that is slightly less narrow, take the next steps very deliberately. Advance the tip of the sheath up to the expanded end of the stent and catch the edge of the stent and support it so that it cannot move. That can often be done right over the balloon catheter that delivered the stent. This is a common maneuver in renal stenting that helps avoid problems from getting out of hand. Also, many times after placement of a balloon-expandable stent, the balloon wings will stick a bit, perhaps getting caught under the tines of the stent. If this is the case, and more than a gentle pull does not solve it, use these steps. Do a super-aspiration, implosion level negative pressure on the balloon. Support the stent by advancing the sheath as described earlier. Try rotating and/or advancing the balloon catheter before withdrawing it. Sometimes, reinflating the balloon will loosen the balloon material, and then go through these steps again.

Precise stent deployment is challenging. The stent may be difficult to visualize in larger individuals, especially if it is in a location with a lot of ventilatory motion, such as the visceral and renal arteries where balloon-expandable stents are used quite often. A difference in location of a few millimeters may be the difference between a perfect placement and a misplaced stent. Bony landmarks may be useful, especially the vertebral bodies or some identifiable vascular calcification. If there are no suitable landmarks, use an external marker, such as a stent guide. This is an adherent, radiopaque measuring tape that can be placed on the patient parallel to the guidewire. These are particularly useful when treating longer lesions. Be cautioned that external markers are susceptible to parallax error if the field of view is modified. They are also in error if there is any change in angle of view, any catching of the tape on the image intensifier, or any significant ventilatory motion. When you use external markers, recheck the lesion before you deploy the stent. Road mapping may also be used for deployment of stents but the roadmap image degrades with time and motion.

A method for precise placement of balloon-expandable stents is as follows. Position the image intensifier and set the field of view in a manner that provides the best view of the lesion. Typically, there is one edge of the stent to be placed that will be the deciding factor as to its accuracy and precision. For example, provided the selected stent is long enough, when performing a stent of the renal artery orifice, the trailing end of the stent should protrude into the aorta about 1 mm to claim adequate treatment of aortic plaque that is spilling over into the renal artery. This same general scenario repeats itself with other aortic branch orifice lesions with spillover plaque that is creating a circumferential napkin ring of atherosclerosis. Balloon-expandable stents work well in these scenarios and all of these situations involve deep imaging (in a body cavity) with significant ventilator motion. A smaller field of view, such as a 6-in. field, is often best since it provides magnification. Choose bony landmarks or place external markers. Perform an arteriogram. Once the image intensifier is positioned, do not move it until after the stent is deployed. Perform a road map with the patient having taken a half breath in (not a deep sea diver breath that can change all the positions and the landmarks). Advance the stent into the lesion, have the patient take the exact same half breath in and hold it, as the patient had done during the angiographic run. During the breath hold, the road map should match up and the stent is deployed. After the stent is in place across the lesion, but before it is deployed, if there is any doubt about correct placement, puff contrast through the sheath to reconfirm the position, or do another road map. Sometimes, this process is repeated a couple of times until the operator is satisfied with the position for stent placement. Have a contingency plan for what to do if the stent is placed too far one way or the other with respect to the lesion.

Guidewire control must be maintained across the stent until the reconstruction is complete. If additional stents are required, the dilator is placed back through the sheath and the dilator and sheath combination is advanced into the appropriate position. If numerous overlapping stents are required, the distal stent is placed first and built proximally to create a "telescope" effect (Fig. 4). If dilation to a larger diameter is required, the deployment balloon is exchanged. A balloon-expandable stent does not taper well but can be dilated to a slightly larger size on one end if necessary to match vessel size and taper. This is especially true of the newer balloon-expandable stents that are constructed of lighter metal.

A completion arteriogram is performed by placing the tip of the sheath at the distal end of the stent and injecting contrast so that it refluxes through

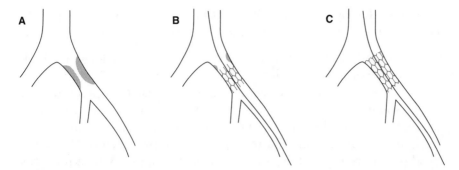

Fig. 4 Telescope effect using balloon-expandable stents. (**A**) A long iliac artery stenosis requires more than one stent for coverage. (**B**) The distal stent is placed first. (**C**) The second stent overlaps the first and fits inside to create a telescope effect. This technique avoids a prominent metal edge protruding into the flow stream.

the area of stent placement. Another option is to place a 5-Fr straight catheter through the sheath, over the guidewire, and position the tip of the catheter at the location proximal to the stent. A 4- or 5-Fr flush catheter may also be placed in the same manner and positioned upstream from the stent site.

Placement Technique for Self-Expanding Stent

Self-expanding stents must be oversized by 1 to 3 mm so that they exert continuous outward radial force at the site of deployment. Placing a stent that is too small in diameter is to be avoided since these stents cannot be dilated beyond their maximum list diameter. If there is doubt about the appropriate diameter stent to use, consider balloon angioplasty first with an evaluation of the inflated balloon profile. If in doubt, go a little bigger on the diameter. This is the opposite of balloon-expandable stents. Placement of a self-expanding stent is performed by withdrawing a covering layer that encloses the stent on a prepackaged catheter. The prepackaged stent delivery catheter is placed through a 6-Fr, 7-Fr, or 9-Fr sheath, as recommended by the manufacturer. Stent length choice varies significantly from one stent type to another. Self-expanding stents are manufactured in multiple lengths, from 20 to 120 mm in fully expanded form. The self-expanding Nitinol stents, which are the most commonly used stents in the noncoronary arteries, do not shorten much upon placement. They are generally simple to place, and they adapt to tortuosity, calcification, and ectopic atherosclerosis.

Wallstent length changes significantly at deployment depending upon the final resting diameter. The constrained length of the Wallstent (in the package) is longer than the deployed length (partially constrained by the artery), which in turn is longer than the stent would be if it were to be completely expanded (unconstrained). For example, a 10 × 42 Wallstent (10-mm diameter × 42-mm length) placed in a 9-mm iliac artery is 50- to

52-mm long after deployment. The Wallstent in practice is never completely expanded, since it is oversized for the artery into which it is placed.

The self-expanding stent catheter is removed from its package, flushed, and wiped with heparin–saline solution. The end stopcock is closed and the catheter is advanced over the guidewire (Fig. 5). Because the apparatus and the stent are somewhat flexible, it can be passed over the aortic bifurcation. The stent is marked by radiopaque markers on its proximal and distal ends, which are observed using fluoroscopy. To deploy the stent, the metal pushing rod is held steady and the valve body is withdrawn, which removes the covering membrane. Fluoroscopy is used because it is easy to move the stent with minimal force. As the metal pushing rod is held stationary and the valve body is withdrawn, the proximal end of the stent begins to expand. The position of the stent is continually assessed. A road map can be used to assist in placement. Self-expanding stents are more likely to be used for lesions in conduit arteries (e.g., iliac artery, superficial femoral artery) that may be longer and that have some degree of tortuosity (e.g., carotid artery, iliac artery), but less ventilator mobility than when balloon-expandable stents are placed at branch artery origin lesions, such as the renal or subclavian arteries.

Self-expanding stents have the disadvantage that only the leading end of the stent, usually the end toward the tip of the catheter, can be placed with a high degree of accuracy. The back end, trailing end, or end of the stent that is closer to the hub end of the catheter, will land with much less placement accuracy than the leading end of the stent. Somewhere in the course of self-expanding stent deployment, but before that there is full engagement of the stent with the artery wall, the stent can be moved and position can be readjusted. When the leading end of the stent starts to open it "flowers". Once that blossom gets big enough to touch the wall of the artery, the stent cannot be advanced, but usually can still be withdrawn. Most self-expanding Nitinol stents can deploy about 15% to 20% of their length or 1 cm (whichever is less) and still be possible to withdraw the whole stent to readjust position. If there is too much adherence of the stent to the wall already in play, when the catheter is withdrawn, the stent just hugs the wall and hangs on to the wall and the stent deploys.

There is a reconstrainable Wallstent that can be covered up again by its covering membrane, provided the release process has stopped short of a certain point that is marked right on the delivery catheter. The stent can then be moved to a different place and then deployed. The Wallstent is a closed cell structure. This permits a relatively smooth outer surface without any "v" shaped stent joints extruding beyond the profile of the open or partially open stent. This facilitates recovering of the outer surface of the stent if desired. This recapturability will probably not be possible with open cell Nitinol self-expanding stents in the near future. The design allows the

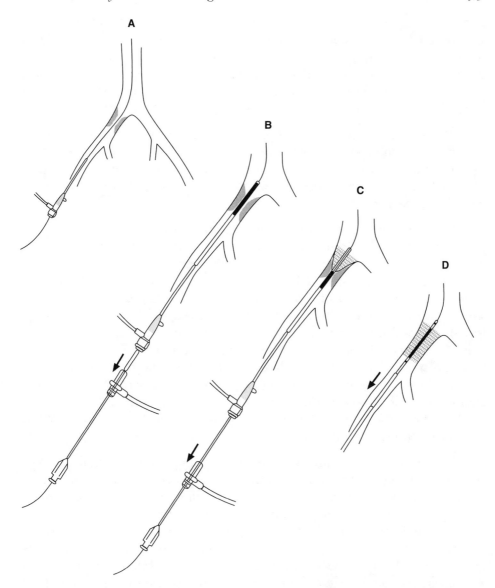

Fig. 5 Placement technique for self-expanding stents. (**A**) The guidewire is placed across the lesion. (**B**) The stent delivery catheter is placed over the guidewire so that the proximal radiopaque marker on the catheter is proximal to the lesion. The metal pushing rod is held stationary while the valve body is slowly withdrawn. (**C**) The position of the stent is continuously monitored using fluoroscopy. As the stent opens, it can be "dragged" distally but not advanced. As the valve body is withdrawn along the length of the pushing rod, the covering sheath that constrains the stent is removed and the stent expands. (**D**) After stent deployment, the stent delivery catheter is removed.

stent to spring all the way open when one end is deployed and one end is still constrained in the delivery catheter. In other words, the open cell stents contour well and they are able to go from a very small diameter to a large diameter over a very short longitudinal distance. This property is needed for the management of tortuous or tapered arteries. But it also creates rough edges where stent joints are under stress and protrude into the lumen.

The self-expanding stents deploy in a similar manner to each other: holding a pushing rod in a stationary position while withdrawing the covering membrane and allowing the stent to expand. Some have fancy handles and knobs to turn for better control, possibly accuracy, but it is the same underlying mechanism.

Take the slack out of the guidewire and catheter. It is best to have an assistant hold the access sheath during deployment. Any withdrawal of the catheter for placement accuracy will also tend to pull the sheath out. Built-up energy in the stent delivery catheter, when released, tends to make the stent pop forward a bit (toward the tip end) during deployment. After stent deployment, the delivery catheter is removed and balloon angioplasty is performed of the length and ends of the stent, especially in sections where there is residual crimping of the stent by the lesion. It is sometimes difficult to assess whether the stent is fully expanded. Keep the balloon within the stent if injury is to be avoided to neighboring artery segments. When balloon angioplasty is to be used within the Wallstent, the central part of the stent is dilated first. The ends of the stent are dilated last because the tines of the stent may rupture the balloon.

The guidewire is maintained across the stented segment until after satisfactory completion studies are performed. Completion arteriography is performed in the same manner as with balloon-expanded stents. If guidewire control of the stent is relinquished prematurely, advance a J-tip or very floppy-tip guidewire back through the stent using a small field of view for magnification. This is done to avoid passing the guidewire through the struts of the stent. This is easy to do, especially prior to postdeployment balloon angioplasty. If you have to cross a fresh stent and you are not sure if you are under the tines of the stent, pass a straight or simple curve catheter over the guidewire. If the guidewire goes under one of the stent struts, the catheter will hang up instead of passing freely.

QUESTION: WHAT TO CONSIDER WHEN SELECTING A STENT

1. Can you visualize the stent in this position?
2. What are the length and diameter requirements of the diseased segment?
3. What is the location of the lesion and what type of lesion is it?

4. Are there delivery restrictions posed by diseased access arteries, sheath size, vessel tortuosity, working room, or distance to the lesion?
5. Can the number of required stents be minimized?
6. Is it in your inventory?

Which Stent for Which Lesion?

Table 4 offers a practical comparison of the working properties of a balloon-expandable stent, a foreshortening self-expanding stent, and a nonshortening Nitinol self-expanding stent. In general, orifice lesions and those that are heavily calcified are best treated with balloon-expandable stents. Lesions located in flexible arteries or tortuous arteries or that are more than several centimeters in length are usually treated with self-expanding stents.

Either balloon-expanding or self-expanding stents may be used in the aorta (Table 5). Short focal lesions may be treated with balloon-expanding stents. Placement is precise and the single stent is less expensive. Self-expanding stents are well suited to longer aortic lesions (longer than 2–3 cm). Placement of a single longer self-expanding stent is usually simpler, faster, and less expensive than placing multiple balloon-expandable stents. Just be careful to make sure that the trailing end of the stent clears the aortic bifurcation and opens fully within the aorta. The other advantage of self-expanding stents in the aorta is when there is a heavily calcified, shelf-like, or iceberg-like lesion; the stent can be laid in and the lumen gradually enlarged with successively enlarging angioplasty balloons. This is done to avoid rupture.

Lesions in the aortic bifurcation are treated by "raising" the aortic flow divider with balloon-expandable stents. Precise, "kissing," and side-to-side placement is possible with self-expanding stents but difficult. Aortic bifurcation plaque usually extends through the common iliac artery orifices. Self-expanding stents don't have as much hoop strength, which is desirable for the aortic bifurcation and other orifice lesions.

Garden-variety common and external iliac artery lesions may be treated with either type of stent. Focal lesions are treated with balloon-expandable stents, and self-expandable stents are used for longer lesions and those located in tortuous arteries or those with significant taper. Distal iliac artery lesions that are close to the groin should be treated with self-expanding stents.

Self-expanding stents are better for stenting in flexible arteries, such as the superficial femoral, popliteal, and distal subclavian arteries. Lesions in an aortic branch orifice, such as the proximal innominate, common carotid, subclavian, visceral, or renal arteries, are best treated with balloon-expandable

Table 4 Practical Stent Comparison: Working Qualities of Palmaz, Wallstent, and Smart Stents[a]

Working quality	Balloon-expandable	Self-expanding (Elgiloy)	Self-expanding(Nitinol)	Advice
Method of expansion	Balloon-expandable	Self-expanding	Self-expanding	Requirement for balloon expansion to deploy makes balloon-expandable stent placement a little more complicated but self-expanding stent always require postexpansion balloon dilatation.
Maximum length	>5 cm	>9.4 cm	20 cm	Balloon-expandable stent length limited; lesions more than 3 cm need more than 1; adds complexity, time, and cost to the case; Self-expanding stents provide longer length.
Length changes during placement	Shortens by 5% to 25%, depending upon final diameter	Shortens by more than 30% of constrained length	Less than 8% does not depend upon final diameter	Final resting Wallstent length can be difficult to predict; Nitinol stents have minimal shortening.
Hoop strength	High	Low	Low to medium[d]	Balloon-expandable stent is a better choice for orifice lesions.
Flexibility	None	High	High	Self-expanding stents are better choices for tortuous or tapered arteries.
Contourability	None	Moderate	High	
Maximum diameter	>24 mm	24 mm	14 mm	Self-expanding stents a better choice for vessels > 12 mm in diameter; balloon-expandable stents can be pushed to larger sizes, but with severe foreshortening.
Precision of placement	Precise	Precise only on one end	Precise on one end	Proximal end (first end to be deployed) of self-expanding can be placed precisely and can be moved a bit prior to full deployment; location of second/distal end of stent is not precise.
Delivery sheath	6–9 Fr	6–9 Fr	6–8 Fr	Balloon-expandable stent requires that a long sheath be placed through the lesion, which adds risk of instrumenting lesion and creates problems for remote delivery. Self-expanding stents are on delivery catheters.
Biohazard	Sharp edges. Cannot be clamped; can tear balloon	Loose wire ends are sharp; can be clamped in emergency	No sharp edges; can be clamped in emergency	In an emergency, self-expanding stents can be clamped with shodded clamp.

Table 5 Which Stent to Use?

Angioplasty site	Lesion type	Stent to use	Reason
Aorta	Focal lesion	Balloon-expandable	Length match
	Bulky lesion	Self-expanding	Gradual expansion, avoid rupture
	Long (>2–3 cm)	Self-expanding	Fewer stents required
Aortic bifurcation	Iliac origin	Balloon-expandable	Hoop strength
Iliac	Focal	Balloon-expandable	Length match; simple
	Tortuous	Self-expanding	Flexible
	Long (especially external iliac)	Self-expanding	Fewer stents required; handles tortuosity well
SFA-popliteal	Long	Self-expanding	Fewer stents required
	Across joint	Self-expanding	
	Focal, short	Self-expanding	Flexible
			Better patency
Renal	Orifice	Balloon-expandable	Hoop strength, rigid
	Body of artery	Either	
Subclavian	Tortuous	Self-expanding	Flexible
	Orifice	Balloon-expandable	Hoop strength

stents. The combination of placement accuracy and hoop strength is better in this setting.

How Do You Select the Best Stent for the Job?

Although there are multiple considerations when selecting a stent for a given case, there is substantial overlap in the capabilities of the various stents. Most specialists develop a short list of one or two favorites in each stent category, balloon-expandable and self-expandable. One trend of note is that self-expanding stents are being used more widely than before. They are becoming more versatile, better engineered, provide more choices, and there is better data on results. What follows is a discussion of some of the issues that drive stent preferences in clinical practice.

Most practices have at least some restriction on the variety of stents stocked and the number of different stent sizes available. Specialists with a limited inventory will ask the question sooner, but everyone must face the availability issue at some point. Work with what is available or plan ahead well enough so that specific items are anticipated and ordered. The development of various sizes, lengths, designs, profiles, and qualities of stents has been significant over the past few years. Although it is difficult to make clear and discerning recommendations, having too many options is a good problem to have.

The single most important thing to do when selecting a stent is to visualize the stent in the intended location. Will it expand to oppose the wall of the artery? Can it handle the tortuosity and/or diameter changes? Does it have the hoop strength to stand up to the amount of calcification present in the lesion? Will the distal end of the stent be floating free in a segment of poststenotic dilatation? Will it cover the segment of artery most in need of treatment? Can the stent be passed safely to the target site?

The length and diameter requirements of the lesion must be taken together with the type and location of the lesion to come up with a stent choice. Lesion type and location were discussed in the earlier section. It is not always apparent how long a length of artery should be stented if there is mild or even moderate disease juxtaposed to the lesion. The operator must make an arbitrary decision in many cases. The diameter may be sized the same way as for balloon angioplasty, but the consequences of a bad guess are greater. If a balloon-expandable stent is undersized, it may not be securely adherent to the artery. If it is oversized too much, the artery may split. One method of dealing with this dilemma is to undersize the balloon-expandable stent just slightly. Deploy the stent so that it is held in place by the newly dilated lesion. Then dilate the stent again to the desired size using a larger balloon if necessary. The diameter choices for self-expanding stents provide more leeway since the stents are oversized from 1 to 3 mm. Nevertheless, if too small a stent is used, it may become free-floating. Required stent lengths can be challenging. All external marking methods have some degree of parallax.

Finally, delivery restrictions may be posed by diseased access arteries, the sheath size of the selected stent, vessel tortuosity, inadequate working room, long distance to the lesion, or branch points between the access point and the lesion. The risk of puncture site thrombosis increases when a large sheath is passed through a diseased common femoral artery. Sheath size may influence the choice of stent, since relatively larger-diameter self-expanding stents may be placed through 6-Fr sheaths. Vessel tortuosity or a branch point on the way to the lesion can usually be overcome with longer, sometimes guiding access sheaths. Occasionally, a more flexible stent is required to make these turns and a self-expanding stent is used instead of a balloon-expandable stent. The distance to the lesion is an important variable. Balloon-expandable stents must be mounted on a balloon with an adequate shaft length and self-expanding stents must be delivered on a catheter of adequate length. Both balloon-expandable and self-expanding stents are generally available on two different lengths of catheter, either 80 cm or 120 cm. If an 80-cm shaft is opened when the longer shaft is required, it will have to be discarded. These challenges can usually be solved by using the balloon shaft length to estimate distance if the lesion was dilated prior to stent placement. If not, a standard arteriographic catheter with a bright tip may be placed over the guidewire and advanced close to the lesion and used to estimate the length from the access to the lesion. If the distance from the access to the lesion is farther, there are some devices up to 150 cm but care must be taken to ensure that these are available. If not, or if the longest devices are inadequate, the operator must make a plan for an alternative access closer to the treatment site.

Tricks of the Trade

RAISING THE FLOW DIVIDER WITH KISSING STENTS

A bifurcation can be reconstructed by modifying the flow divider with kissing stents. Two stents are placed simultaneously with the leading edge of each stent abutting the other at a point proximal to the location of the native flow divider. The need for kissing stents arises most commonly at the aortic bifurcation (see chap. 19 for a detailed discussion of this technique). The atherosclerotic disease that occurs at the aortic bifurcation tends to be extensive and circumferential. With kissing stents, the aortic bifurcation can be reconstructed.

TAPERING A STENT

The various self-expanding stents tend to taper naturally with diminishing distal arterial diameter. Nitinol stents should be dilated with the appropriately sized balloon. The Wallstent may be tapered by slightly overdilating the proximal end. The upper body of the Wallstent is usually dilated first (Fig. 6). The Wallstent shortens with expansion. The very end of the Wallstent is dilated last since it may lead to rupture of the balloon.

The shorter, more rigid balloon-expanding stents can also be tapered, but to a lesser degree (1–2 mm maximum). One end of the stent is selectively dilated using only the shoulder of the balloon (Fig. 7).

MOVING A SELF-EXPANDING STENT

Self-expanding stents can be withdrawn or pulled back but not advanced forward after partial deployment. The entire deployment catheter apparatus must be withdrawn in a retracted position to move the stent (Fig. 8). An assistant should hold the access sheath since it will come out if not secured. Moving the stent can be helpful in achieving very precise placement of its proximal end. It is not possible to move a stent after it has been fully deployed. If the stent has not been deployed in the correct location, the best solution is to place another stent at the desired location.

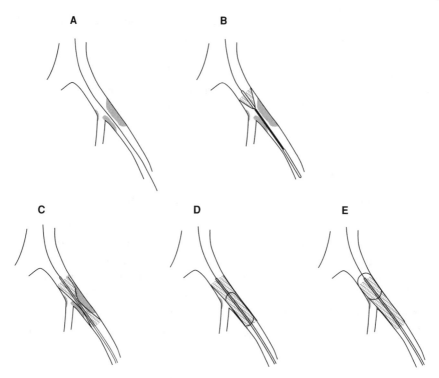

Fig. 6 Tapering a self-expanding stent. (**A**) The guidewire is passed through an iliac artery stenosis. (**B**) The self-expanding stent is deployed across the lesion. (**C**) The self-expanding stent tends to taper naturally with decreasing distal arterial diameter. (**D**) The distal end of the stent is ballooned to the diameter appropriate for the external iliac artery. (**E**) Angioplasty is performed in the larger proximal end of the stent that lies in the common iliac artery.

CROSSING A STENT

Once a stent has been deployed, the guidewire position across the stent is not relinquished until the procedure is completed. If the guidewire position is lost, or if a repeat study is necessary in a patient who has a stent, it is best to cross the stent using a J-tip guidewire (Fig. 9). The elbow of the J-tip guidewire is less likely to pass through the struts of the stent. If there is any doubt about the position of the guidewire, it should be withdrawn and a repeat crossing should be performed. The J-tip guidewire should be able to twirl and bob freely within the lumen of the stent. After the guidewire is across the stent, intraluminal position can be checked using a 5-Fr straight angiographic catheter passed over the guidewire. Any resistance as the catheter passes through the stent indicates a false passage. Use a small field view for magnification, and oblique views if needed. Passing the guidewire through the interstices of the stent will lead to complications if it is not recognized that this has occurred.

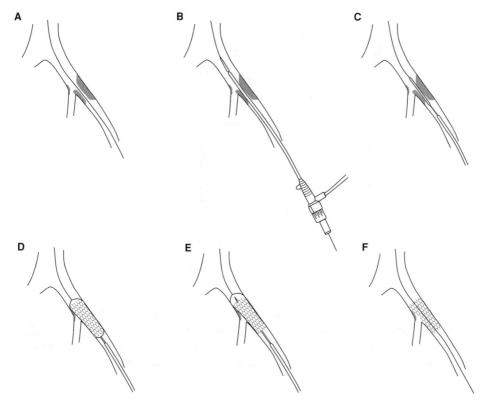

Fig. 7 Tapering a balloon-expandable stent. (**A**) The guidewire is passed through an iliac artery stenosis. (**B**) The sheath and dilator are advanced through the lesion. (**C**) The balloon and mounted stent are advanced through the lesion and the sheath is withdrawn. (**D**) The balloon-expandable stent is deployed to a size appropriate to the diameter of the external iliac artery. (**E**) A larger diameter angioplasty balloon is used to enlarge the proximal end of the stent. (**F**) A slight taper of the stent is created across the iliac bifurcation.

GOING NAKED: PLACEMENT OF A BALLOON-EXPANDABLE STENT WITHOUT A SHEATH

Placement of balloon-expandable stents was designed to be performed with a sheath. Occasionally, however, placement of the sheath into the desired location across the lesion is difficult, dangerous, or both, especially with highly tortuous approach arteries or when the sizable sheath hangs up on the lesion itself (Fig. 10). One option is to use a short-access sheath. Advance the balloon and stent over the guidewire and through the lesion without a sheath to protect them. Use a premounted stent, which comes in a package with the stent already sealed onto the balloon (Cordis, a Johnson & Johnson Co., Miami, Florida, U.S.A.). If treating a critical stenosis, predilate the lesion so that the stent will pass through without being dislodged from the balloon.

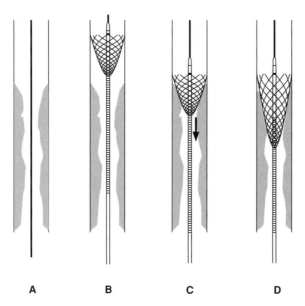

A   B   C   D

Fig. 8 Moving a self-expandable stent. (**A**) The guidewire is placed across the lesion. (**B**) Stent deployment is initiated more proximally than its final intended location. (**C**) The entire delivery apparatus is withdrawn to move the proximal expanded end of the stent into the lesion. (**D**) After correct positioning, deployment continues.

TECHNIQUE: BAILOUT MANEUVERS FOR BALLOON-EXPANDABLE STENTS

1. Sheath won't advance across the lesion: Dilate the lesion, and then advance again. Consider using a stiffer guidewire.
2. Balloon with stent will not pass through the sheath: The sheath may have kinked (Fig. 11). Consider pulling the kinked part of the sheath back into a straighter segment of the artery and try again to pass the balloon and stent. If unsuccessful, pull out the balloon and stent with the sheath but leave the guidewire in place. Change the sheath and start again. Consider using a self-expanding stent for tortuous arteries (Predilate the lesion; use a larger sheath and stiffer wire)
3. Loose stent inside the sheath: Pull out the sheath, balloon catheter, and stent. Leave the guidewire, if possible. Use fluoroscopy to ensure that the stent comes out with the sheath.
4. Loose stent on the catheter shaft: Pull the balloon back into the stent using the tip of the sheath to pin the stent. Pull the stent back into the sheath, if possible. Use a partially inflated balloon to pull the stent and remove the sheath. If the stent cannot be pulled back into the sheath, pin the back end of the stent with the tip of the sheath and deploy in a neutral location (Fig. 12).

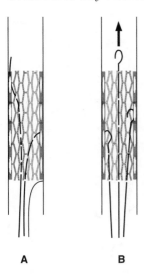

A   B

Fig. 9 Crossing a stent. (**A**) After deployment of a stent, there are many potential routes of false passage. (**B**) Passage through the struts of a stent is usually avoided with a J-tip guidewire.

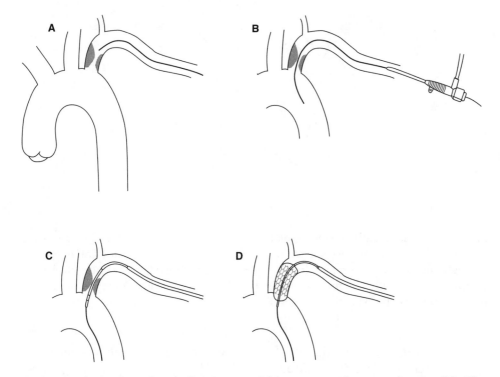

Fig. 10 Placement of a balloon-expandable stent without a sheath. (**A**) The guidewire is placed across a lesion at the origin of the subclavian artery. (**B**) A transbrachial sheath is placed but the artery is too tortuous to permit safe passage of the sheath through the lesion. (**C**) The angioplasty balloon with premounted stent is passed beyond the sheath and through the lesion. (**D**) The stent is deployed.

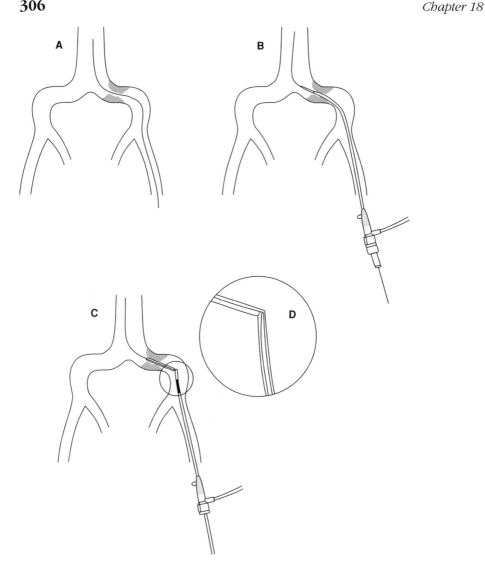

Fig. 11 Kinked sheath prevents passage of a stent. (**A**) The guidewire is passed through a lesion in a tortuous iliac artery. (**B**) The sheath and dilator are advanced through the lesion in preparation for stent placement. (**C**) After the dilator is removed, the sheath becomes kinked. (**D**) The balloon with mounted stent cannot pass because the sheath is kinked.

5. Loose stent on the guidewire: Advance small balloon into the stent to flare the end and stabilize. Deploy in a neutral location (Fig. 13).
6. Stent embolizes: Use a long sheath and cardiac biopsy forceps or a loop snare to pull or push into a favorable location to abandon (internal iliac, deep femoral, or tibial arteries) or to retrieve surgically (common femoral artery).

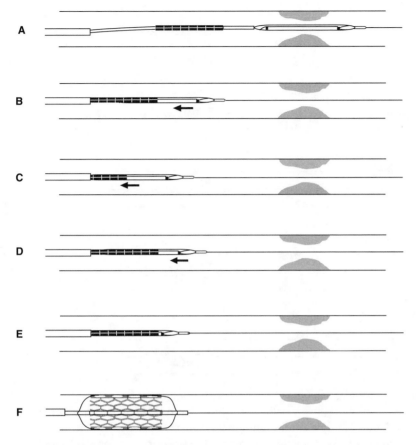

Fig. 12 Balloo-expandable stent is loose on the catheter shaft. (**A**) A stent becomes dislodged from its position on the balloon catheter during passage through the sheath. (**B**) An attempt is made to pull the stent back into the sheath. (**C**) The entire sheath is removed with the stent inside. (**D**) If the stent cannot be dragged back into the sheath, the end of the stent is pinned with the tip of the sheath. (**E**) The balloon is pulled back into the stent to reload. (**F**) The sheath is withdrawn and the newly remounted stent is deployed in a neutral location.

7. Balloon ruptures during deployment of balloon-expandable stent: Perform high-pressure, hand-powered balloon inflation with saline solution in an attempt to overwhelm the hole in the leaky balloon (Fig. 14). Advance the sheath to pin the stent so that it is not withdrawn with the balloon. Rotate and remove the ruptured balloon, cross the stent with another balloon, and inflate.
8. Dissection at the end of the stent: Place a new overlapping stent (Fig. 15).
9. Stent tilts: Some balloon-expanding stents are too rigid for tortuous arteries. Self-expanding stents are often a better choice (Fig. 16). Place another stent to straighten the curve.

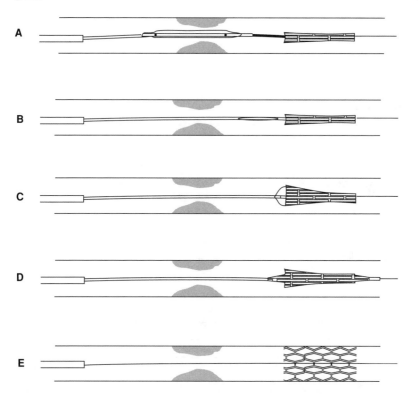

Fig. 13 Balloon-expandable stent is loose on the guidewire. If improperly mounted, the stent may shoot forward off the balloon during inflation. The end of the stent may be partially flared and dangling on the guidewire. (**A**) The guidewire is advanced to allow room to maneuver. (**B**) A smaller, lower profile balloon is exchanged. (**C**) One end of the stent is flared further. (**D**) The appropriately sized balloon is substituted. (**E**) The stent is deployed in a neutral position.

10. Balloon sticks in the expanded stent: Material is caught in the struts. Do not yank because the material may fragment. Rotate the catheter, reinflate, push in to advance, and then withdraw. If that does not work, advance the sheath so that the tip of the sheath can at once hold the stent in place and act as a funneling device to accept the torn balloon.
11. Stent requires surgical removal: If the stent is fully deployed, the artery probably requires reconstruction. An artery cannot be occluded with a clamp at the location of a stent. The ends of the stent are sharp!
12. Avoid deployment of stent in the sheath: Be sure that the tip of the sheath has been withdrawn adequately to avoid capturing the end of the stent.

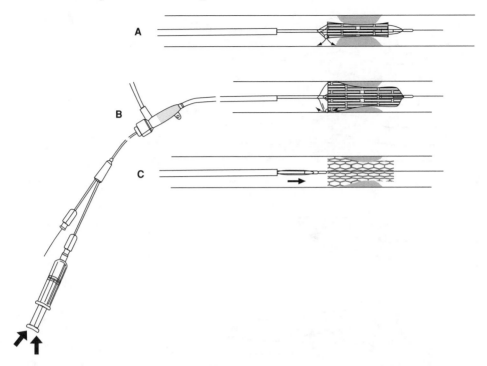

Fig. 14 Balloon ruptures during deployment of balloon-expandable stent. (**A**) The angioplasty balloon ruptures on the sharp edge of the stent during deployment. (**B**) A high-pressure, hand-powered inflation attempts to overwhelm the leak in the balloon. The ends of the stent flare enough to prevent immediate migration. (**C**) A new balloon is placed to complete the deployment.

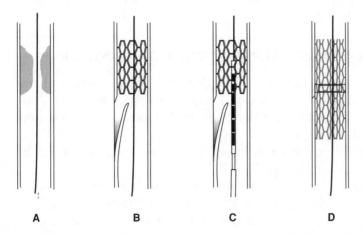

Fig. 15 Dissection at the end of the stent. (**A**) A guidewire is placed across the lesion. (**B**) A stent is placed but a dissection flap develops at the interface between the lesion and the adjacent nondiseased segment. (**C**) Another stent is advanced into position with a slight overlap of the previously placed stent. (**D**) Stent placement repairs the dissection.

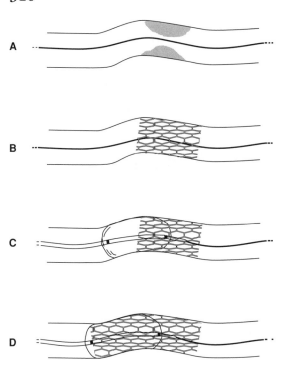

Fig. 16 Tilted balloon-expandable stent. (**A**) A guidewire is passed through a stenosis along a curve in the artery. (**B**) A stent is placed across the lesion. The combination of the curvature of the artery and the location of the lesion prevents the edge of the stent from being well opposed to the arterial wall. (**C**) Balloon angioplasty of the protruding end of the stent is performed. (**D**) If angioplasty is not successful, another stent is placed to decrease the curvature of the artery and force the edge of the stent against the wall.

TECHNIQUE: BAILOUT MANEUVERS FOR SELF-EXPANDING STENTS

1. End of the stent is not fully expanded: The hoop strength of the self-expanding stent may not be adequate to compress the lesion. Dilate the body of the stent to make sure it is properly seeded, and then dilate the ends (Fig. 17).
2. Stent is undersized for given artery: The chosen stent is too small. There is no good solution.
3. Stent extends into undesired location: Dilate the stent to foreshorten it (Fig. 18). This works well with a Wallstent. Other types of self-expanding stents can sometimes be moved a very short distance by inflating a balloon and pulling gently on the catheter.
4. Stent location is inaccurate: The only way to avoid this is to deploy the end of the stent first that has the greatest precision requirement (Fig. 19).
5. The end of the stent extends into the hemostatic introducer sheath: The stent will not deploy. If the tip of the sheath does not have

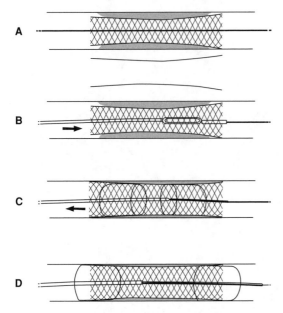

Fig. 17 End of the self-expanding is not expanded. (**A**) A self-expanding stent is placed but one end does not fully expand to meet the vessel wall. (**B**) A balloon catheter is passed. (**C**) Angioplasty is performed along the entire length of the stent. The body of the stent is dilated first to ensure that it is well embedded into the vessel wall. As the stent is dilated, the length may change slightly. (**D**) The ends of the stent are dilated last because the balloon may rupture on the sharp wire ends of the stent.

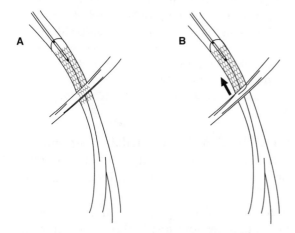

Fig. 18 Self-expanding stent extends into undesired location. (**A**) A Wallstent is placed in the distal external iliac artery. The distal end of the stent extends into the common femoral artery. The Wallstent is flexible enough to be placed across joints but it should be avoided when possible. (**B**) Slight overdilation along the length of the stent with angioplasty causes the stent to shorten a few millimeters.

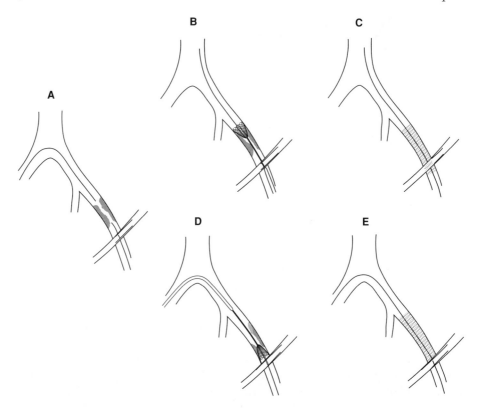

Fig. 19 Self-expanding stent location is inaccurate. Deployment should be initiated at the end where the most accuracy is required. (**A**) An external iliac artery lesion can be approached either antegrade or retrograde. (**B**) Wallstent placement through a retrograde approach ensures precise placement of the proximal end of the stent. (**C**) The final length of the stent may be difficult to predict. The distal end of the stent extends into undiseased common femoral artery. (**D**) Wallstent placement through an antegrade approach places the distal end of the stent first because the working room between the inguinal ligament and the lesion is limited. (**E**) The excess length of the upper end of the stent extends into the proximal external iliac artery.

a radiopaque marker, it may be difficult to visualize. Puff contrast through the sheath. Pull the sheath back slightly while holding the stent delivery catheter in place to release the crimped stent (Fig. 20).

6. Stent collapses in its midsection: Repeat angioplasty. If that is unsuccessful, place a balloon-expandable stent inside the self-expanding stent (Fig. 21).

7. Balloon breaks on the end of the stent: Balloon the end of the stent last or use a thicker polymer balloon.

8. Artery with stent in it requires clamping: Use large, shodded arterial clamp. The artery can be clamped enough to occlude inflow but may damage the stent.

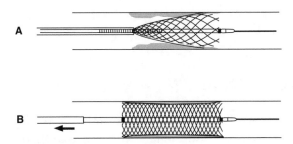

Fig. 20 Partially deployed self-expanding stent extends into hemostatic introducer sheath. (**A**) Stent deployment begins but the second end of the stent cannot be deployed because the tip of the access sheath impinges on the stent. This occurs when working room between the deployment site and the arterial entry site is limited. (**B**) The hemostatic access sheath is withdrawn enough to permit the stent to expand. A sheath with a radiopaque tip may help avoid this problem.

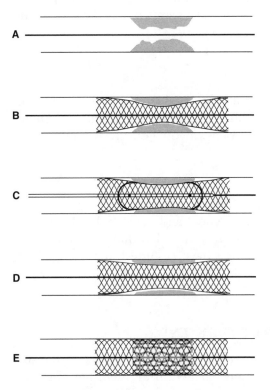

Fig. 21 Self-expanding stent collapses in its midsection. (**A**) A guidewire is placed across the lesion. (**B**) A Stent is placed but remains partially constrained in its midsection. (**C**) Balloon angioplasty is performed. (**D**) Because self-expanding stent hoop strength is low, a recalcitrant lesion may impinge on the stent, which results in incomplete expansion. A central stent narrowing can also occur if the stent is placed across a segment with too sharp a turn. (**E**) If angioplasty is unsuccessful, a balloon-expandable stent is placed to resolve the stenosis.

9. Stent requires surgical removal: The stent may be extracted by squeezing it, which narrows the whole stent.

Acute Complications of Stent Placement

Complications that occur during stent placement or immediately thereafter include arterial dissection and/or occlusion, arterial rupture, migration or embolization of the stent, or embolization of atherosclerotic material.

ARTERIAL DISSECTION

If acute arterial dissection occurs in juxtaposition to a stent, an additional stent is placed in this location (Fig. 15). The lead point for arterial dissection associated with stent placement is usually within a centimeter of the end of the stent. A stent is placed in this segment even if it is not clear exactly where the lead point of the dissection is located.

ARTERIAL OCCLUSION

The stented site may occlude as a result of arterial dissection or as a result of placement of a stent that is not fully expanded. After stent placement, additional balloon dilatation is usually performed to ensure full expansion of the stent.

ARTERIAL RUPTURE

If arterial rupture occurs during stent placement and the stent has been fully deployed, a balloon catheter is inserted and placed within the stent along the area where the rupture is thought to have occurred and the balloon is inflated. A covered stent is placed in the same location or emergency operative repair is undertaken.

MIGRATION OR EMBOLIZATION OF THE STENT

Migration of the stent may occur during deployment, usually because the size of the stent that was required was underestimated. If the stent has migrated enough that the area of interest has not been adequately stented, another stent is placed in this location.

EMBOLIZATION OF ATHEROSCLEROTIC MATERIAL

Distal embolization may occur as a result of instrumentation of a friable atherosclerotic lesion. It is unusual for further embolization to occur after the entire lesion has been covered with stents.

Chronic Complications of Stent Placement

Chronic complications from stent placement that may develop over time include intimal hyperplasia, recurrent stenosis, infection, and damage to the stent from external forces.

INTIMAL HYPERPLASIA

Intimal hyperplasia can be treated with repeat balloon dilatation, additional stents, directional atherectomy, or surgery.

RECURRENT STENOSIS

If recurrent stenosis occurs in juxtaposition to a stent, an overlapping stent is placed.

INFECTION

Infection of a stent is rare and is managed by excising the stent and the arterial segment.

STENT DAMAGE

Stents can be damaged by external forces. Chronic repetitive shoulder motion with compression of a stented subclavian artery against the first rib leads to stent fracture. Stents can also be crushed, especially the balloon-expandable stents, by arterial clamps, blood pressure cuffs, motion at joints, and external blunt trauma.

Selected Readings

Dotter CT. Transluminally placed coilspring endarterial tube grafts: Long-term patency in canine popliteal artery. Invest Radiol 1969; 4:327–332.

Krankenberg H, Schlüter M, Steinkamp HJ, et al. Nitinol stent implantation versus percutaneous transluminal angioplasty in superficial femoral artery lesions up to 10 cm in length: The femoral artery stenting trial (FAST). Circulation 2007; 116(3):285–292.

Perera GB, Lyden SP. Current trends in lower extremity revascularization. Surg Clin North Am 2007; 87(5):1135–1147.

Sarwar S, Al-Absi A, Wall BM. Catastrophic cholesterol crystal embolization after endovascular stent placement for peripheral vascular disease. Am J Med Sci 2008; 335(5):403–406.

Schmehl J, Tepe G. Current status of bare and drug-eluting stents in infrainguinal peripheral vascular disease. Expert Rev Cardiovasc Ther 2008; 6(4):531–538.

19

The Infrarenal Aorta, Aortic Bifurcation, and Iliac Arteries: Advice About Balloon Angioplasty and Stent Placement

Balloon angioplasty and stents have had a profound impact upon the management of atherosclerotic occlusive disease of the aortoiliac segment. The long-term results of endovascular intervention are not quite as good as with open surgery, but they are reasonable. The long-term success of aortoiliac intervention is closer to the results of open surgery than any other endovascular intervention. In addition, the short-term risk of percutaneous intervention is so much less than with open surgery that endovascular approaches have become the treatment of choice for most patients. Open surgery is reserved only for patients who have failed endovascular intervention or in whom a percutaneous approach is not technically feasible. Chapter 9 provides a step-by-step approach for crossing the aortic bifurcation. Chapter 10 provides information about aortoiliac arteriography. Supplies for aortoiliac intervention are listed in Table 1. Aortoiliac occlusive disease is usually treated with coaxial catheters on a 0.035 in. platform. Most aortoiliac lesions can be treated using 6- or 7-Fr sheath access.

Aorta

Isolated, focal stenoses of the infrarenal abdominal aorta often respond to balloon angioplasty alone (Fig. 1). However, the availability of stents permits the treatment of more complex lesions with endovascular intervention. If the aorta is suspected as a source of emboli or the aorta is inflow for more distal reconstruction, a primary stent should be considered. Selective stenting should be performed for inadequate results of balloon angioplasty. Stents provide the opportunity to approach lesions that would not be expected to respond to balloon angioplasty alone. Aortic lesions that extend to the bifurcation also require kissing balloons or kissing stents placed through each iliac artery.

Lesions that are limited to the infrarenal aorta may be accessed through a unilateral femoral approach on either side. Lesions of the aorta that extend near or into the aortic bifurcation should be accessed with a guidewire placed through each iliac artery. This is discussed in more detail in the next section. If there is coincidental, nonbifurcation, unilateral iliac disease that also requires treatment along with a separate aortic lesion, the access should be ipsilateral to the iliac lesion. This permits treatment of both the aortic and iliac lesions through the same approach without passing guidewires and sheaths over the aortic bifurcation.

Retrograde passage of the guidewire is performed from the femoral puncture site and an aortogram is performed using a flush catheter. After appropriate arteriography is completed and the decision is made to proceed with treatment, 50 to 75 U/kg of heparin is administered. The operator may consider a larger bolus of heparin when treating very complex or embolizing lesions or preocclusive stenoses or if longer indwelling catheter times are

Table 1 Supplies for Aortoiliac Intervention

Category	Subtype	Description	Length/Size	Fr/in.
Guidewire	Starting guidewire	Bentson	145 cm, length	0.035 in. diameter
	Selective guidewire	Glidewire	150 cm	0.035 in. (angled tip)
	Exchange guidewire	Amplatz super-stiff	180 cm	0.035 in.
Catheter	Flush catheter	Omni-flush	65 cm, length	4 Fr
	Selective catheter	Angled glide cath	65 cm	5 Fr
	Exchange catheter	Straight	70 cm	5 Fr
Sheath	Access sheath	Standard hemostatic access	12 cm length	6 Fr, 7 Fr, 9 Fr
	Straight sheath	Long straight with radiopaque tip	30, 35 cm	7 Fr, 9 Fr[b]
	Selective sheath	Over bifurcation	40 cm, 45 cm, 55 cm	6 Fr, 7 Fr
Balloon	Balloon angioplasty catheters	Balloon diameter	6, 7, 8, 10, 12, 14, 16, 18 mm	
		Balloon length	4 cm	
		Catheter shaft	75 cm	5 Fr
Stent[a]	Balloon-expandable	Stent diameter	6–22 mm	
		Stent length	25–50 mm	
		Delivery on 75-cm-length angioplasty balloon catheter		
	Self-expanding	Nitinol or elgiloy diameter Stent length Stent	8, 10, 12, 14 mm	
		Delivery catheter	40, 60, 80 mm	
		Length	80 cm	

[a] A 9- or 10-Fr sheath is used to introduce large-diameter balloons for aortic angioplasty (>12-mm diameter) or a Wallstent larger than 14 mm.

[b] A 9-Fr sheath is used to introduce a large Palmaz stent (P308) for diameters of 10 to 12 mm.

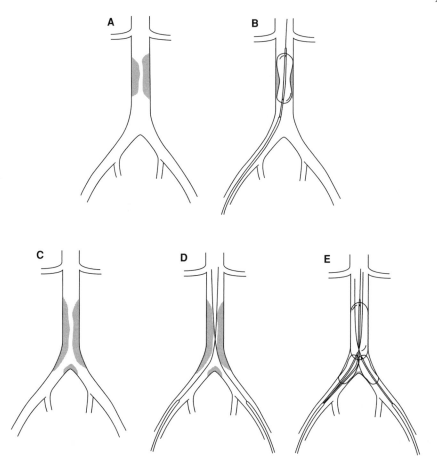

Fig. 1 Endovascular approaches to aortic lesions. (**A**) A significant but focal lesion is isolated within the infrarenal abdominal aorta. (**B**) Balloon angioplasty of the aortic lesion is performed. (**C**) A more extensive lesion involves the infrarenal aorta and its bifurcation. (**D**) The complex lesion is approached by placing a guidewire retrograde through each femoral artery. (**E**) Balloon angioplasty is performed in the aorta and kissing balloons are used to dilate the bifurcation.

anticipated. The catheter is removed and the appropriately sized sheath is placed through the femoral entry site (Fig. 2). If there is significant tortuosity, the lesion is very complex, or a particularly large sheath is anticipated, the operator should consider placing an Amplatz guidewire to provide extra support during the intervention. Standard-length hemostatic access sheaths of 10 to 12 cm may be used for simple balloon angioplasty and placement of stents. However, it is also useful to consider a 30- or 45-cm sheath with a radiopaque tip to treat aortic lesions. Through this type of sheath, interval arteriography may be performed with contrast administered in proximity to the target lesion site. The size of the sheath depends upon the intended diameter to which the aorta is to be dilated and whether a stent will be placed. Balloon angioplasty may be performed up to 10-mm diameter using

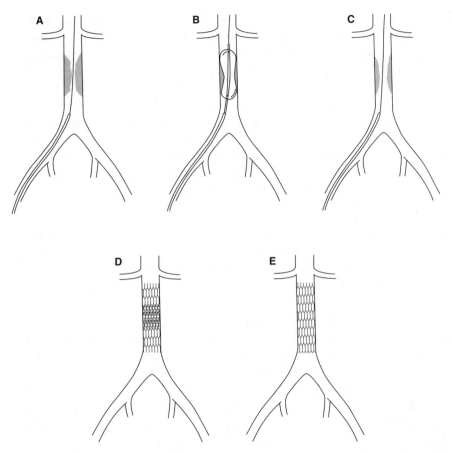

Fig. 2 Balloon angioplasty of the aorta. (**A**) A guidewire is placed through a stenosis in the infrarenal aorta. (**B**) Aortic balloon angioplasty is performed. (**C**) A residual stenosis requires additional therapy. (**D**) Palmaz stent placement requires the use of two overlapping stents to cover the entire lesion. (**E**) A single self-expanding stent placed in the infrarenal aorta is another option.

a 5-Fr catheter shaft through a 6-Fr sheath. Self-expanding nitinol stents up to 12 mm in diameter can also be placed through a 6-Fr sheath. Dilatation to 12 or 14 mm is performed using a 5-Fr catheter shaft through a 7-Fr sheath. A 9-Fr sheath is required for 16- to 20-mm balloons. Balloon-expandable stents up to 9 or 10 mm in diameter may be placed through 7-Fr sheaths. A 9-Fr sheath is required for balloon-expandable stents up to 12 or 14 mm. Larger diameters require 10- or 12-Fr sheaths. Self-expanding stents up to 14 mm in diameter may be placed using 7-Fr sheaths, with larger stents placed through 9-Fr sheaths.

Accurate sizing of an artery for balloon angioplasty is usually simpler for other arterial segments since the usual range of diameter sizes varies from 2 to 4 mm in most vascular beds. Aortic angioplasty is performed with balloons ranging from 8 to 18 mm in diameter. Sizing the intended diameter of the aorta may be challenging because of the broad range of potential sizes, but there are several options. A flush catheter with 1-cm markers may be used for the aortogram, and the known distance between markers may be used to calculate the desired diameter of the aorta for angioplasty. If intravascular ultrasound is available, this method probably provides the most accurate representation of vessel diameter. This modality requires a moderate-sized sheath that would also be required for aortic angioplasty. Another method is to proceed with balloon angioplasty using a balloon that is an underestimation of the probable aortic diameter and compare the inflated balloon profile to the preintervention aortogram. The selected balloon is advanced over the guidewire and into position using externally placed or bony markers.

The balloon is inflated under fluoroscopy. The aorta may rupture at lower pressure than smaller-diameter vessels so inflation is performed cautiously. Initial inflation with a slightly undersized balloon may be performed to evaluate how the lesion will respond to dilatation. Less than 8 atm of pressure is usually required to dilate aortic lesions. Larger balloons tend to have longer shoulders that extend a centimeter or more beyond the location of the radiopaque marker. The shoulders of the balloon must be placed so that they do not extend into an area not intended for dilatation, such as the proximal iliac artery. Balloon inventory for diameters larger than 10 mm is usually limited, so catheter availability should be confirmed prior to the procedure. If the appropriately sized balloons are not available, two equally sized balloons of half the desired diameter are placed retrograde, one through each femoral artery, and inflated together.

The balloon is brought to full profile and is then deflated. Repeat inflations may be performed if the waist has not resolved. The balloon catheter is withdrawn. Balloon deflation takes longer because the large balloon must empty through a relatively small lumen. Completion aortography is performed by exchanging the balloon catheter for an arteriographic catheter or by administering contrast retrograde through the sheath.

Because the infrarenal aorta is a large vessel, clinical success is often achieved despite an angiographically suboptimal appearance. In practice, a lumen of 10 to 12 mm is usually sufficient to support bilateral iliac flow. A major risk of aortic angioplasty, especially with a large plaque burden, is lower-extremity embolization. A lesion that presents with embolization or appears to be prone to embolize can be treated with primary stent placement or stent–graft placement with outflow control (Fig. 3). However, it is important to ensure that the lesion is not contained within a small aneursym.

A large plaque load also increases the likelihood of a residual stenosis. The pressure is measured if it is not clear whether a bulky, residual plaque constitutes a hemodynamically significant lesion. If the lesion is significant,

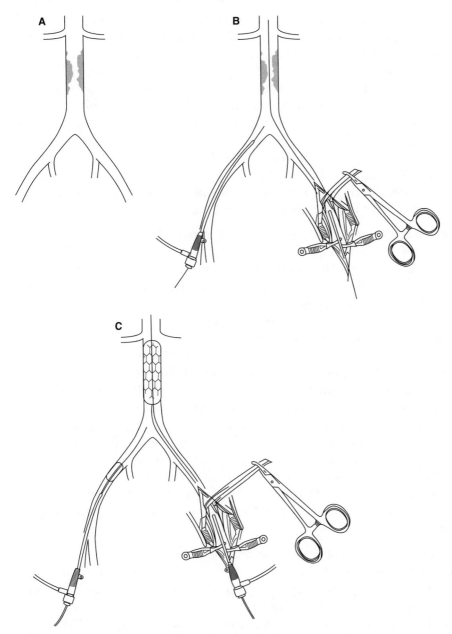

Fig. 3 Management of an embolizing aortic lesion. (**A**) An ulcerated aortic lesion presents with embolization. (**B**) Percutaneous access is obtained through one femoral artery and open access is obtained through the other femoral artery. (**C**) An occlusion balloon is placed in the proximal right external iliac artery using percutaneous access to prevent distal embolization. A stent is placed through the open left femoral access. The left lower-extremity outflow is clamped to prevent embolization.

stent placement is a reasonable option (see chap. 18). Many operators favor primary stent placement for aortic lesions, especially if there is a high degree of irregularity of the surface or a substantial amount of plaque. Primary stent placement permits the plaque to be caged by the stent and may decrease the likelihood of embolization or fragmentation during angioplasty. Choosing which stent to use can be a challenge. Self-expanding stents offer the advantage that the final resting diameter may be estimated to within 2 to 3 mm, as long as the selected stent is oversized and not too small in diameter. The balloon-expandable stents have better hoop strength and the precision of placement is slightly better. However, the diameter size must be accurate. Too small a stent diameter upon placement will leave the stent in an unstable position and it may migrate before it can be fully expanded.

When planning stent placement, a super-stiff guidewire may be used to take slack out of the system and improve placement accuracy. The appropriately sized sheath should be placed. A long sheath (35 cm) with a radiopaque tip is useful. Supplemental arteriography may be performed through the sheath during stent deployment. Landmarks must be carefully considered and distances measured. Distance from the renal arteries and the aortic bifurcation should be considered. If the lesion extends to the aortic bifurcation, and this segment also requires treatment, it is probably best to place the aortic stent first, with single-guidewire access in the aorta (Fig. 4). A sheath is placed in the proximal common iliac artery on the contralateral side. After the aortic stent is placed, the contralateral guidewire is advanced very carefully through the aortic stent. Kissing iliac stents can then be placed, advancing inside the distal end of the aortic stent if necessary. Be careful to make sure the guidewire is in the lumen and not passing behind the struts of the aortic stent. Placement of the stent too close to renal arteries should be avoided. If the patient requires an aortofemoral bypass at a later time, stents placed in the very proximal infrarenal aorta will necessitate suprarenal cross-clamp of the aorta.

Self-expanding stents offer the advantage of a relatively larger stent diameter for a given sheath size. For example, a 7-Fr sheath accommodates 12- to 14-mm diameter self-expanding stents, whereas the largest balloon-expandable stent that can be placed through this sheath is 8 to 10 mm. Self-expanding stents should be oversized for the intended final diameter by about 2 to 3 mm. Nitinol stent length shortens by a few percent when expanded but Wallstent length changes significantly with placement. The final resting length must be carefully estimated to ensure that the distal end of the Wallstent does not extend beyond the aortic bifurcation. Any location along the length of the Wallstent that does not reach its estimated final diameter causes the length of the stent to increase. When placing a self-expanding stent across a ledge-like lesion, place the leading end of the stent 2 cm or more proximal to the ledge. This allows the proximal end of the stent to be opposed to the aortic wall proximal to the lesion. If

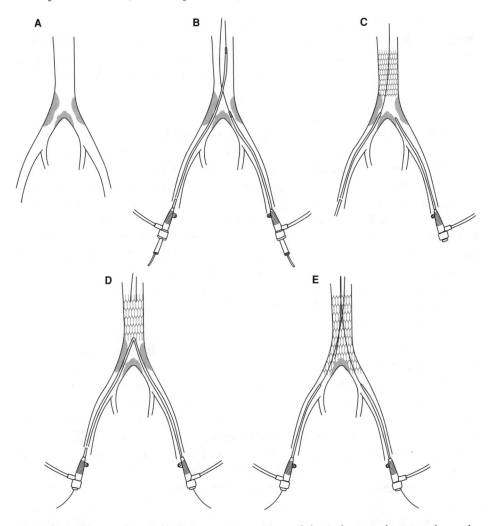

Fig. 4 Endovascular aortoiliac reconstruction. (**A**) A lesion that involves the infrarenal aorta and the iliac arteries can be treated with a multistent reconstruction. (**B**) Sheaths and guidewires are placed through each iliac artery. The sheath intended for delivery of the aortic stent (*the right side in this example*) is advanced into the aorta. (**C**) The guidewire is withdrawn from the contralateral (*left*) side so that it will not be trapped behind the aortic stent. A stent is placed in the aorta. (**D**) The contralateral guidewire is advanced through the aortic stent and both sheaths are advanced. (**E**) Kissing stents are placed with their leading edges up to or even inside the aortic stent.

the stent is placed too low, it will be constrained by the lesion and may even pop down distal to the lesion before it can be fully dilated. Self-expanding stents have an advantage at the larger diameters of 20 mm or more. In this range, self-expanding stents are available up to 28 mm that can be placed through an 11-Fr sheath. The only corresponding balloon-expandable stent available is a large Palmaz stent that is 5 cm in length and requires a large sheath, at least 12 Fr, which can accommodate the large-diameter balloon and the stent simultaneously. Chapter 18 contains a detailed discussion of stent placement technique. After placement of a self-expanding stent, balloon angioplasty fully dilates the stent and embeds it into the aortic wall.

Treating a heavily calcified lesion poses a risk of rupture if overdilation is performed. The best approach in this case may be to place an oversized self-expanding stent that is well opposed to the aortic wall proximal and distal to the lesion, and then to gradually dilate the lesion with progressively larger diameter balloons. If the patient starts to have severe pain, the procedure can be stopped safely, even if there is some residual stenosis. The challenge with self-expanding stents is that the trailing end of the stent lands in a less easily predictable location. Most aortic stents are placed from a femoral approach. The tip end of the stent will deploy first. The hub end, or trailing end, will deploy on the basis of the location of the whole stent; if the length requirements are misjudged, the lower end of the self-expanding stent could deploy in the iliac artery, rather than be proximal to the aortic bifurcation.

When using a balloon-expandable stent, the operator must decide whether to advance the dilator and sheath through the aortic lesion. Initial recommendations included this maneuver so that the stent was not rubbed off the balloon catheter. If a hand-mounted stent is being used, as is sometimes the case with the larger diameter stents, placing the sheath through the lesion in order to deliver the stent in a protected manner is advisable. If a premounted stent is being used, which is a stent that is mounted on the balloon at the factory, this step is probably not necessary. If sheath passage is indicated and the residual lumen within the lesion is inadequate to permit sheath placement, predilatation is required. A 9-Fr sheath requires at least a 3-mm lumen for placement. A slightly undersized balloon may be used to place a balloon-expandable stent initially, as long as the stent expands enough to be held in place by the lesion. The stent can then be further expanded with a larger balloon. Some balloon expandable stents, such as the Palmaz stents, can be pushed beyond the limit of their stated diameters. However, the length will shorten further. For lesions longer than 2 cm, more than one balloon-expandable stent is used or a self-expanding stent is selected. After placement of a balloon-expandable stent, each end of the stent is dilated to be sure that it has assumed a cylindrical shape. If the lesion is close to aortic bifurcation, the stent will tend to lean toward the side opposite the femoral access when deployed because of the guidewire bias induced by coming from one side or the other. Consider placing a guidewire through a contralateral femoral access and using kissing balloons in the lower end of the stent. These balloons should be one-half the diameter of the stent. A 16-mm stent can be dilated with bilateral 8-mm balloons. Completion arteriography is performed by placing a flush catheter over the guidewire and administering contrast proximal to the stent site or by administering contrast retrograde through the sheath.

Aortic Bifurcation

Aortic bifurcation stenoses that extend into the proximal common iliac arteries are treated with a kissing-balloon technique (Fig. 5). This is usually aortic plaque, concentrated especially along the posterior wall, which has extended into the common iliac arteries. A guidewire is placed through each femoral artery and advanced into the aorta. If the femoral arteries are pulseless, use can be made of the techniques described in chapter 3 for percutaneous puncture of a pulseless femoral artery. A micropuncture approach may be used, as described in the same chapter. Systemic heparin administration is not absolutely required for simple balloon angioplasty, but 25 to 50 U/kg should be considered. If a complex reconstruction, prolonged catheter time, or stent placement is anticipated, 50 to 75 U/kg of heparin should be administered. Starting guidewires are exchanged for Amplatz guidewires (0.035-in. diameter, 180-cm length) through a straight exchange catheter.

Sheaths are selected as described in the earlier section. If balloon angioplasty with selective stenting is planned, 6-Fr, standard-length access sheaths are adequate for balloons up to 8 mm in diameter, and 7-Fr sheaths are used for 9- or 10-mm-diameter balloons. Appropriately and equally sized balloons are advanced over the guidewires. The balloons are positioned so that the proximal radiopaque markers on each balloon overlap each other. The balloons are simultaneously inflated to the same pressure using dual inflation devices. This allows the entire aortic bifurcation and proximal iliac segments to be dilated simultaneously to the same pressure. This approach facilitates

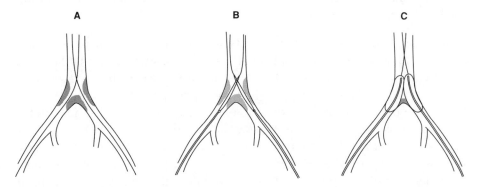

Fig. 5   Management of a lesion in the aortic bifurcation using kissing balloons. (**A**) Bilateral guidewires are placed across a stenosis in the aortic bifurcation. (**B**) One balloon catheter is placed retrograde through each femoral artery and the proximal radiopaque markers are placed so that they overlap. (**C**) The equally sized balloons are inflated simultaneously to the same pressure to dilate the lesion in the bifurcation.

fracture of the often circumferential cast of plaque that develops at the aortic bifurcation.

The kissing-balloon technique is usually performed with balloons in the range of 6 to 10 mm in diameter. The size of the balloon must match not only the proximal common iliac arteries, but also the distal aorta. If there is significant narrowing in the distal aorta, it is important to remember that two separate balloons expanded simultaneously reach a large additive diameter. If 10-mm kissing balloons are used, the distal aorta must be 20 mm. If the aorta cannot quite accommodate that diameter, the balloons can be withdrawn just slightly to decrease the overlap between the two balloons in the distal aorta. In this case, most of the length of each balloon will be in the iliac artery, rather than in the aorta.

If results are not satisfactory, or if residual stenosis is significant following angioplasty, or if the operator believes that these lesions are best to be stented, then kissing-stent placement can be used to reconstruct the aortic bifurcation (Fig. 6). This technique raises the aortic flow divider by a few millimeters to a centimeter. Although either self-expanding or balloon-expandable stents may be used, balloon-expandable stents provide the advantage of better hoop strength to treat these orifice lesions. In addition, the proximal ends of the stents, which create the new aortic flow divider, are easier to match up during deployment since accuracy of balloon-expandable stent placement is excellent. Self-expanding stents are a better choice if there is a lot of contour change, diameter mismatch, or tortuosity between the aorta and the proximal iliac arteries. The accuracy of placement has improved with the addition of markers on the ends of the stents and the delivery catheters are also improved. The self-expanding stents, however, do not create a rigid flow divider if the bifurcation is being raised. Bilateral 6- or 7-Fr sheaths are usually adequate in size to handle either self-expanding or balloon-expanding stents.

Matching balloon-expandable stents are mounted on the same size balloons as were used for the angioplasty. Bilateral long sheaths, with dilators in place, are advanced into the distal aorta. Using fluoroscopy, the unexpanded stents are positioned so that the proximal radiopaque markers on the balloon catheters are parallel to each other, but not quite overlapping, as they are for kissing balloons alone. Examine the stents under fluoroscopy to be sure that they have not migrated on their respective balloons. The sheaths are gently withdrawn to expose the bilateral stents. The proximal ends of the stents are usually 2 to 10 mm proximal to the aortic flow divider, depending upon the amount of aortic plaque that must be treated. Road mapping may be used to outline the aortic bifurcation so that the stents are not placed more proximally than desired. Often times, the aortic outline can be observed on plain fluoroscopy because of the presence of calcification. Careful consideration should be given to the length of distal aorta to be stented. If the lesion extends more than a centimeter up into the aorta, a separate aortic stent secures inflow for the kissing stents at the bifurcation.

Kissing stents are best deployed with an assistant because balloon expansion must be performed simultaneously. Although an inflation device is not required to place all balloon-expandable stents, it is essential in this situation to maintain the balloon pressure at an equal level bilaterally. After

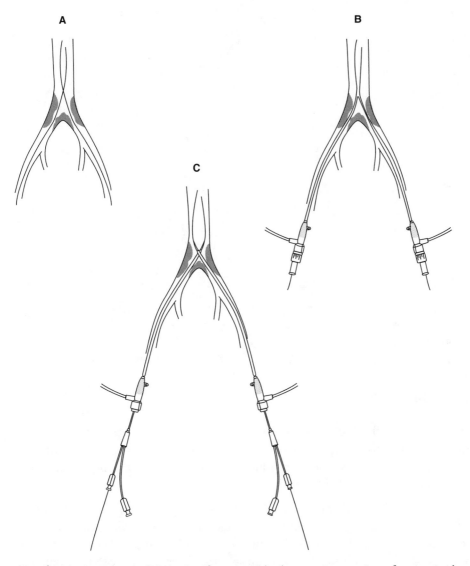

Fig. 6 Kissing stents. (**A**) A significant residual stenosis remains after angioplasty. (**B**) Long access sheaths are advanced into the distal aorta. (**C**) The dilators are removed. (**D**) Equally sized balloons with mounted stents are advanced through each sheath. (**E**) The stents are deployed bilaterally by inflating the balloons simultaneously to the same pressure. (**F**) Kissing stents can raise the aortic flow divider to reconstruct the bifurcation.

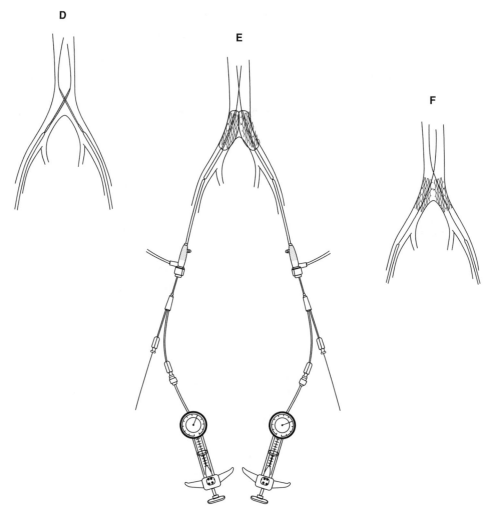

Fig. 6   (*Continued*)

stent placement, the balloons are reinflated at more proximal and distal positions to be sure that the stents have fully expanded. The balloon catheters are removed. A flush catheter is placed through one side and completion arteriography is performed.

The placement of self-expanding stents may be performed either with or without predilation. Predilating the lesion is usually advisable for the following reason. If the residual lumen is severely restricted, the stent may not expand sufficiently in order to allow placement of a poststent balloon angioplasty catheter. Because the metal mesh of the self-expanding stent does not have a lot of hoop strength, don't place exposed bare metal any higher into the aorta than is necessary. The stents are deployed gradually and simultaneously by the operator and an assistant and then postdilated with kissing balloons.

Iliac Artery

Iliac artery balloon angioplasty is *the* index endovascular procedure. It is a common procedure and has had a profound impact upon the management of atherosclerotic occlusive disease. This procedure has a three-decade track record and has been refined and improved along the way. Technical modifications, such as stents, have dramatically expanded the complexity of the pathology that can be treated with endovascular intervention. It has superceded its surgical predecessor, aortofemoral bypass, and has largely replaced this operation. In appropriately selected patients, overall results are quite good and risks are acceptable. The durable results of this operation have been extrapolated to angioplasty of other vascular beds in hope of justifying the broader use of balloon angioplasty at sites where there is much less long-term evidence of success. Failure of this procedure can often be treated with secondary endovascular procedures, and these rarely if ever take away later surgical options if they should become necessary.

An iliac artery lesion can be approached either retrograde, through the ipsilateral femoral artery, or antegrade, through the contralateral femoral artery or an upper-extremity puncture site (Fig. 7). The location of the lesion determines the approach. Lesions of the aortic bifurcation, which are discussed in the earlier section, are treated with kissing balloons. Nonorifice lesions of the proximal common iliac artery are treated with a retrograde approach. There is not adequate working room between the aortic bifurcation and the lesion to treat these with a contralateral, up-and-over approach. Midiliac lesions, from the middle section of the common iliac artery to the middle section of the external iliac artery, may be treated by using either an ipsilateral retrograde approach or a contralateral antegrade approach. Lesions of the distal several centimeters of external iliac artery must be treated with an antegrade approach, usually through the contralateral femoral artery, since there is not enough working room to maneuver through an ipsilateral femoral access.

A retrograde approach is performed by puncturing the common femoral artery distal to the iliac artery lesion. The femoral artery pulse may be diminished or absent (see chap. 3 for a detailed discussion and specific maneuvers for percutaneous access of the pulseless femoral artery). The ipsilateral retrograde approach is the most simple and direct once access has been obtained. The retrograde approach is useful for all iliac artery lesions except those in the very distal external iliac artery.

Standard, single-balloon angioplasty can be performed on iliac artery stenoses that begin a centimeter or more distal to the origin of the common iliac artery. Lesions that begin in the orifice of the common iliac artery pose a risk of pushing plaque into the contralateral iliac artery during balloon angioplasty. The kissing-balloon technique protects the contralateral side,

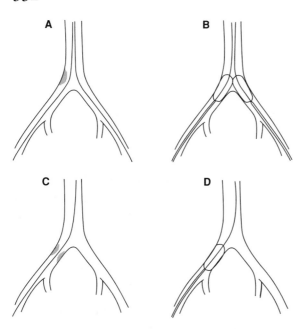

Fig. 7 Approaches to angioplasty of the iliac artery. (**A**) A very proximal common iliac artery lesion is present that requires treatment. (**B**) Proximal lesions are treated with kissing balloons, even if there appears to be minimal disease in the proximal contralateral iliac artery. (**C**) Proximal common iliac artery lesions that are distal to the iliac artery origin by a centimeter or more are also treated through an ipsilateral retrograde femoral approach. (**D**) This type of proximal common iliac artery lesion does not require a contralateral or kissing balloon. A balloon placed through the contralateral iliac artery and passed over the aortic bifurcation is not a good option for dilatation of this lesion, since there is not adequate working room between the aortic bifurcation and the lesion. (**E**) Midiliac lesions are located between the mid–common iliac artery and the mid–external iliac artery and may be treated through a choice of multiple approaches. (**F**) These lesions may be treated through an ipsilateral retrograde femoral approach. There is adequate working room for an ipsilateral femoral access and the lesion is not too near the aortic bifurcation. (**G**) Midiliac lesions may also be treated through a contralateral approach. The guidewire and balloon catheter are passed over the aortic bifurcation. This may also be performed through an up-and-over sheath with the tip placed in the proximal common iliac artery. (**H**) Distal external iliac artery lesions are located so that there is inadequate working room for an ipsilateral femoral approach. (**I**) Distal external iliac artery lesions are approached through the contralateral femoral artery using an up-and-over sheath.

even if there is no significant stenosis in the contralateral iliac origin. The challenging situation that often arises is a nonorifice proximal common iliac artery lesion that requires dilatation and the adjacent iliac artery origin is mildly or moderately diseased. In these cases, if the origin of the common iliac artery requires dilatation, kissing balloons should be used.

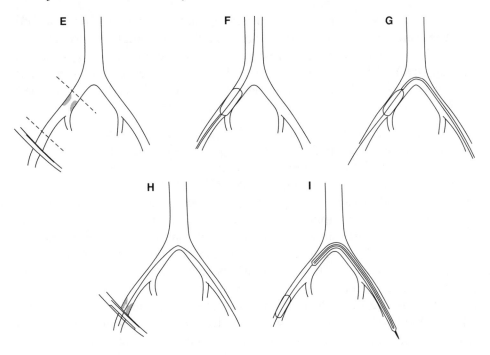

Fig. 7 (*Continued*)

Ipsilateral Retrograde Approach to the Iliac Artery

After the strategic arteriogram has been evaluated and the approach is selected, the lesion is crossed with a guidewire if it has not already been traversed. When arteriography has been performed through the ipsilateral femoral artery, the guidewire has already been placed across the lesion just to achieve sheath access. When arteriography has been performed through a contralateral femoral puncture, the operator has the option of passing the guidewire over the aortic bifurcation or placing a retrograde guidewire through a new ipsilateral puncture site. If the lesion is complex, the approach is tortuous, the femoral access is difficult, or a multilevel intervention is anticipated, consider placing a super-stiff guidewire. Guidewires that are 0.035 in. in diameter and 150 to 180 cm in length are used. The appropriate sheath is selected and inserted using the same guidelines as in the earlier section. Usually a 6- or 7-Fr sheath is adequate depending upon whether a stent is required. Short access sheaths of 10 or 12 cm are adequate for balloon angioplasty and for placement of stents. A radiopaque tip on the sheath is desirable. Sheaths that are long enough to reach the lesion, usually 25 cm or more, are inserted if balloon-expandable stent placement is likely or if extra support is needed. Heparin may be administered at 25 to 75 U/kg at the discretion of the operator.

There are occasions when it is appropriate to avoid placing a sheath over the aortic bifurcation. When the aortic bifurcation angle is very narrow, or heavily calcified, or severely diseased, it may make more sense to avoid this maneuver. If the groin in which the sheath is inserted is heavily calcified or scarred, this will also add to the friction, poor trackability, and diminished maneuverability.

If there has been a significant change in the location of the image intensifier since the strategic arteriogram was performed, or the landmarks need to be rechecked, retrograde arteriography can be performed through the sheath. The image intensifier is placed in the best position and the appropriate field of view is used to get the optimal degree of magnification. The image intensifier is placed close to the abdominal wall. External iliac artery lesions and sometimes those in the distal common iliac artery are often well visualized using a contralateral anterior oblique projection. Radiopaque markers such as tape with 1-cm markers may be placed parallel to the guidewire on the patient's abdominal wall after the location of the image intensifier has been established. This type of external marker is particularly helpful when a small field of view is used for more magnification, since this field size tends to exclude some of the surrounding bony landmarks. The linear centimeter-length markers will not be accurate for exact length at the angioplasty site due to parallax.

The balloon is selected and passed over the guidewire through the lesion (Fig. 8). Common iliac artery angioplasty is performed with balloons between 6 and 10 mm in diameter. The balloons are usually either 2 or 4 cm in length and are mounted on 5-Fr catheters that are 75 or 80 cm in length. External iliac artery angioplasty is usually accomplished with 6- to 8-mm balloons. If it is difficult to pass the balloon catheter, the guidewire is exchanged with an Amplatz super-stiff. Occasionally, predilatation with a lower-profile, smaller-diameter balloon is required. This may occur in the setting of a heavily calcified but preocclusive lesion. The balloon is centered so that the radiopaque markers straddle the lesion. The location of the worst stenosis should be along the central segment of the balloon.

Iliac balloon angioplasty often causes flank discomfort, which should resolve when the balloon is deflated. Overdilatation may cause rupture. Lesions of the external iliac artery, especially origin lesions, are more likely to result in dissection following angioplasty. Completion arteriography can be performed through the sheath or with a flush catheter placed in the aorta proximal to the lesion.

Stents are placed for specific indications (see chap. 18 for a detailed discussion of the indications for stents) (Fig. 9). There is more clinical experience and better results with stent placement in the iliac artery than at any other location. Most iliac artery lesions may be treated satisfactorily with either balloon-expandable or self-expanding stents (see chap. 18). Long

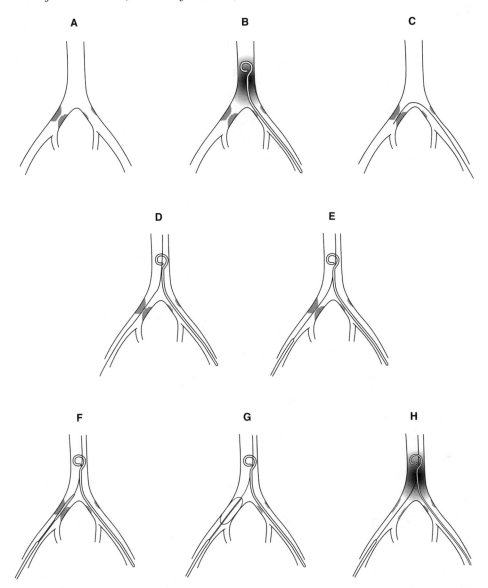

Fig. 8 Options for angioplasty of the iliac artery. (**A**) A significant right iliac artery stenosis requires treatment. (**B**) Aortography is performed through a contralateral femoral artery approach if the location of the lesion is not known precisely prior to arteriography. (**C**) A lesion of the middle iliac artery segment is dilated by passing the guidewire and catheter over the aortic bifurcation. (**D**) Another option is a second puncture site on the side ipsilateral to the lesion. If the location of the stenosis is known before arteriography, an ipsilateral retrograde puncture is used as the initial approach. (**E**) An access sheath is placed to simplify catheter passage for angioplasty. (**F**) A balloon catheter is passed across the lesion. (**G**) The balloon is inflated to dilate the lesion. (**H**) A contralateral catheter from the initial arteriogram is used for completion arteriography.

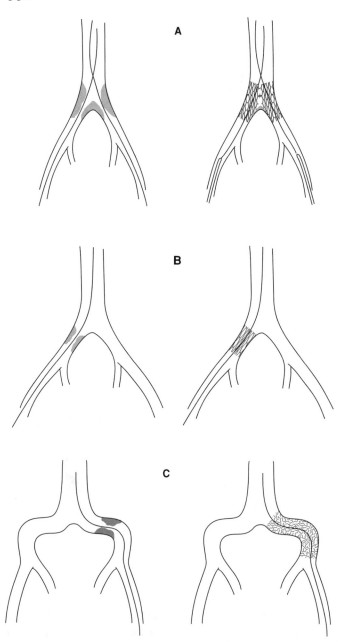

Fig. 9 Placement of an iliac artery stent. (**A**) Aortic bifurcation lesions that spill over into the proximal iliac artery require kissing balloon stents. (**B**) A short, focal iliac artery stenosis is treated with a single expandable stent. (**C**) A lesion in a tortuous iliac artery is best treated with a flexible self-expanding stent. (**D**) A long iliac artery stenosis is treated with a single self-expanding stent. (**E**) A lesion that requires stent placement from over the aortic bifurcation is best treated with a self-expanding stent. The delivery catheter is passed over the aortic bifurcation.

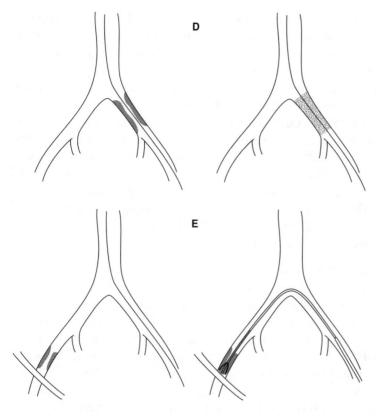

Fig. 9 (*Continued*)

lesions and arteries with significant taper or tortuosity are best treated with the self-expanding stents. Focal lesions or lesions located at the origin of the common or external iliac arteries are treated with balloon-expandable stents. After the stent is selected, double-check the size of the sheath in place to be certain that it is adequate in caliber. The appropriately sized sheath is placed. The intended location for stent placement is identified by external markers or bony landmarks or road mapping. The area to be covered by the stent may be slightly different than for the preceding balloon angioplasty, especially if there has been a dissection that requires treatment. Greater precision is required for stent deployment than for balloon angioplasty alone.

After placement of either stent type, additional balloon angioplasty is performed. A stent can be placed across the origin of the internal iliac artery and patency is usually maintained (see chap. 18 for a detailed discussion of the techniques of stent placement).

Contralateral Approach to the Iliac Artery

The usual scenario for the contralateral approach is the setting of a contralateral puncture for a strategic aortoiliac arteriogram that then proceeds to treatment. The locations of the lesions are considered and an approach is selected (Fig. 7). A hook-shaped catheter is placed in the infrarenal aorta and used to direct the guidewire over the aortic bifurcation. This maneuver is described in some detail in chapter 9. The guidewire is passed over the aortic bifurcation and into the contralateral femoral artery. The catheter is advanced into the femoral region and the guidewire is exchanged for a stiffer one, such as a Rosen guidewire or an Amplatz guidewire, which is used to support the passage of a sheath over the aortic bifurcation. Heparin is administered. Insertion of a sheath over the aortic bifurcation is detailed in chapter 14. These sheaths are 40 cm or longer in length and the caliber is selected in the same manner as for an ipsilateral retrograde approach, usually 6 or 7 Fr. The up-and-over sheath has a radiopaque tip and can be advanced well into the contralateral iliac if the lesion is distal. The sheath should not be inadvertently advanced into the lesion.

After sheath placement, a repeat iliac arteriogram is usually performed after the image intensifier has been optimally positioned. External marking tape may also be placed. Arteriography is performed through the sheath. The appropriate balloon catheter is selected, as described in the earlier section. Catheters 75 to 80 cm in length are usually adequate to reach to the contralateral groin. Balloon angioplasty is performed. The contralateral femoral area should be prepped into the field and the pulse is available for palpation. The balloon catheter is withdrawn but guidewire position is carefully maintained. Completion arteriography is performed through the sheath.

Self-expanding stents can be placed through a 6- or 7-Fr sheath placed over the aortic bifurcation. The sheath must be held in place as the stent is deployed since traction on the stent delivery catheter tends to pull the sheath back. Balloon-expandable stents are more of a challenge to pass over the aortic bifurcation because of their rigidity. If a balloon-expandable stent is desired, it is still possible, but the following should be considered. Use a shorter stent, 2 or 3 cm, instead of 4 cm. Use a balloon-expandable with less metal in it, for example, Corinthian instead of standard Palmaz. Use a larger sheath, 8 Fr instead of 7 Fr.

Balloon angioplasty of nonorificial proximal common iliac artery lesions is difficult with an up-and-over sheath in place since the tip of the sheath requires several centimeters of purchase in the proximal contralateral iliac system to maintain its curvature. A short distance of clearance, about 1 cm, is required distal to the end of the sheath to accommodate the shoulder of the angioplasty balloon. Contralateral iliac angioplasty was performed for many years without an up-and-over sheath. The balloon catheter is placed over the guidewire and angioplasty is performed without a guiding sheath. The disadvantage of this approach is that there is no simple way to obtain a completion arteriogram. The usual method is to replace the balloon catheter with a multi-side-hole straight catheter. The guidewire is removed but the straight catheter still maintains control at the angioplasty site. Arteriography through the catheter shows the velocity of forward flow distal to the angioplasty site. If it is satisfactory, the catheter is gently withdrawn and arteriography is repeated to illuminate the angioplasty site. The risk with this approach is that control of the lesion may be lost prematurely and could be difficult to regain while working from the contralateral side. It is even more challenging to place stents into the proximal contralateral iliac system. Self-expanding stents are the only option in this setting and the concern is that the second end or trailing end of the stent may be deployed too close to the bifurcation.

Selected Readings

Björses K, Ivancev K, Riva L, et al. Kissing stents in the aortic bifurcation—a valid reconstruction for aorto-iliac occlusive disease. Eur J Vasc Endovasc Surg. 2008; 36(4):424–431.

Hood DB, Hodgson KJ. Percutaneous transluminal angioplasty and stenting for iliac artery occlusive disease. Surg Clin North Am 1999; 79:575–596.

Lin PH, Weiss VJ, Lumsden AB. Stented balloon angioplasty in aortoiliac arterial occlusive disease. In: Moore WS, Ahn SS, eds. Endovascular Surgery. Philadelphia, PA: W. B. Saunders, 2001:233–242.

Schneider PA, Rutherford RB. Endovascular interventions in the management of chronic lower extremity ischemia. In: Rutherford RB, ed. Vascular Surgery. Philadelphia, PA: W. B. Saunders, 2000:1035–1069.

Sharafuddin MJ, Hoballah JJ, Kresowik TF, et al. Long-term outcome following stent reconstruction of the aortic bifurcation and the role of geometric determinants. Ann Vasc Surg 2008; 22(3):346–357.

Tsetis D, Uberoi R. Quality improvement guidelines for endovascular treatment of iliac artery occlusive disease. Cardiovasc Intervent Radiol. 2008; 31(2):238–245.

20

The Infrainguinal Arteries: Advice About Balloon Angioplasty and Stent Placement

Balloon angioplasty and stents expand the scope of patients who are eligible for treatment of infrainguinal occlusive disease. Several newer techniques are developing that substantially increase the spectrum of treatment options and these are detailed in chapter 25. Endovascular infrainguinal techniques are most useful in patients who are poor candidates for open surgery and in those with focal, short segment disease. The long-term results of femoropopliteal angioplasty are not generally as good as those for surgery and vary significantly based upon the severity and extent of the occlusive disease. The current practice of infrainguinal intervention may differ substantially from institution to institution based upon the level of enthusiasm for these techniques. Infrainguinal arteries may be approached through an ipsilateral antegrade femoral puncture or a contralateral femoral puncture followed by passage of the catheter over the aortic bifurcation. Chapter 3 shows how to perform an antegrade puncture. Chapter 9 provides methods for antegrade passage into the ipsilateral superficial femoral artery (SFA) and also crossing the aortic bifurcation. Chapter 10 details techniques for including the lower extremity in an arteriographic runoff study and for performing femoral arteriography and selective lower-extremity and pedal arteriography.

Superficial Femoral and Popliteal Arteries

Table 1 compares the over the bifurcation approach to infrainguinal disease to the ipsilateral, antegrade approach. The ipsilateral, antegrade approach provides better control of guidewires and catheters and excellent access to distal infrainguinal arteries. The inventory is simple, and once the guidewire is in the SFA, the procedure tends to be fairly straightforward. The antegrade puncture can be a challenge, and entering the SFA from the common femoral artery often requires patience. Aortoiliac disease must be ruled out prior to this approach. The antegrade approach is not appropriate in obese patients due to the risk of puncture site complications. It is not used in patients with common femoral or proximal SFA disease because of the proximity of the puncture site to the disease. The over the bifurcation approach to infrainguinal disease from the contralateral femoral is advantageous in obese patients, those with proximal SFA disease, and those in whom aortoiliac disease must be evaluated prior to infrainguinal intervention. Entering the SFA is usually simple with this approach, but tortuous aortoiliac anatomy or occlusive disease can make the up-and-over catheterization difficult or even dangerous. The up-and-over approach requires an inventory of longer catheter sizes. Control of longer catheters and guidewires after they take multiple turns is not as satisfactory but most cases can be performed using this method at the discretion of the surgeon.

Table 1 Approaches to Infrainguinal Interventions: Ipsilateral Approach Versus Up-and-Over Approach from Contralateral Femoral

	Up-and-over approach	Antegrade approach
Puncture	Simple retrograde femoral	More challenging, less working room
Catheterization	Up-and-over catheterization is challenging with tortuous arteries, narrow, or diseased aortic bifurcation; easier to catheterize SFA when going up and over	Entering SFA from antegrade approach requires proximal femoral puncture and selective catheter
Guidewire/catheter control	Fair	Excellent
Catheter inventory	Need more supplies	Minimal, shorter catheters
Specialty items	Flexible sheath, long balloon catheters	None
Indications	Proximal SFA disease, CFA disease ipsilateral to infrainguinal lesion, obesity	Intrapopliteal disease, patients with contraindication to up-and-over approach

Abbreviations: SFA, superficial femoral artery; CFA, common femoral artery.

Ipsilateral Antegrade Approach to the Superficial Femoral and Popliteal Arteries

After antegrade puncture, the guidewire is directed into the origin of the SFA with a bent-tip selective catheter (see chap. 9). The guidewire must be advanced far enough into the artery to secure the access. If a Glidewire has been passed into the SFA, advance a 4- or 5-Fr dilator over it and exchange for a stiffer guidewire and then pass the access sheath. If there is concern that the guidewire will cross the lesion prior to arteriography (e.g., with a lesion in the proximal or mid-SFA), follow the advancing guidewire carefully using fluoroscopy, then pass a 4- or 5-Fr dilator and perform a femoral arteriogram. A radiopaque ruler or external marker is placed on the drapes to mark the location of the lesion.

A 5-Fr sheath can be placed after secure guidewire access to the SFA has been obtained (Fig. 1). After femoral arteriography, which includes distal runoff, the guidewire is passed antegrade through the lesion. Large collaterals are juxtaposed and often parallel to femoropopliteal lesions and should be avoided. A steerable guidewire is often required. After the guidewire is placed, a repeat arteriogram through the sidearm of the sheath is performed to ensure that the lesion has been appropriately crossed. Heparin is administered for infrainguinal angioplasty. Consider 50 to 75 U/kg for

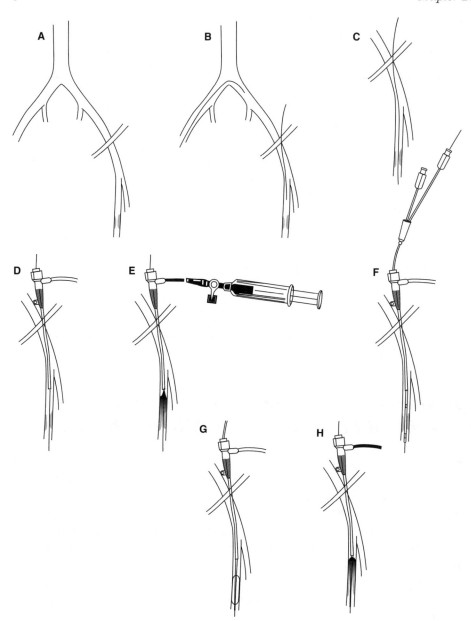

Fig. 1 Balloon angioplasty of the superficial femoral and popliteal arteries. (**A**) A stenosis of the SFA is deemed suitable for angioplasty. (**B**) The stenosis is approached antegrade through an ipsilateral femoral artery puncture or across the aortic bifurcation. (**C**) An ipsilateral antegrade femoral artery puncture is usually the most simple. The guidewire is placed across the stenosis. (**D**) A hemostatic access sheath is placed over the guidewire into the proximal SFA. (**E**) Femoral arteriography through the sidearm of the sheath evaluates the lesion and confirms guidewire position. (**F**) The angioplasty balloon is selected and passed through the stenosis. (**G**) The stenosis is dilated. (**H**) The balloon is removed but the position of the guidewire is maintained. Completion arteriography is performed through the sidearm of the sheath.

simple, focal lesions. When the catheter is in the artery for a short time, no stent is required, and flow is interrupted for only a few seconds, a lower dose of heparin usually suffices. Consider higher heparin doses for more complex cases.

Guidewires in the range of 145 to 180 cm in length are used with angiographic catheters that are 65 to 70 cm in length (Table 2). Balloon angioplasty catheters that are 75 or 80 cm in length are adequate to reach the mid-tibial level in most patients through an antegrade approach. If a longer balloon catheter is used, a longer guidewire may be required. Once the intended site of intervention is marked with an external marker or road map, the distance can be measured outside the limb to estimate the length required. Balloon diameters range from 4 to 7 mm in the SFA and 3 to 6 mm in the popliteal artery. A 5-Fr sheath will accommodate balloons up to 6 mm in diameter. The rare case that requires a 7-mm-diameter balloon will require a 6-Fr sheath to pass the balloon catheter. It is usually best to begin with a balloon of lesser diameter than will probably be required, rather than over-size. Self-expanding stents up to 6 mm in diameter may be placed through a 4-Fr sheath. An 8-mm self-expanding stent requires a 6-Fr sheath.

The tip of the guidewire is usually placed in the distal popliteal artery. If the balloon angioplasty site is below the knee, the guidewire should be advanced into the tibial arteries. During exchanges of catheters, occasional fluoroscopy of this area is performed to ensure that the guidewire is not allowed to move from its position. Always confirm guidewire position in the true lumen of the artery distal to the lesion prior to performing balloon angioplasty. Once the balloon angioplasty catheter is in place, the balloon is inflated using fluoroscopy. Following deflation, the balloon is withdrawn and completion arteriography is performed through the sidearm of the sheath. If a 5-Fr balloon catheter shaft is used with a 5-Fr hemostatic sheath, the sheath lumen is completely obstructed by the catheter. The balloon catheter must be completely withdrawn before arteriography is performed. If the sheath is 6 Fr or larger, the balloon catheter is withdrawn from the angioplasty site and contrast is injected around the shaft of the balloon catheter through the sidearm of the sheath. When a deflated 6-mm-diameter balloon is removed through a 5-Fr sheath, the fit is very snug. The balloon should be aspirated continuously with a syringe to decrease its profile.

Completion arteriography is used to assess the size of the lumen after balloon angioplasty and the flow through the intervention site and to look for extravasation, contrast trapping in the vessel wall, or evidence of extensive dissection. Best results are obtained with angioplasty of focal, critical lesions. Long-segment femoropopliteal angioplasty is complicated by a higher incidence of acute occlusion, dissection, and lower long-term patency rates.

Angioplasty of the SFA, especially at the adductor canal, almost routinely produces some evidence of a dissection plane on completion images,

Table 2 Supplies for Antegrade Femoral Approach to Infrainguinal Intervention

Guidewire	Starting/selective guidewire	Bentson	145 cm, length	0.035 in. diameter (steerable, shapable tip)
	Selective guidewire	Glidewire	180 cm	0.035 in. (angled tip)
	Exchange guidewire	Rosen	180 cm	0.035 in. (J tip)
Catheter	Selective	Kumpe	40 cm	5 Fr (short, bent tip)
	Exchange	Straight	70 cm	5 Fr
Sheath	Access	Standard hemostatic access	12 cm	4 Fr, 5 Fr, 7 Fr[a]
Balloon	Balloon angioplasty catheters	Balloon diameter	3, 4, 5, 6 mm	
		Balloon length	2, 4 cm	
		Catheter shaft	75 cm, distal tibial may require 90 cm	
Stent		Self-expanding		
		Stent diameter	6, 8 mm	
		Stent length	20–120 mm	
		Delivery catheter length	80 cm	

[a] Use 4-Fr sheath for tibial balloon angioplasty with 3.8-Fr catheters. Use 5-Fr sheath for balloon angioplasty up to 6 mm on a 5-Fr shaft. A 6-Fr sheath is required for stent placement using a 0.035-in. system.

and most dissections heal. A stent is placed if an acute dissection has caused an occlusion or threatens imminently to occlude the artery (Fig. 2). A 6-Fr sheath is required for self-expanding stent placement using a standard 0.035-in. system. If a stent must cross the knee joint, a self-expanding stent is appropriately flexible. A standard 12-cm length access sheath is used with an 80-cm delivery catheter. The stent is oversized 2 mm from the intended placement site. An 8-mm stent is usually placed in a 6-mm-diameter artery to maintain constant outward radial force. The constrained stent is passed beyond the lesion by a few millimeters. The leading end of the stent is allowed to flare. The delivery catheter is then withdrawn slightly to land the stent in the appropriate location. Poststent balloon angioplasty is routinely performed and often reveals a residual waist. Most operators prefer self-expanding stents because of their ease of placement, longer available lengths, flexibility within the artery, and contourability along a tapering artery. It is possible to crush balloon-expandable stents with external compression so these are generally avoided. Completion arteriography is performed through the sidearm of the sheath.

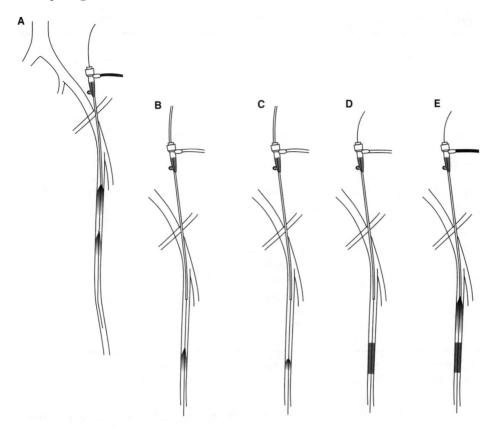

Fig. 2 Stent placement in the SFA. (**A**) Postangioplasty dissection is present on completion arteriography. (**B**) A self-expanding stent is delivered to the site. (**C**) The stent is deployed from the distal end of the lesion to its proximal end. (**D**) Poststent balloon angioplasty is performed to bring the stent to its appropriate profile. (**E**) Completion arteriography is performed through the sheath while maintaining guidewire access.

Up-and-Over Approach to the Superficial Femoral and Popliteal Arteries

Selective catheterization of the aortic bifurcation and antegrade passage of a catheter into the contralateral iliac artery are discussed in chapter 9. Details of the passage of an up-and-over sheath are presented in chapter 14. Equipment required for an up-and-over approach to infrainguinal intervention is listed in Table 3.

Contralateral intervention can be performed without an up-and-over sheath but there are substantial disadvantages and this is no longer a reasonable approach. Guidewires and catheters passed over the aortic bifurcation without a guiding sheath lose pushability. After intervention, guidewire control of the lesion must be relinquished in order to obtain a completion

Table 3 Supplies for Up-and-Over Approach to Infrainguinal Intervention

Guidewire	Starting	Bentson	145 cm, length	0.035-in. diameter
	Selective	Glidewire	150 cm	0.035 in. (steerable)
		Glidewire	260 cm	0.035 in. (steerable)
	Exchange	Rosen	180 cm	0.035 in. (J tip)
		Amplatz Super-Stiff	180 cm	0.035 in.
Catheter	Flush/selective	Omni-flush	65 cm	4 Fr
	Exchange	Straight	90 cm	5 Fr
Sheath	Selective sheath	Up and over	40, 55, 70 cm	5.5 Fr, 6 Fr, 7 Fr
Balloon	Balloon angioplasty catheters	Balloon diameter	3–6 mm	
		Balloon length	2, 4 cm	
		Catheter shaft	75, 90, 110 cm[a]	
Stent		Self-expanding		
		Stent diameter	6, 8 mm	
		Stent length	20–120 mm	
		Delivery catheter length	80, 120 cm	

[a] A 75-cm catheter shaft for balloon angioplasty to mid-SFA. Longer catheters are required for contralateral approach to distal SFA, popliteal, and tibial intervention.

arteriogram. A variety of acceptable sheaths are available and one can almost always be placed.

The length of the sheath can be estimated based on the length of diagnostic catheter that is required to reach close to the lesion. Usually, it is best to place the tip of the sheath as close to the lesion as possible. If balloon angioplasty alone is anticipated, a 5-Fr sheath is adequate for angioplasty up to 6 mm in diameter. If stent placement is anticipated or it becomes necessary to treat a postangioplasty complication, a 6-Fr sheath is required to place a self-expanding stent using a 0.035-in. guidewire system. A femoral arteriogram may be performed through the sidearm of the sheath (Fig. 3). If the amount of contrast administration must be limited, a straight catheter may be passed through the sheath and into the proximal SFA and an arteriogram may be performed. The exchange guidewire over which the sheath has been passed is exchanged for a steerable guidewire, usually a 260-cm angled-tip Glidewire, which is used to cross the infrainguinal lesion. Heparin is administered, 50 to 75 U/kg.

The length of the balloon catheter shaft is selected based upon the location of the lesion. The proximal SFA can be reached with a 75- or 80-cm length catheter. In a patient of short stature, it will reach the mid-SFA. More distal lesions require a 90- or 110-cm catheter. An estimate of the required catheter length can be made using the straight exchange catheter, which

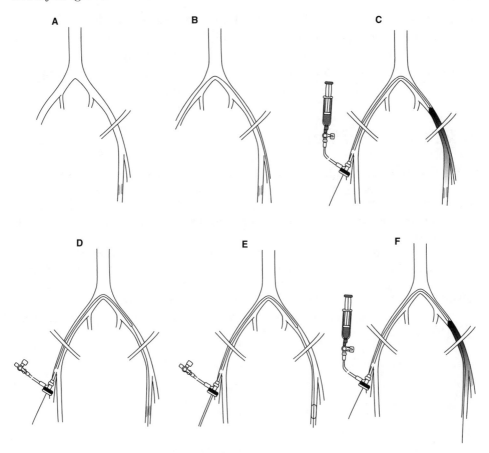

Fig. 3 Balloon angioplasty of the femoral and popliteal arteries through an up-and-over approach. (**A**) A SFA lesion is identified. (**B**) A guidewire is introduced through the contralateral femoral artery and placed over the aortic bifurcation. The guidewire may be placed in either the profunda femoris or superficial femoral arteries. If the guidewire is placed in the SFA, care should be taken to prevent unintended encounters between the guidewire and the lesion during sheath placement. (**C**) An up-and-over sheath is placed and arteriography is performed. (**D**) The guidewire is advanced across the lesion. (**E**) Balloon angioplasty is performed. (**F**) Completion arteriography is performed through the sheath.

is used to exchange the guidewires. The exchange catheters are usually 70 or 100 cm in length. Care must be taken to maintain the guidewire in a stationary position so that its leading edge does not advance into the distal infrageniculate runoff arteries during passage of long catheters. Intermittent fluoroscopy is required.

After balloon angioplasty, the catheter is withdrawn while the guidewire is maintained in place. A completion arteriogram is performed through the sidearm of the sheath. The angioplasty site is assessed in the same way as described in the earlier section. If a stent is required, the sheath must be upsized to 6 Fr if not already in place. Most self-expanding stents are delivered on catheters that are either 80 or 120 cm in length. The required distance may be estimated based upon the length of the balloon catheter required. After stent placement, balloon angioplasty is performed along the length of the stent followed by completion arteriography.

Selected Readings

Baril DT, Marone LK, Kim J, et al. Outcomes of endovascular interventions for TASC II B and C femoropopliteal lesions. J Vasc Surg 2008; 48(3):627–633.

Davies MG, Saad WE, Peden EK, et al. Impact of runoff on superficial femoral artery endoluminal interventions for rest pain and tissue loss. J Vasc Surg 2008; 48(3):619–625.

Schneider PA, Rutherford RB. Endovascular interventions in the management of chronic lower extremity ischemia. In: Rutherford RB, ed. Vascular Surgery. Philadelphia, PA: W. B. Saunders, 2000:1035–1069.

Zeller T, Tiefenbacher C, Steinkamp HJ, et al. Nitinol stent implantation in TASC A and B superficial femoral artery lesions: The Femoral Artery Conformexx Trial (FACT). J Endovasc Ther 2008; 15(4):390–398.

21

Advice About Endovascular Salvage of Previous Reconstructions

Endovascular intervention is essential in the salvage of previous endovascular and open surgical reconstructions. The mechanisms of failure of previous reconstructions, whether open or endovascular, are similar. These include failure of inflow due to new or residual lesions, failure at the site of previous intervention, or new lesions involving the outflow. Failure at a site of previous balloon angioplasty or surgical bypass may be due to intimal hyperplasia during the early phase or recurrent atherosclerosis if it occurs later. Although the record of endovascular intervention for intimal hyperplasia is variable, this may be the method of choice in patients who are poor candidates for open surgery. Cutting balloons may play a future role in the endovascular treatment of intimal hyperplastic lesions. These are discussed in more detail in chapters 22 and 25.

Previous Endovascular Reconstruction: Balloon Angioplasty, Stents

When recurrent stenosis occurs at a site of previous balloon angioplasty, it can usually be treated with repeat balloon angioplasty and stent placement. Arteriograms from the previous procedure should be reviewed for evidence of untreated residual stenosis that may have been evident at the completion of the initial procedure. Care should be taken to avoid passing the guidewire into an area of partially healed dissection at the intervention site. If the lesion is heavily calcified, a stiff exchange guidewire should be used for control of the lesion.

Patients with failing endovascular sites may require surgery, and care should be taken to avoid compromising surgical options. Avoid large-bore or repeat punctures in femoral areas that may require surgery. Failing endovascular sites are more likely to acquire fresh thrombus or other material that could form an embolus. Consider administering adequate heparin and avoid crossing lesions that appear likely to embolize.

When the previous reconstruction was a stent, the key maneuver in repeat treatment is to be certain that the guidewire is placed across the stent within the lumen and not under the struts of the stent. Guidewires in general and Glidewires in particular may pass through the struts of a stent and potentially lead to a stent-deforming balloon angioplasty. Passing a guidewire through a previously stented segment is discussed in chapter 18. If the operator cannot be certain about the guidewire position, a catheter may be passed over the guidewire to be certain that the catheter does not catch on the sidewall of the stent. If the end of a previously placed stent is at the origin of an artery, such as the common iliac or the renal artery, additional care should be taken when crossing the stent. A soft-tipped guiding catheter or sheath may be used to encounter the end of the stent. Repeat balloon angioplasty within a previously placed stent may cause balloon rupture, especially if it is a stainless steel, balloon-expandable stent with sharp metal edges. The balloon may occasionally catch on the stent, which prevents the balloon from being withdrawn. If additional stents need to be placed, consider overlapping slightly with the previously placed stent.

Infrainguinal Bypass Graft

Failing infrainguinal bypasses present a common application of endovascular intervention for salvage. One of the most difficult facets of bypass graft angioplasty is locating and entering the graft from its proximal end, especially if the stenosis is severe and is at the proximal anastomosis (see chap. 9 for a detailed discussion of the technique for entering an infrainguinal graft). If the graft is placed subcutaneously, such as an in situ graft, a percutaneous puncture of the graft in the subcutaneous position can be performed using micropuncture technique with ultrasound guidance. If this is chosen as the access method, a 4-Fr sheath and a 0.014-in. guidewire system should be used. Most grafts are entered through the proximal anastomosis.

The method for approaching an infrainguinal bypass graft is dependent upon the location of its proximal anastomosis. Grafts that originate from the anterior wall of the common femoral artery are accessed through a contralateral femoral artery puncture and passage of the guidewire and catheter over the aortic bifurcation (Fig. 1). Grafts originating from the superficial femoral artery, popliteal artery, or deep femoral artery are usually cannulated after an antegrade ipsilateral femoral artery puncture (Fig. 2).

A steerable, hydrophilic-coated guidewire is useful to enter the orifice of the graft. If the stenosis is preocclusive, it may be difficult to identify the proximal origin of the graft because of very low flow. Since most anastomoses are placed on the anterior side of the artery of origin, steep oblique views may be helpful in localizing the area of interest. A stump or hood of graft is sometimes visible when local contrast is injected. This area should be probed with a steerable guidewire.

Arteriography and confirmation of guidewire placement is performed through the sidearm of the hemostatic sheath, which has been placed to provide an antegrade approach to the infrainguinal bypass. Heparin is administered (50–75 U/kg) prior to passage of the balloon catheter, since the catheter itself may stop flow in the graft. Consider placing the guidewire through the length of the bypass graft before beginning balloon angioplasty,

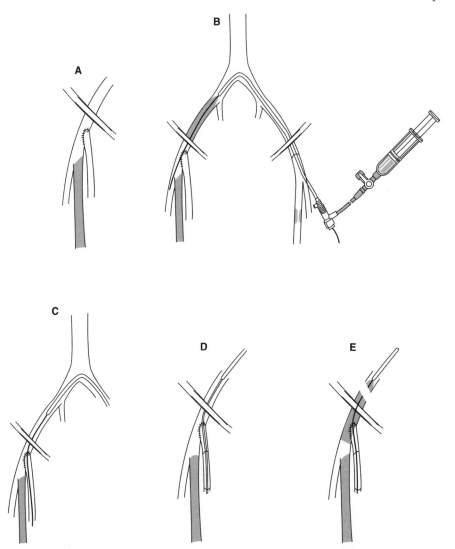

Fig. 1 Balloon angioplasty of infrainguinal bypass graft through an up-and-over approach. (**A**) An infrainguinal bypass graft that originates from the common femoral artery has developed a proximal graft lesion. (**B**) An up-and-over sheath is placed and arteriography is performed. (**C**) The guidewire is passed through the graft lesion. (**D**) Balloon angioplasty is performed. (**E**) Completion arteriography is performed through the sheath.

just in case low flow in the graft progresses to thrombosis of the graft. After the graft is entered, the balloon angioplasty catheter is passed over the guidewire.

High pressures (up to 20 atm) may be required to reopen a segment of intimal hyperplastic disease. Stenoses within the graft or at an anasto-

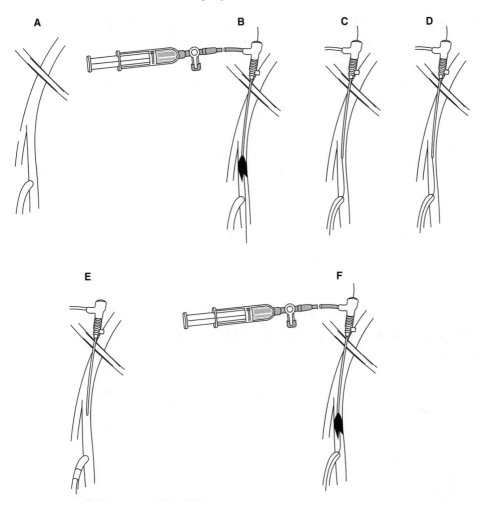

Fig. 2 Balloon angioplasty of infrainguinal bypass graft through an antegrade ipsilateral approach. (**A**) This approach is useful for interventions in infrainguinal bypass grafts that originate from the superficial femoral, popliteal, or profunda femoris arteries. (**B**) An antegrade femoral sheath is placed and arteriography is performed. (**C**) The guidewire is directed into the vein graft using a selective catheter and passed across the vein graft lesion. (**D**) The selective catheter is removed. (**E**) Balloon angioplasty of the infrainguinal bypass graft is performed. (**F**) Completion arteriography is performed while maintaining guidewire access.

mosis generally require higher pressures and longer inflation times. The likelihood of a localized dissection is low but the graft may rupture if it is overdilated. After angioplasty, the balloon is removed while the guidewire is maintained and completion arteriography is performed through the sheath.

Extra-Anatomic Bypasses: Axillofemoral and Femoral–Femoral Bypasses

Extra-anatomic bypass grafts may be evaluated arteriographically by direct puncture and catheter placement or through entry into the native vasculature proximal or distal to the graft. Selective catheterization of prosthetic grafts is detailed in chapter 9. Interventions to salvage axillofemoral grafts usually involve distal lesions, either at the femoral anastomosis or in the runoff. After arteriography, an access sheath is placed. Dilators must be used to permit the entry of the sheath, and the smallest caliber sheath that is adequate for the intervention should be placed. A balloon catheter is passed over the guidewire and angioplasty is performed. After the intervention, pressure is held at the site of the puncture so that the graft itself maintains flow and a platelet plug is permitted to form.

Reconstructions for Aortoiliac Disease: Aortofemoral, Iliofemoral, and Aortoiliac Bypasses

Most failing in-line grafts that were originally performed for aortoiliac occlusive disease should be treated with repeat surgery. The most common lesions affecting these grafts are at the distal anastomoses. Nevertheless, endovascular intervention is well suited to treat lesions that are at the proximal anastomosis and would be difficult to reach surgically. Figure 3 demonstrates an aortic graft that is failing due to progression of aortic disease. Balloon angioplasty and stent placement in the infrarenal aorta are used to prevent repeat open aortic surgery.

Inflow disease may also occur proximal to an iliofemoral bypass graft. This may be reached through an ipsilateral or contralateral femoral puncture, depending upon the site of the proximal anastomosis. Grafts that end in the iliac arteries may be difficult to cannulate through an ipsilateral femoral puncture (Fig. 4). The guidewire naturally tends to remain within the native circulation. An oblique view and steerable guidewire and angled-tip selective catheter are used to locate and enter the graft. Aortofemoral bypass graft bifurcations are manufactured at a fairly narrow angle, and crossing the graft bifurcation may be a challenge. It is much simpler to cross with an angiographic catheter than with an access sheath, since the catheter is more flexible. A selective catheter with a tight hook, such as a Rim catheter, may be used with a steerable 0.014-in. guidewire. However, if a graft limb must be treated and cannot be reached by an ipsilateral puncture, it is usually best to approach from a proximal puncture in the upper extremity to benefit by the relatively straight pathway to the groin.

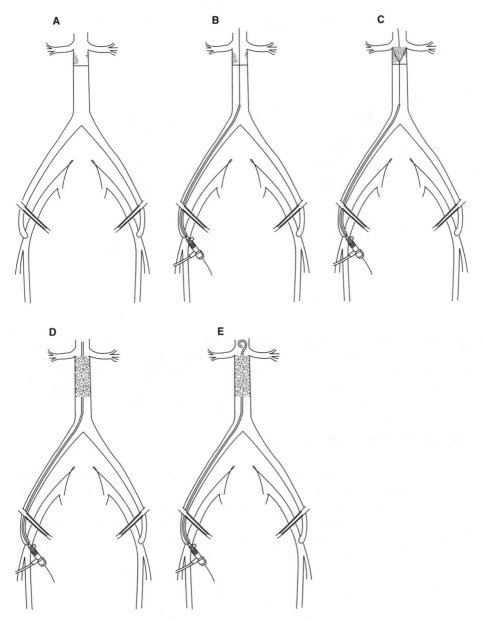

Fig. 3 Endovascular salvage of an aortofemoral bypass graft. (**A**) Disease has progressed in the residual infrarenal aorta after prior aortofemoral graft placement. (**B**) A femoral sheath and guidewire are placed. (**C**) Stent placement is performed distal to the renal arteries. (**D**) Poststent balloon angioplasty expands the stent to its correct profile. (**E**) Completion arteriography is performed through a proximally placed flush catheter.

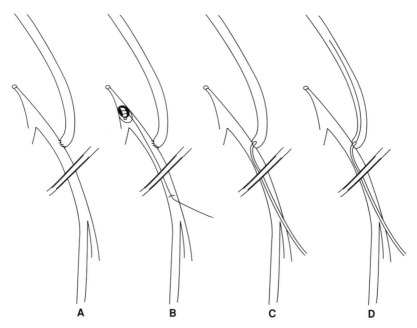

Fig. 4   Retrograde guidewire placement after iliac anastomosis. (**A**) The iliac artery is the recipient artery of a previously placed bypass graft and the common iliac artery has been ligated. (**B**) The tendency of a guidewire placed retrograde is to remain in the native circulation. (**C**) A selective catheter is placed and is used to direct the guidewire. (**D**) The guidewire is passed across the anastomosis.

Selected Readings

Anain PM, Ahn SS. Femoral-popliteal-tibial graft occlusion: Thrombolysis, angioplasty, atherectomy, and stent. In: Moore WS, Ahn SS, eds. Endovascular Surgery. Philadelphia, PA: W. B. Saunders, 2001:393–398.

Criado FJ. Technical approaches for endovascular intervention below the knee and vein graft stenosis. In: Criado FJ, ed. Endovascular Intervention: Basic Concepts and Techniques. Armonk, NY: Futura, 1999:115–122.

Part III

Advanced Endovascular Therapy

22

New Tools and Devices and How to Use Them

Microcatheters

Microcatheters are small, lengthy, and flexible catheters that are compatible with small caliber guidewires. They may be used for strategic angiography, to exchange guidewires, and to provide support for a guidewire system in a challenging situation. Microcatheters may also be used to provide therapy, such as when small caliber coils are delivered or therapeutic medication is administered. Thrombolytic agents may be delivered through microcatheters, for example. Microcatheters are generally 2.3 to 3.8 Fr in caliber, in comparison to the standard 5-Fr catheter used with a 0.035-in. system (Fig. 1).The tip of the catheter may be floppy or stiff and may be either straight or have angles at the tip. These catheters may be designed to accept a 0.10-in., a 0.014-in., or a 0.018-in. diameter guidewire. They are generally 120 to 150 cm in length but may be even longer. The longer and smaller caliber the catheter becomes, the more the friction increases during guidewire passage through the catheter and also during catheter passage over the guidewire. There are some microcatheters which have radio opaque tips, which make them more readily visible, and also some microcatheters that have stiff tips. The microcatheters with the stiff tips may be used for crossing occlusions. The catheter and the guidewire can be used in a hopscotch manner to get across

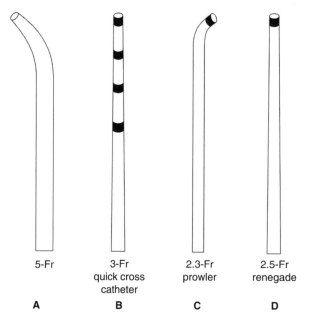

| 5-Fr | 3-Fr quick cross catheter | 2.3-Fr prowler | 2.5-Fr renegade |
| A | B | C | D |

Fig. 1 Microcatheters are used regularly as an adjunct in small vessel intervention. (**A**) A standard 5 Fr angiographic catheter. (**B**) A Quickcross catheter (Spectranetics) has a stiff tip and markers and is used to push across occlusions. (**C**) A Prowler (Cordis) is a soft, floppy neurovascular catheter with an angled tip. (**D**) A Renegade (Boston Scientific)is a low profile neurovascular catheter with a straight tip and a marker.

an occlusion, each providing support to the other. Microcatheters may be used to provide support to a guidewire system where support is inadequate due to the lack of strength of the guidewire shaft itself. The relationships of the guidewire to the surrounding tissues may be changed significantly by adding a microcatheter.

Microcatheters have significantly changed the practice of vascular in several areas including neurovascular applications and delivery of thrombolytic medication for stroke and also in terms of tibial artery interventions and crossing tibial occlusions with a microcatheter with a stiff tip. Microcatheters have also provided a whole new dimension in terms of opportunities for wire exchange, visualization, passage of guidewire–catheter apparatus into tortuous, and extremely remote locations and in terms of options for getting out of trouble. Several of the major companies make an array of microcatheters and these are mostly geared toward neurovascular but their applications may be possible throughout all of the vascular systems.

Subintimal Angioplasty

Subintimal angioplasty refers to passage of the guidewire in the wall of the artery to get past an occlusion and then performing balloon angioplasty in this space (Fig. 2). This has been a major advance in the treatment of occlusions and it is being applied to many different vascular beds. Because it is not always possible to pass through an occlusion from a transluminal standpoint, techniques have been developed wherein a guidewire and catheter combination may be passed around the lesion. It is unlikely that the passage is actually subintimal for any significant distance along the artery; the passage probably varies from just deep to the plaque to just inside the adventitia. In practice, the actual location of guidewire passage probably does not matter.

Subintimal angioplasty has had its broadest application in the infrainguinal arteries including the superficial femoral, popliteal, and tibial vessels. Subintimal angioplasty has also been performed in other areas such as the coronaries, iliac arteries, the infrarenal aorta, and other vessels. The adventitia acts as a fairly tough outer casing with excellent tensile strength and it only rarely results in perforation. In the lower extremity where the superficial femoral and popliteal arteries have surrounding soft tissue, muscle, and venous structures, a perforation is usually not clinically consequential and usually does not require treatment. Subintimal passage may be created either intentionally or unintentionally. For many years, short occlusions of the superficial femoral artery were treated by forcing a guidewire or even a stiff guidewire end across the lumen of the artery that was occluded. No one knew whether the pathway was intimal or subintimal. At the present time, it is quite common to enter the subintimal space intentionally and there are specific tricks for doing this.

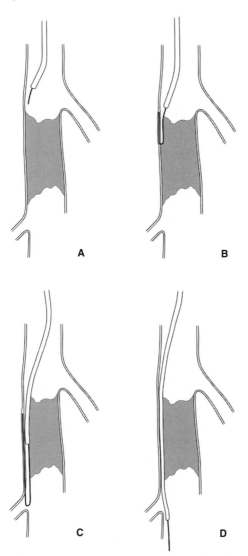

Fig. 2 Method of subintimal recanalization. (**A**) A sheath is placed close to the origin of the occlusion and a braided catheter with an angled tip is pointed opposite to the largest proximal collateral. (**B**) The Glidewire tip probes the interface between the plaque and the artery wall until the guidewire tip buckles and forms a loop. (**C**) The loop in the guidewire is maintained and pushed forward until the knuckle of guidewire pops back into the true lumen. (**D**) The catheter is advanced to support the guidewire and to advance into the true lumen.

The key technical points have to do with getting into the subintimal space and then getting from the subintimal space back into the true lumen and are summarized in Table 1.

To perform a subintimal angioplasty, one needs a solid treatment platform. Go into the subintimal space with the concept that the treatment will definitely be carried out and will require a sheath to do so. Pick the

Table 1 Technical Point About Using the Subintimal Space

How to get into the subintimal space
Use a braided catheter with a stiff angled tip
Aim the tip of the catheter at the plaque/artery interface
Point toward the stump of the occluded artery, or if no stump, point opposite the largest
 end-collateral
Advance an angled Glidewire until it catches and forms a loop
Follow the loop of guidewire with the catheter

How to get back into the true lumen
Advance guidewire loop into the reconstituted stump of distal artery
If loop does not pop back into the true lumen:
 Perform balloon angioplasty in the area to break plaque
 Direct a stiff, angled-tip catheter toward reconstituted artery segment and probe
  with wire
 Use reentry catheter

right-sized sheath for treatment and advance the sheath to within a few centimeters of the origin of the artery. Use a stiff tip angled catheter such as a vertebral catheter to point into the stump of the occluded artery and angle the catheter toward the wall on the side that's opposite the best collateral which is keeping the stump open. Advance the Glidewire through the tip of the catheter; allow it to form a loop and force the loop into the subintimal space. Once the loop is formed and advanced for several centimeters, advance the catheter over the guidewire. Pull the guidewire back ever so slightly to again form the appropriate-sized loop, which is not too wide in its trajectory, and advance the guidewire and then the catheter over it in a step-by-step fashion. As the guidewire loop approaches the reconstituted distal true lumen, make sure the catheter is close behind the loop to support it and to keep the loop as narrow as possible. Usually the loop pops into the true lumen. When the advancing loop does not pop into the true lumen, it is usually due to severe calcification of the reconstituting artery. If the advancing catheter and guidewire in the subintimal space reach an area where there is a heavy calcification that can be seen on fluoroscopy and/or where the catheter cannot be adequately advanced because of the constriction of the tight subintimal space onto the catheter, then a balloon angioplasty catheter may be passed to start to break the plaque a little bit and this frequently helps to create a space through which to reenter into the true lumen. The catheter itself pointed toward the true lumen with the Glidewire is another way to reenter the true lumen. If this is not possible, then reentry catheters may be used and some operators prefer to use reentry catheters preferentially.

Subintimal angioplasty has also provided a new method of managing occlusions, which has substantially improved the entire field but specifically has changed lower extremity revascularization. There is more about subintimal angioplasty in the aorta, iliac, and lower-extremity arteries in chapter 25.

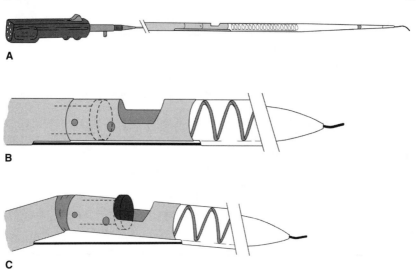

Fig. 3 The Silverhawk atherctomy catheter (EV3). (**A**) The catheter handle contains the motor controls. The tip is tapered. The nosecone contains the cutting device and space to collect plaque specimen. (**B**) Close up of the nosecone showing the cutting chamber in the open position. (**C**) When engaged for cutting plaque, the tip of the catheter becomes angulated. This allows eccentric positioning of the cutting chamber against the wall of the artery.

Atherectomy

Atherectomy is performed by a device that removes a portion of the atheroma from the lumenal surface using a cutting technique. There are different types of atherectomy devices, such as directional shaving devices (as pictured in Fig. 3) and rotational devices. The advantage of these devices is the potential to remove some of the plaque and create more space in the lumen, rather than just pushing the plaque aside as all the other methods do. The problem with these devices is the risk of distal embolization during the procedure and the incidence of recurrent stenosis on later follow-up. The most common commercially available device at this time is the Silverhawk™. At the present time, the main application for available atherectomy devices is in the lower extremity arteries. New devices are being prepared for market and some of these will use rotational atherectomy.

The Silverhawk atherectomy device comes in different sizes depending on the lumen of the artery, which is going to be treated. The larger devices used for treatment of arteries proximal to the tibial vessels are passed over a 0.014-in.-diameter guidewire. The size of the sheath required is either a 6 or 7 Fr depending on the size of the lumen of the artery, which is being treated. The atherectomy device is passed through the sheath to a point where the cutting chamber is visible fluoroscopically just proximal to the location of the lesion to be treated. When the catheter is properly positioned, the motor handle is engaged and the motor is turned on which can be heard turning and the catheter is slowly advanced over the guidewire with the cutting chamber up against the plaque. As the motor is engaged, the catheter itself assumes an angulated configuration, which helps to force the cutting chamber up against the wall of the artery. The pass of the atherectomy catheter is performed under fluoroscopy. The guidewire is carefully held in place while the atherectomy cutting chamber is advanced. After the atherectomy catheter is advanced and it is advanced at a fairly slow rate of approximately 1 cm every 5 to 10 seconds. The atherectomy cutting chamber eventually passes the lesion and the motor is disengaged. With disengagement of the motor, the cutting chamber is closed and tamps down the atherectomy specimens that have accumulated. The wire is held steady as the atherectomy catheter is withdrawn until it is proximal to the lesion. The atherectomy catheter has on its shaft a device which helps to assist in rotation of the catheter head. By holding the shaft or handle of the cath steady, the catheter may be rotated or pivoted and approximately six to nine clicks of the rotation will allow the cutting device to turn approximately 90 degrees. If it is not possible to see that the catheter is rotating with the clicks, then the catheter may have to be withdrawn and readvanced slightly. Sometimes the potential energy of twisting is built up within the catheter and not expressed by movement at the level of the cutting chamber. After the catheter has been rotated approximately 90 degrees, the motor is reengaged opening the cutting chamber and starting the motor and this allows the motor and cutting chamber to be advanced again across the lesion and another quadrant of cutting is performed. After each cut, the catheter is rotated approximately 90 degrees. When the cutting chamber becomes full or nearly full, the tamping device will only reach across the opening to the cutting chamber and will not reach all the way into the nose of the cutting chamber. When this is the case, the entire catheter is withdrawn. The cutting chamber is opened and the cutting chamber is flushed so that the atherectomy specimens can be removed. Once all the atherectomy specimens are removed, the atherectomy catheter is then passed again along the guidewire to the location of the lesion and additional atherectomy may be performed.

Clinically significant embolization is uncommon although it is common to produce emboli. It is quite common to have the impression that the lesion removed in terms of the actual specimens is much less than the amount of the lumen that has been created. There are some possible explanations for this. One is that the atherectomy specimens as they are removed are compressed into the cutting chamber thus making them look smaller than they might otherwise have been while in situ. There may also be some rigid catheter dilatation effect from the atherectomy device itself. Another concern is that the atherectomy cutting device works at a fairly constant rate of speed while the plaque being cut is heterogeneous. Some plaque is more solid and calcific and some is softer and more malleable. Therefore, as the atherectomy device is being pushed across the lesion, no matter how steady and gradually this is performed, there is the sense of skipping or hopping a little bit as the cutting chamber moves across the more calcified or difficult areas to cut. Atherectomy in the lower extremity is particularly useful at locations where stents are undesirable, such as locations where the artery will bend with flexing of the knee or the hip. In addition the origin of the superficial femoral artery, the origin of the tibial arteries and possibly the common femoral artery are other locations which are undesirable for stenting that may possibly be well treated with atherectomy.

Cryoplasty™

Cryoplasty is the use of cooling of the inflated angioplasty balloon in an attempt to induce apoptosis. The idea behind cryoplasty is that cell division can be interrupted and potentially even the process of recurrent stenosis could be diminished or prevented using cooling of the artery and the surrounding tissues. There is a substantial amount of science behind this but whether or not it actually decreases long-term rates of recurrent stenosis has not been conclusively shown. Cryoplasty is another potential option that may be used in locations where stenting is undesirable. It has been developed and priced to be used in lieu of a stent. Cryoplasty appears to be quite useful in the arteries of the lower extremities and may well be of value in other vascular beds.

The cryoplasty apparatus includes a balloon catheter that has multiple layers (Fig. 4). When the balloon is inflated, the multiple layers are designed to prevent leakage of nitrous oxide. Because the balloon has multiple layers, the caliber of the sheath required is either 6 or 7 Fr depending on the size of the balloon diameter which is desired. The balloon catheter is connected to a pump and when the balloon is located within the lesion, the balloon catheter is aspirated to clear the lumen of any air or nitrogen that may be there. The pump is then set into action and at the press of a button. Nitrous oxide is pumped into the balloon catheter and then cooled to $-10°C$. The balloon is inflated gradually over a course of several seconds and is inflated to a very reproducible level of 8 atm. This helps to decrease the likelihood that the balloon could be punctured or ruptured and also helps to achieve a very even type of dilatation. The gradual inflation and the very steady pressure increase over the course of a couple of minutes helps to minimize dissection. This minimization of dissection is something that is apparent when using the cryoplasty apparatus. The other piece of the system is a nitrous oxide canister, which may be placed within the pump at the appropriate time. After angioplasty is done, the catheter must be vented and after it's vented a negative aspiration is drawn. This helps to empty the balloon and as the balloon empties the blood flows around it and rewarms the balloon. Once the balloon is rewarmed, it may be repositioned for an additional inflation. Cryoplasty has been used quite extensively in the lower extremities in the

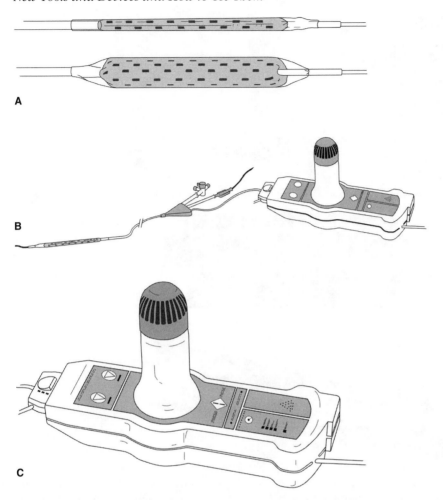

Fig. 4 Apparatus for performing Cryoplasty (Boston Scientific). (**A**) The multilayered cryoplasty balloon in its deflated and inflated states. (**B**) The control panel connects to the cryoplasty catheter. (**C**) A nitrous oxide canister is used to inflate the balloon.

superficial femoral, popliteal, and tibial arteries, especially in locations where stenting is undesirable.

Laser

There are several types of lasers that are being marketed currently for vascular disease. Lasers are being used both in the coronary and noncoronary arteries and in the venous system. A laser may be used to open a pathway through an occlusion and then have that pathway assumed by some other modality to achieve reconstruction. Laser may also be used to perform

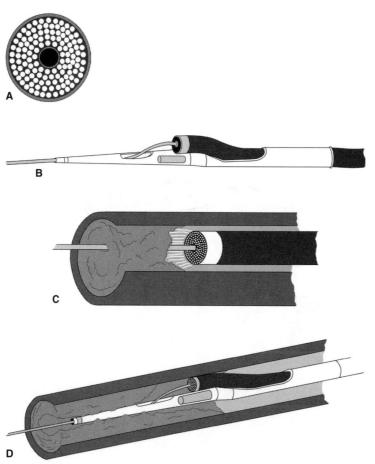

Fig. 5 Laser for peripheral artery use (Spectranetics). (**A**) The tip of the laser catheter. (**B**) Laser atherectomy is being performed over a guidewire. (**C**) The laser booster is a cradle that allows a broader sweep of the arterial lumen for the tip of the catheter.

debulking of plaque by means of laser atherectomy. Quite often, laser is used as an adjunct along with some other method. The laser catheters are in different sizes and each of the different sizes has a range of diameters of arteries for which it can be used (Fig. 5). The laser is passed over a wire. The tip of the laser catheter is advanced to within less than a centimeter of the lesion for crossing and the laser is turned on and it then vaporizes the lesion. The laser is advanced very slowly to perform even treatment of the plaque. In addition, there is a sled or booster which can be used to carry the laser catheter and this device may be rotated within the artery to create a larger borehole, and to use the same laser to create a larger passageway. The laser may be used to perform a translumenal recanalization by vaporizing either a chronic compacted thrombus, acute thrombus, or plaque. When embolization occurs, especially in the lower extremity, the laser may be used to chase that debris into the runoff vessels. The laser has been used with success in the superficial femoral arteries to reopen occlusions and is frequently used in combination with angioplasty and/or stenting. The laser is another device which is in the midst of a resurgence after previous efforts had not been found to be substantially valuable. The utility of this tool will be determined sometime in the next few years as additional data is accumulated.

Drug Eluting Stents

Drug eluting stents have had a significant impact in the care of coronary artery disease but have not as of yet had a significant impact in the treatment of noncoronary artery disease. Several trials are evaluating drug eluting stents in the superficial femoral and tibial arteries. The concept of drug eluting stents is to coat the stent with a drug which is gradually delivered to the artery wall. The drug is intended to cause a diminishment if not inhibition of cell division at this location so that intimal hyperplasia may be prevented. Studies in the coronary arteries using drug eluting stents have shown just such an effect. The drug delivery, however, is for a finite period of time and at some point the drug will be completely dissolved and there is an incidence of coronary stent thrombosis. The coronary arteries are of course much smaller than the superficial femoral and popliteal arteries and the same mechanisms of action may not take place in these locations. At the present time, there is no noncoronary indication for drug eluting stents but many operators are evaluating the potential for use of drug eluting stents in various locations, especially with recalcitrant or recurrent lesions and the tibial arteries.

Cutting Balloons

The concept of a cutting balloon is to place a cutting device on the side of the balloon so that when the balloon is inflated the blade will cut the lesion (Fig. 6). This will provide the potential for a fairly predictable cleavage plane when balloon angioplasty is performed. Cutting balloon angioplasty was developed to treat coronary in-stent restenosis but it has been only moderately successful in this application. The cutting angioplasty balloons are approved for both coronary and noncoronary usage. The smaller diameter balloons are in increments 0.5 mm steps up to 4.0 mm in diameter. These are monorail platform, 0.014 in. compatible. The larger balloons are in 1 mm incremental steps from 5 to 8 mm. Because the atherotomes make the balloon relatively rigid, these balloons are fairly short. The blades have T-shaped notches in them to assist with flexibility, although they still remain somewhat rigid. When the balloon is inflated, it's usually not possible to

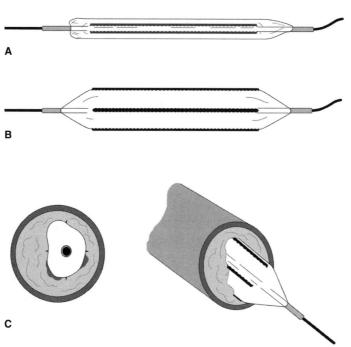

Fig. 6 Cutting balloon (Boston Scientific). (**A**) The cutting balloon has blades or atherotomes on its side. (**B**) When the balloon is inflated, the cutting blades dig into the plaque. (**C**) The blades create an impression on the lumenal surface of the plaque.

see a waist since the balloon sides are fairly rigid and expand all at once. The cutting balloon usually expands at fairly low pressures since the blades do in fact incise the tissue and allow expansion of the balloon. It's rare to proceed to a nominal pressure of approximately 8 atm without expanding the balloon. These balloons are semicompliant. Caution should be exercised in avoiding overinflation of the balloon for fear that a rupture of a balloon may cause loss of an atherotome. The smaller caliber balloons are 1.8 cm in length and the atherotome is 1.5 cm in length. Care is exercised when inserting the balloon into the sheath. Avoid cutting a finger by supporting the relatively stiff balloon catheter at the back end of the balloon with a pincer grasp as it's pushed into the sheath. After that, it advances in a manner much the same as any other monorail platform balloon.

The cutting balloon has applications in in-stent restenosis, recurrent stenosis due to intimal hyperplastic tissue, vein graft stenosis, stenosis within dialysis grafts, central vein stenoses, and pulmonary artery stenoses. When infrainguinal vein bypass grafts or central vein stenoses are treated, consider undersizing the cutting balloon; large enough to cut the lesion but not large enough to cut the juxtaposed normal vein tissue. Then follow up with a balloon sized to the desired final diameter. Cutting balloon angioplasty has also been used for focal infrainguinal artery lesions. This is especially useful with focal tibial artery lesions where standard angioplasty is somewhat limited because of the undesirability of placing stents in the tibial arteries. When the balloon is inserted into the correct location, the balloon is inflated slowly over the course of approximately half of a minute to a minute. This is done so that the atherotomes may correct themselves and to separate themselves along the inner circumference of the blood vessel wall. Avoid inflating the balloon twice in one location if at all possible. It is usually appropriate if further angioplasty is required to follow it with a standard angioplasty balloon and to open the caliber of the blood vessel further since the cleavage planes have been made within the plaque or within the scar tissue that represents a lesion. After balloon inflation, the balloon catheter is aspirated aggressively to attempt to shrink it down to its smallest possible size prior to removal. A cutting balloon may be used more than once but should be used with caution.

Peripheral Stent–Grafts

Stent–grafts have broad applications in relining the aorta and iliac arteries when treating aneurysm disease. There are other conditions that occur outside the aortoiliac system, which may require stent–graft placement. Stent–grafts available for peripheral use include the Viabahn™ (Gore, Inc.) stent–graft, the Fluency™ (Bard, Inc.) stent–graft, the Wallgraft™ (Boston Scientific), and the Icast™ (Atrium). None of these is a perfect system. All of these devices have a certain bulkiness and rigidity beyond standard stents and require larger sheaths for placement. The uses for stent–grafts are being evaluated and their indications for use in the treatment of occlusive disease of the lower extremity is an active area of investigation.

The most commonly implanted stent–graft outside the aortoiliac system is the Viabahn stent–graft which has an indication for use in the superficial femoral artery (Fig. 7). The Viabahn stent–graft is a nitinol mesh with polytetrafluoroethylene (PTFE) covering. It is relatively flexible and floppy. It is deployed using a ripcord style deployment system. The Viabahn stent–grafts may be obtained in lengths from 5 to 15 cm. The diameters in which they are available range from 4 to 10 mm. Viabahn stent–grafts require sheath sizes anywhere from 6 to 9 Fr and the sheath sizing charts and specific catheter availability should be consulted prior to any case. When treating a lesion with Viabahn stent–grafts one wants to achieve a seal within the artery and in a graft-to-graft fashion of approximately 3 cm. Occasionally, 2 cm is adequate; 3 cm is better, especially in a flexible system like the extremity. Viabahn stent–grafts may be oversized slightly but if they are oversized too much there will be wrinkling and corrugation of the material within the area of the lumen of the blood vessel. The Viabahn stent–graft is prepackaged on a delivery catheter that is placed through the sheath and then when the Viabahn stent–graft

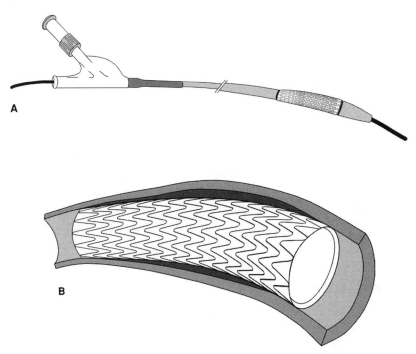

Fig. 7 Viabahn (Gore) peripheral stent-graft. (**A**) The stent-graft has a nitinol skeleton and a PTFE cover and is delivered on a catheter. The handle of the catheter contains a rip-cord type mechanism which is pulled to release the graft. (**B**) After deployment, the graft is self-expanding and somewhat flexible.

is in its proper location, the ripcord is pulled and the graft is deployed. Appropriate measuring should be performed prior to placement of the graft of both the length and the width required. Viabahn stent–grafts have been used to treat peripheral artery aneurysms throughout the body including carotid, renal, visceral, iliac, and popliteal vessels. They have also been used to treat occlusive disease in the superficial femoral artery and in the iliac artery and occasionally in other locations. After the stent–graft is placed, balloon angioplasty is performed of the stent–graft connections and at the ends of the graft to ensure that it is fully expanded. Patients who are treated with stent grafts are typically maintained on antiplatlet agents or anticoagulation and occasionally both.

Other types of stent grafts in the peripheral arteries include the aforementioned three grafts. The Fluency graft is a nitinol stent covered with a PTFE. It is stiffer than the Viabahn stent–graft and is more of a metal stent with a PTFE scaffold rather than PTFE with a metal scaffold. Because it is more rigid, it is only useful for relatively straighter conduit arteries. This is a particularly useful device for iatrogenic or traumatic injuries to the subclavian, superficial femoral, and other arteries. The Wallgraft is also somewhat rigid, and has handling and placement properties similar to the Wallstent but it has PTFE covering. There is some length variability at the time of deployment since the final deployed length is dependent upon the diameter to which it is deployed. The contourability is poor as it remains relatively rigid. The Icast is a balloon expandable metal stent with graft material covering it. These are short and rigid and accuracy of placement is quite good since it's balloon expandable and they are useful for vessel artery origin lesions such as renal, subclavian, or common carotid arteries. Regardless of one's practice, it is a good idea to have some stent–grafts available in the case of an injury, traumatic or iatrogenic, which may present in the course of usual vascular practice.

Thrombolysis

The intent of both chemical and mechanical thrombolysis is the removal of thrombotic material from the vascular system. In the case of chemical thrombolysis, the thrombolytic agent is delivered directly into the thrombus. Chemical thrombolysis has been available for several decades and has been through various iterations with different agents and approaches. The development of mechanical thrombectomy devices has prompted efforts to optimize treatment by combining chemical and mechanical thrombolysis in each case for a faster and more complete thrombus removal.

Chemical thrombolysis calls for pulse spray administration of thrombolytic agent directly into the thrombus, followed by an infusion of the same agent over a period of hours. In the case of mechanical thrombolysis, there are various churning type devices which may be used to disrupt thrombus and to dissolve or remove it. The relative advantage of chemical thrombolysis is the avoidance of injury to surrounding tissues, access of the medication to the thrombus regardless of other nearby lesions. In general, this is a more gentle process than mechanical thrombolysis, but it often takes too long. Longer procedures are not feasible in the setting of acute ischemic pain or ischemic organ damage and they expose the patient to longer intensive care stays and higher doses of thrombolytic agents. The advantage of mechanical thrombolysis is the ability to quickly debulk the clot burden and speed the procedure along. The disadvantage of mechanical thrombolysis is mostly logistical; investment in equipment and time is required, during the procedure larger sheaths are needed, each device has its learning curve, and the thrombus cannot always be reached. Most thrombolysis procedures are preformed with a combination of both chemical and mechanical thrombolysis; these two techniques are used in concert to achieve a faster and safer result.

If thrombotic problems occur during an endovascular procedure, the best initial step is aspiration thrombectomy. That is, place a catheter in proximity to the identified thrombus and aspirate. This is a useful adjunct and is required at sometimes unexpected occasions. Aspiration may be performed using a specifically designed aspiration catheter or using a small sheath or diagnostic catheter.

A commonly used chemical thrombolytic agent is tissue plasminogen activator (TPA). TPA is mixed in normal saline at a specific concentration and administered in a variety of ways. One common method is as follows. Place a sheath close to the thrombus. Enter the thrombus with a guidewire and pass a catheter over the guidewire and through the thrombus. Lace the clot with lytic agent using rapid injection of thrombolytic agent directly into the thrombus. This is performed with a 1-cc syringe injected into multiple locations along the length of a thrombus while gradually withdrawing the catheter over the guidewire so that the thrombolytic agent can be evenly distributed. This is the pulse spray technique. After this is performed, a soaker hose type catheter with multiple side holes is advanced into the thrombus and the guidewire is removed in exchange for an end-hole guidewire, which can be used to infuse thrombolytic agent into the distal runoff. Put the guidewire through the lumen of the soaker hose catheter. That forces the thrombolytic agent out the side holes of the soaker hose catheter. Two drip infusions are set up: one through the soaker hose catheter itself and one through the end-hole guidewire so that the tip of the guidewire is also infusing TPA. The tip of the guidewire is infused so that the runoff blood vessel whether it's in the kidney or in the lower extremity or other locations may be protected from thrombus accumulation. Soaker hose catheters can also be obtained that have a valve on the end so that the lytic agent does not all run off into the distal vasculature and miss the thrombosed segment of artery. Through the sidearm of the entry sheath, heparin is infused at a subtherapeutic level to prevent thrombus from accumulating in association with the sheath.

During infusion with thrombolytic agent, the patient undergoes intermittent laboratory analysis, including hematocrit, platelet level, thrombin level, protime, and partial thromboplastin time. If the thrombin level drops below 100, the lytic agent should be stopped. The complications of chemical thrombolysis increase with the time required for the infusion and the overall dose. A typical dosing regimen for TPA for an occluded lower extremity bypass is to lace the clot with several milligrams of TPA, anywhere from 2 to 6 mg, and then to run the infusion at 1 mg/hr for four hours and then to decrease the infusion to $\frac{1}{2}$ mg/hr after that. Most of the improvement that can be expected will be seen within the first eight hours. Typically, if there is a change clinically or if several hours have gone by, then it's time to repeat the angiogram and check the progress. Chemical thrombolysis may be combined with aspiration thrombectomy. A standard aspiration catheter may be placed over the guidewire and used to aspirate any thrombus which can be removed in this manner.

There are several devices available for mechanical thrombolysis. One commonly used device with a broad variety of applications is the AngioJet™ device (Fig. 8). When this device is used, a rapid spray of heparinized saline is infused and simultaneously aspirated. This creates a Bernoulli-type effect, which emulsifies the clot, converts it into very small particulate, and allows it to be removed with the effluent from the catheter. The device has several

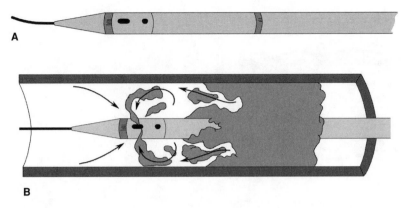

Fig. 8 The Angiojet™ (Possis) mechanical thrombectomy catheter. (**A**) the catheter is passed over the guidewire. (**B**) When engaged, the catheter tip simultaneously provides administration of fluid and aspiration of effluent.

different types of catheters which are geared for blood vessels of a variety of diameters. Care must be taken to choose the appropriately sized catheter and to advance it over the guidewire. As the catheter approaches the thrombus, the machine is engaged, the catheter is advanced slowly, and the clot is gradually removed.

This device may be used alone or in conjunction with chemical thrombolysis to help remove clot. Very often, a thrombolysis case will be initiated with pulse spray using the AngioJet™. This is done by temporarily occluding the effluent from the catheter so that a very small amount of infusion of lytic agent is placed at high speed and efficiency directly into the clot. After waiting a pre-set time, usually 15 to 30 minutes, the AngioJet™ is passed over the guidewire several times to remove thrombus. After several passes, interval arteriography is performed. If thrombus removal is incomplete, catheter-based chemical thrombolysis is established. One major limitation of the AngioJet™ is hemolysis; continued usage causes ongoing damage to circulating red blood cells and this is manifested by patient's blood-colored urine, decreased hematocrit, and even hemodynamic instability. The patient is maintained on full anticoagulation during mechanical thrombectomy.

Distal Protection Devices

Distal protection devices, or embolic protection devices, were developed for use in the carotid vascular bed (Fig. 9). Other applications may also be developed, such as protection during renal stenting or complex lower-extremity revascularization. Available data are not clear about whether distal protection devices have been an advance in the carotid circulation. These devices have some risk and cost of their own and only some data shows a trend toward lower stroke rates with protection devices. Nevertheless, the

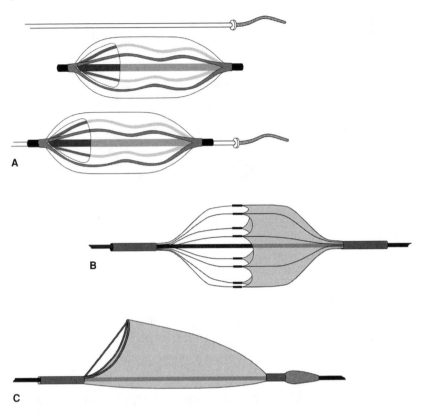

Fig. 9 Distal embolic protection devices. (**A**) The Emboshield (AbbottVascular) is a freewire system comprised of a 0.014 guidewire with a 0.019 knob on it near the tip, and the self-expanding filter held open with nitinol struts. (**B**) The AngioGuard™ (Cordis) is a fixed wire system with a short landing zone and an umbrella-like structure. (**C**) The Filterwire (Boston Scientific) is a fixed wire system with an eccentric nitinol hoop and a wind sock.

anecdotal finding of major embolic debris in a filter following a carotid stent placement makes the case to anyone who has had this experience. Distal protection devices were approved first for use in the coronary circulation when there is stenosis within a previously placed coronary vein graft. There are several approved distal protection devices for carotid stenting. Some of them are approved for use along with a concurrently used stent such as the Emboshield™ and the Acunet. Other devices, such as the Spider filter, are approved for use with any of the approved stents.

Distal protection devices function by being placed beyond the lesion prior to treatment. There are two competing design concepts; one is a fixed wire system (filter is fixed to the guidewire and they are placed together) and one is a free wire system (wire and filter are separate, first the wire is placed and then the filter). The Acunet and the Filterwire™ are examples of fixed wire systems, where the filter is fixed in place along a guidewire. A short segment of soft directional wire which is used to cross the lesion extends from the tip of where the filter is fixed on the shaft of the guidewire. Once the tip wire is across the lesion, the filter delivery catheter is advanced until the filter, which is compacted tightly into the filter delivery catheter, is also across the lesion. After the filter has crossed the lesion, a covering membrane is withdrawn and this allows the self-expanding filter to deploy and set its position. The alternative design, the free wire systems, includes the Emboshield and the Spider filters. With the use of the Emboshield, a specially designed guidewire is passed across the lesion. This guidewire has a shapable tip and comes in several different wire body strengths. There is a 0.019-in. diameter knob on the body of the 0.014-in. wire close to the tip and this knob is used as a stop for the filter to prevent it from going off the end of the guidewire. In this case, the wire is placed first, separate from the filter. The guidewire behaves more like a traditional guidewire, without the bulky filter on the guidewire during passage. After the guidewire is across the lesion, the filter delivery catheter is advanced and the filter is deployed along the wire. The Spider filter is different in that it allows the usage of any choice of guidewire that is 0.014 in. in diameter or less. Subsequently, a microcatheter is passed over the initial guidewire of choice and that guidewire is removed and then through the microcatheter is placed the filter itself. The filter is then deployed. During the procedure the filter is maintained in place. With the free wire filter systems, it is possible to have minor wire movement without significant filter movement. With the fixed wire system any movement of the wire will also cause a movement of the filter. The fixed wire systems permit crossing of the lesion and placement of the filter in a single step whereas the free wire systems require separate maneuvers for each of these steps.

In each of these systems there is some component of nitinol scaffolding which provides for the self-expanding properties of the filters. The filters have a specific pore size or a range of pore sizes. There is a range of expanded filter diameters, generally from 3 to 8 mm and a range of filter lengths. At the conclusion of the procedure the filter is recaptured. In each case, the filter recapturing catheter is larger than the delivery catheter with the rationale being that once the lesion is treated the lumen will accommodate a somewhat larger catheter in order to pass through and capture the filter. In addition, it is not desirable to squeeze the filter into as small a diameter as when it is an empty new filter, just in case the filter is full of debris.

Filters may prevent a disastrous case of untreatable distal embolization. However, filters also have pitfalls. There is the potential that with the release of embolic material that filtration will not be complete or that the embolic material may spill out of the filter prior to retrieval of the filter. An additional concern is that if the pore sizes in the filter itself are too large, then embolic material may pass through the filter but if the pore sizes are too small that it will induce thrombus formation and may cause a slow flow situation. The support structure for the filter is in the direction of the lesion. When a stent delivery catheter is advanced over the guidewire, if the tip of the stent delivery catheter encounters the filter support system, it may become entangled and may become irreversibly caught and necessitate some other type of drastic action to complete the procedure. Damage to artery may occur during filter placement for recapturing. Placement of the filter delivery catheter itself could cause embolization. Recapturing the filter may be very challenging in tortuous anatomy.

Lesions of significant complexity are being revascularized using endovascular techniques in many different vascular beds. The potential benefit of using filters in other locations is being explored. Indications for filters may include renal angioplasty and stenting, complex lower-extremity revascularization, atherectomy cases, subintimal angioplasty cases, treatment of acute or chronic thrombus formation with mechanical thrombectomy devices, and during coil embolization cases to prevent distal embolization of coils. There is a risk–benefit ratio associated with the filter when used as an adjunct. Most of the existing filters have been designed for coronary or carotid circulations and have not been designed for renal, lower-extremity, or other applications. The filter systems are somewhat restrictive with respect to the strength of the guidewire, which is used to support the filter. The filter has a length that requires a specific landing zone, varying from 2 to 4 cm. This distance of nondiseased artery distal to the lesion may not be available in every anatomical bed. The filter has a specific intended diameter and these were designed for the internal carotid artery. Outside that diameter range, there are no appropriate filters. The filter itself may cause damage to the artery in the runoff bed and manipulation of the wire in this area may also cause damage.

Most of the earlier discussion is in regard to distal protection devices. There are two other types of protection devices, which are not filters but are occlusive devices. These devices provide protection by using occlusion to either stop prograde cerebral flow or to reverse it. An example of a distal occlusion device is the Percusurge balloon. The Percusurge is approved for coronary vein grafts. The guidewire is a hypotube with a lumen in it. A balloon is mounted on the tip of the wire and is passed across the lesion. Using a special device, the hypotube is opened and fluid is administered to fill the balloon until occlusion of the distal artery is achieved. Treatment is undertaken and after this is done, an aspiration catheter is passed over the guidewire with flow at a standstill. The area is aspirated of any potentially embolic material. After multiple aspirations, the balloon is deflated and the guidewire with the balloon on it is removed. There is also a proximal occlusion balloon system which may be combined with reversed flow to achieve distal protection. This is performed with a transfemoral sheath that is quite sizable, up to 9 to 11 Fr. The sheath is advanced into the common carotid artery. The balloon is inflated to stop forward flow in the common carotid artery. Backbleeding flow from the external carotid artery is occluded with an occlusion balloon. Cerebral flow is reversed through the sheath by connecting to a low-pressure venous cannula. There is continuously reversed flow during the time of the treatment.

23

Brachiocephalic Interventions

Brachiocephalic interventions are being performed with increasing frequency. Endovascular approaches have replaced open surgery for most cases of arch and subclavian diseases. The role of carotid bifurcation stents is not yet determined, but they will have some role in treatment. In this chapter, these areas are described.

Carotid Bifurcation

Patient preparation for carotid bifurcation stenting includes Clopidogrel (Plavix®) 75 mg/day for five days prior to the procedure and daily aspirin 325 mg. The aortic arch, carotid arteries, and cerebral arteries are evaluated prior to the stent procedure using arteriogram, magnetic resonance angiography (MRA), or computerized tomographic angiography (CTA). The current preferred approach is transfemoral with a minority of patients being more appropriate for a transbrachial approach or a transcervical exposure. The procedure is performed under local anesthesia with minimal or no sedation to facilitate continuous neurological monitoring. An arterial line is placed for continuous pressure monitoring and electrocardiography (EKG) leads for cardiac monitoring. Temporary pacer pads should be available and patients with aortic stenosis should have the temporary pacer pads in place. Antihypertensive medications may be held on the morning of the procedure, especially beta blockers. Bradycardia occurs frequently with balloon angioplasty of de novo carotid bifurcation stenosis and this may be sustained after the procedure.

Femoral access is achieved and heparin is administered, 100 units per kg. An activated clotting time is obtained and is maintained at >250 seconds. The same size femoral sheath access sheath is placed as that anticipated for the procedure, usually either 6 or 7 Fr. A floppy-tip guidewire is placed in the aortic arch and the image intensifier is rotated into the left anterior oblique position to reflect the best angle achieved for viewing as identified on the preoperative study. The cerebral catheter of choice is placed over the guidewire. Chapter 9 offers a discussion of carotid catheterization and chapter 10 discusses carotid arteriography. The image intensifier is maintained in its fixed position left anterior oblique (LAO) and the bony landmarks may be used to guide vessel cannulation. The cerebral catheter is placed in the common carotid artery origin. A hydrophilic, steerable guidewire is advanced through the catheter and into the mid-to-distal common carotid artery. The location of the carotid bifurcation can often be identified on plain fluoroscopy due to the presence of vessel calcification. The guidewire is not permitted to pass into the bifurcation. The cerebral catheter is advanced so that its tip is well seeded in the common carotid artery. A road map of the carotid bifurcation is performed (Fig. 1). The position of the image intensifier may require adjustment to obtain the best image showing the bifurcation and the separation of the internal and external carotid arteries. Multiple views may be needed to best open the carotid bifurcation.

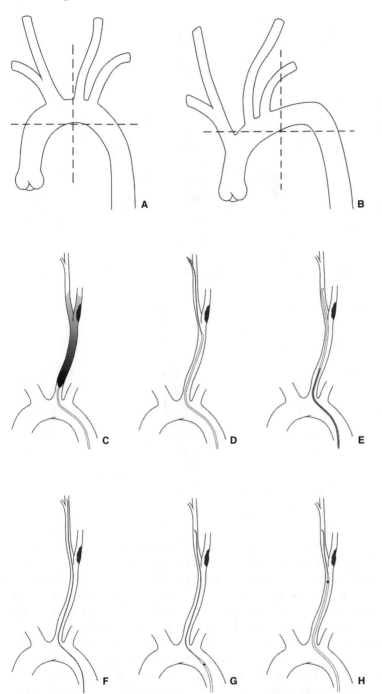

Fig. 1 Carotid bifurcation stent placement. (**A**) Normal aortic arch in segments. The branches originate from the top of the arch. All the branch origins are a substantial distance superior to the horizontal line drawn across the upper, inner aspect of the arch. (**B**) An elongated arch, which is common in the elderly and those with hypertension. A line drawn across the upper inner aspect of the arch readily demonstrates that the origin of the innominate is inferior to the lie and will likely be a challenging catheterization. (**C**) The left common carotid artery is catheterized and a roadmap is

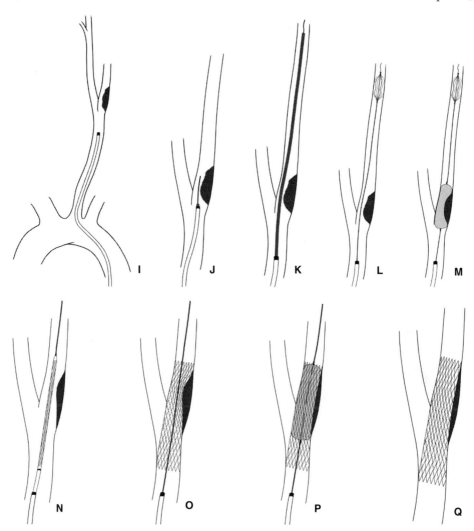

Fig. 1 (*Continued*) created of the bifurcation. (**D**) The Glidewire is advanced into the external carotid artery and the catheter is advanced. (**E**) The stiff exchange guidewire is placed in the external carotid artery. (**F**) The angiographic catheter is withdrawn from the external carotid artery. (**G**) The sheath is advanced over the stiff guidewire. (**H**) The tip of the sheath is placed in the mid- to distal common carotid artery. (**I**) The exchange guidewire is withdrawn from the external carotid artery. (**J**) The leading wire for the distal embolic protection device is placed across the lesion. (**K**) The filter delivery catheter is passed across the carotid stenosis. (**L**) The filter is deployed. (**M**) Pre-dilatation of the lesion. (**N**) The stent delivery catheter is advanced. (**O**) The stent is deployed across the bifurcation. (**P**) Post-stent dilation is performed, keeping the balloon within the stent and only dilating the area of residual lesion within the stent. (**Q**) After completion angiography, the filter is removed.

The next step is selective cannulation of the external carotid artery. Selective external carotid cannulation is performed with a 260-cm-angled Glidewire advanced under road map and the cerebral catheter is advanced into the external carotid artery. When common carotid catheterization is performed with a simple-curve catheter, the advancement of the catheter into the external carotid artery is facilitated. When a complex-curve catheter is used to cannulate the common carotid artery, this complex-curve catheter is sometimes possible to advance into the external carotid artery. However, frequently, it must be exchanged for a simple-curve catheter. An attempt should be made to reach as distally on the external carotid artery as possible. This allows adequate guidewire length beyond the bifurcation for the subsequent placement of the carotid access sheath. The Glidewire is withdrawn from the cerebral catheter and a 260-cm stiff exchange guidewire, such as an Amplatz super-stiff wire, is placed in the external carotid artery. Before placing the exchange guidewire, check to make sure there is backbleeding from the catheter. If the catheter has been advanced into a very small branch or if spasm has occurred and there is no backbleeding, the inner catheter surface may become lined with air bubbles. When the exchange guidewire is introduced, these microbubbles may be pushed into the systems and become emboli. Occasionally, the catheter must be very slightly withdrawn to restore backbleeding. When the stiff exchange guidewire is advanced, it is usually best to position the image intensifier in the left anterior oblique position. The field of view includes the top of the arch on the inferior aspect of the monitor so that the last turn from the arch into the common carotid artery can be visualized as the stiff guidewire rounds the turn. Superiorly on the monitor, the tip of the catheter is visualized and its position is established using bony landmarks. If there is significant arch tortuosity, the last turn from the arch into the common carotid artery may be a challenging angle. As the stiff guidewire enters the common carotid artery, it may start to pull the catheter down from the external carotid artery. If the tip of the catheter starts to migrate inferiorly, this serves as an early warning system that the catheter–guidewire apparatus has too much tension in it and that an alternative plan is required.

After the stiff exchange guidewire is placed, the simple-curve catheter is withdrawn leaving the stiff guidewire in the external carotid artery. The access sheath in the groin is removed. A 6- or 7-Fr 90-cm-long sheath is advanced over the stiff guidewire into the common carotid artery. There are many sheath choices for this maneuver. Two good choices are the Cook Shuttle sheath and the Terumo Destination sheath. As the sheath is advanced, image the distal end of the stiff wire in the external carotid artery, including the last turn exiting the arch and the tip of the guidewire. If the tip of the guidewire starts to back up, it indicates that the sheath is not advancing appropriately over the guidewire.

The dilator for the carotid sheath is several centimeters longer than the sheath itself and could be inadvertently advanced into the bifurcation. The outline of the dilator tip can usually be identified under fluoroscopy even though it does not have a radiopaque marker. When the dilator reaches its desired location in the mid or distal common carotid artery, it is held steady and the sheath may be advanced over the dilator itself. The dilator is withdrawn and the carotid angiogram is performed through the sheath to be sure that the tip of the sheath is optimally placed. The stiff guidewire is removed, and the image intensifier is optimally positioned to road map the bifurcation.

Embolic protection may be performed with one of a variety of distal protection devices. There are a variety of occlusive devices, for either proximal or distal occlusion, that are not covered in this chapter. Several distal filters are available and are used most commonly. Some examples of filters are discussed in chapter 22. As mentioned, the filter may be either a free wire or fixed wire system. Either way, the tip of the 0.014-in. guidewire is shaped appropriately to aid access to the internal carotid artery. After crossing the stenosis, the tip of the guidewire is placed close to the skull base. It is important to not advance the tip of the guidewire any further. The intracranial portion of the carotid artery is prone to dissection with guidewire manipulations. The image intensifier position is then set, with the tip of the sheath visible at the lower margin of the view, the bifurcation in the middle, and the tip of the guidewire upon which the filter is based located at the upper end of the view.

After the guidewire is placed across the lesion, the filter is rapidly deployed. The length of the filter and the location of the stenosis must be taken into account. Each filter require the appropriate landing zone, preferably in a straight and nondiseased artery segment at least 2 cm distal to the location intended for the upper end of the stent. The lesion is predilated with a 2-mm or 3-mm balloon, a monorail based 2-cm or 4-cm length balloon. Prior to specific events, such as predilatation, stent placement, and post-stent balloon angioplasty, some operators prefer administer small doses of atropine (0.25–0.50 mg each time) to prevent or at least to blunt the bradycardic response that may occur. The duration of the predilatation depends on the appearance and behavior of the balloon but is kept as short as possible. The predilatation balloon is inflated only once and the inflation time varies depending on the lesion. The purpose of the predilatation is to create a safe tract for the stent delivery catheter. Some operators practice "primary stenting" without predilatation on a regular basis. However, with any significant stenosis, a 6-Fr stent delivery catheter will have a dottering effect on the lesion unless predilatation is performed.

Carotid bifurcation lesions may be treated with any one of a variety of self-expanding stents that are available for use in this position. The stents vary from 2 to 4 cm in length. The stents may be open cell or closed cell. Most available stents are constructed of nitinol, may be tapered or tube structure, and vary from 6 to 10 mm in diameter. The stent diameter is selected based on the largest diameter that must be fitted to the stent, usually that of the common carotid artery.

The self-expanding stent is deployed using road mapping and/or land-marks, such as the vertebral bodies. The self-expanding stent is postdilated with a 5 mm × 20 mm balloon over the 0.014-in. wire, depending on the size of the internal carotid artery. This is usually easily performed by placing the balloon in the location where any residual stenosis is seen to be crimping the stent. A 5-mm balloon percutaneous transluminal angioplasty (PTA) is often adequate, rarely is a 5.5- or 6-mm PTA required poststent deployment. A mild or even moderate residual stenosis may be accepted, as the self-expanding stents continue to expand with time. The risks of overdoing it with lost-stent balloon dilatation include embolization of plaque contents, severe bradycardia and hypotension, and very rarely vessel rupture. The balloon used for poststent PTA is always maintained within the stent. Nominal pressure is used to fully expand the balloon and the stent and it is not kept inflated any longer than necessary. High pressures are not used. In the majority of cases, the stent is placed across the bifurcation into the common carotid artery, crossing the origin of the external carotid artery.

Occasionally, some flow of contrast is visible outside the stent profile and into an ulcer. No attempt should be made to obliterate this by using larger balloons or higher pressures as this almost always smooths out in the ensuing weeks and is usually of no consequence. Patients with >2-cm-long carotid lesions, dense calcification (seen on plain fluoroscopic images), and large ulcerated plaques are at higher risk for carotid angioplasty and stenting (CAS) complications. Tortuosity of the common carotid, bifurcation, or more commonly the distal internal carotid artery may be challenging to manage during CAS. Tortuous inflow causes problems in creating and maintaining a safe and stable access. Kinks and bends near the lesion and in the distal internal carotid artery may pose a problem with stent implants. Tortuosity cannot be removed, only transferred to another location. As a stent is placed that partially straightens a curved segment, another segment juxtaposed to the stented location usually becomes more tortuous. Deploy stents across bends only if they are isolated and only when necessary. Avoid placing the distal end of the stent into kinks and tortuosities of the internal carotid artery if more than a single bend is noted. A very tortuous internal carotid artery should be considered a relative contraindication for CAS.

The filter is removed only after an arteriogram confirms forward flow through the filter and no filling defect in the stent or filter. The filter is removed and final angiograms are acquired in the projection that had demonstrated the maximum stenosis. Attention is paid to the internal carotid artery immediately cephalad to the stent. Spasm in this segment may be encountered. The best treatment for internal carotid artery spasm is to finish the case and remove the distal protection device. A small dose of intra-arterial nitroglycerine (50–100 mcg) is directly administered into the artery. Post-CAS intracranial angiograms are obtained by most operators as a routine. The sheath is then removed.

Patients are monitored overnight for cardiac and neurologic problems. It is not uncommon, especially in patients with a history of coronary artery disease to have a heightened response to carotid sinus distension. It may require inotropic support for a time before the carotid sinus adapts to the radial force of the self-expanding stents. Avoiding extreme over sizing of the stents helps to decrease the incidence of post-CAS bradycardia and hypotension. The presence of significant hypotension in the absence of bradycardia is unusual in the immediate postprocedure period; it is worth emphasizing that other causes, e.g., retroperitoneal bleed related to access site problems, should also be excluded as the cause. Medications include Aspirin 325 mg each day indefinitely and Clopidogrel 75 mg each day for one month. Follow-up includes duplex scan at intervals just as is performed after carotid endarterectomy.

Innominate and Common Carotid Artery

There are significant differences between interventions in the carotid bifurcation and those in the common carotid and subclavian–axillary arteries. Most symptomatic carotid bifurcation lesions present as a result of cerebral embolization, and the potential for embolization with manipulation is probably higher than for lesions of the arch. Carotid bifurcation stent placement is performed with some type of cerebral protection, almost always is just a single self-expanding stent, and is performed with a 0.014 platform. Lesions of the innominate and common carotid arteries are less common than carotid bifurcation stenoses. Subclavian artery stenoses and occlusions are quite common but they do not often need to be treated. Innominate, common carotid, and subclavian lesions, as compared to the carotid bifurcation, are less likely to present with embolization and are more likely to present with hypoperfusion syndromes. These are usually treated without a cerebral protection device and may be managed with either 0.014 or 0.035 systems and with either self-expanding or balloon-expandable stents. The most common disease to occur in the innominate, common carotid, and subclavian arteries, which requires angioplasty and stent placement, is disease that occurs at the origins of these arteries. These lesions tend to be heavily calcified. They also tend to occur at the origin of the artery where the location of the sheath for delivery of the stent is less stable.

Chapter 9 provides a detailed discussion of selective catheterization of these arteries. Chapter 10 covers arch aortography and selective branch vessel arteriography. Supplies required for interventions of the innominate, common carotid, and subclavian arteries are listed in Table 1.

Focal lesions of the common carotid artery may be approached either antegrade through a femoral access or retrograde through a distal common carotid artery exposure. It is rare to access the common carotid artery from its distal end. However, the occasions for this would be when there is need

Table 1 Supplies for Interventions of the Innominate, Common Carotid and Subclavian Arteries[a]

Guidewire	Starting guidewire	Newton	180 cm length	0.035 in. diameter
	Selective guidewire	Glidewire	260 cm	0.035 (angled tip)
	Exchange guidewire	Amplatz Super-stiff	260 cm	0.035
Catheter	Flush catheter	Pigtail	90 cm length	5 Fr
	Selective cerebral catheter	H_1	100 cm length	5 Fr
		DAV	100 cm	5 Fr
		Vitek	125 cm	5 Fr
		Simmons 1, 2	100 cm	5 Fr
		H_3	100 cm	5 Fr
Sheath	Cerebral guide sheath	Shuttle	90 cm length	6 Fr, 7 Fr
Balloon	Balloon angioplasty catheter	Balloon diameter	5, 6, 7, 8, 9, 10 mm	
		Balloon length	2, 4 cm	
		Catheter shaft	120 cm length	5 Fr
Stent[b]	Balloon-expandable stent	(premounted)	Stent diameter	6, 7, 8, 10 mm
			Stent length	15–35 mm
			Shaft length	135 cm
	Self-expanding stent	nitinol	Diameter	8, 10, 12, 14 mm
			Stent length	20, 40 mm
			Delivery catheter	120 cm

[a] Excluding carotid bifurcation balloon angioplasty and stenting.
[b] No stents are approved by the FDA for routine usage in this vascular bed.

for a concomitant carotid bifurcation endarterectomy or when the arch is too dangerous to cross (in coming from a transfemoral route) but the patient is otherwise a good stent candidate.

Arch aortography is performed through a femoral approach using a pigtail catheter and a pressure injector, as described in chapter 10. The image intensifier is best placed in the LAO position (fig. 1 of chap. 9). An image of the arch, the origins of its branches, and the carotid bifurcation is saved on the monitor and the image intensifier is not moved until the artery origin is cannulated.

Assessment of Arch Branch Lesions

Because these lesions are typically at the origins of the arteries and are associated with the arch of the aorta, imaging of the chest must be performed in order to fully understand the extent of lesions in these locations. An arch aortogram in the left anterior oblique position is one way to evaluate the origins of the innominate, left common carotid, and left subclavian arteries. To visualize the innominate bifurcation, which includes the origins of right subclavian and the right common carotid arteries, a right anterior oblique projection is usually required. If there is associated disease in the arch of the aorta or lesions in middle segments of the arch branches, it may influence catheter placement in an effort to avoid the worst part of the disease and avoid embolization as a result of encountering arch disease. The arch and its proximal branches may also be assessed using MRA or CTA. The results are somewhat limited by the fact that they tend to overemphasize the severity of the lesions. It is not simple to obtain confirmatory information about lesion severity using duplex, as it is with carotid bifurcation lesions. In addition, the CTA while it gives useful anatomical information tends to overemphasize the calcium and these tend to be heavily calcified lesions. Both methods are very helpful at delineating the anatomy of the area.

Prepare for the case by assessing the length of the disease to be treated and choosing the stents or the stents which are most likely to be used during the procedure. Placement of stents from a transfemoral route will require a 70-cm sheath in a short person and a 90-cm sheath in a normal sized to tall person using a transfemoral approach. If there is significant calcium in the aorta, it may influence the type of catheter. Simple-curve catheter choices for crossing these lesions include a vertebral catheter and for a complex-curve catheter a Vitek catheter is frequently useful since this may be pushed into the arch from the descending aorta rather than dragged backward from the right side of the arch to the left side of the arch. There is a choice with arch branch lesions as to whether a 0.014- or a 0.035-in. diameter system would be best. In addition with respect to the planning and treatment of subclavian lesions, it is quite often valuable to approach these lesions either for part of or all of the treatment by using a brachial access and this is discussed more later. This, however, should be decided, to the extent possible, at the beginning of the procedure.

Principal Techniques

Access is usually obtained in the femoral artery. Systemic anticoagulation is administered. A 5- or 6-Fr sheath is placed in the femoral artery and a 100-cm length 5-Fr pigtail catheter is advanced so that the head of the pigtail catheter is in the ascending aorta. An arch aortogram is performed. This demonstrates the location of the lesion as well as its length and its approximate diameter. Subsequently a Glidewire is passed through the pigtail catheter and the pigtail catheter is removed. An angled catheter, usually a simple-curve catheter or a vertebral catheter, is advanced over the Glidewire. The Glidewire is withdrawn into the shaft of the catheter. The catheter is then withdrawn slightly and pointed toward the location of the lesion at the artery origin, which is intended for crossing. The so-called "no touch" technique is used if possible. The catheter is pointed in the appropriate direction. Occasionally, a puff of contrast may be used to assist visualization. The guidewire is used to gently probe the roof of the arch and to probe for the lesion and to get across the lesion. After the Glidewire has crossed the lesion, it is then advanced into the mid-distal common carotid artery. If possible the simple-curve catheter is advanced over the Glidewire and the carotid artery is road mapped to identify the location of the carotid bifurcation and to avoid inadvertently crossing it if crossing the bifurcation is not required. Subsequently, a 0.035-in. diameter stiff exchange wire is advanced through the catheter. The tip of the exchange wire is placed in a way that's consistent with the degree of tortuosity which the sheath must pass. The tip of the wire is usually placed in the distal common carotid artery. For a tortuous arch, it may require placement in the distal external carotid artery. The sheath is then advanced over this system with the stiff exchange wire. Be careful to not inadvertently advance the tip of the dilator for the sheath across the lesion if this is not something that is planned. At some point, the dilator is held steady and the sheath is advanced over the dilator to achieve the last couple of centimeters.

If the planned procedure is to take place using 0.035-in. compatible balloon catheters and stent delivery catheters, the same stiff guidewire is maintained in place and used for treatment. If it is desirable to switch to a 0.014-in.-based system, then this is the time to do it. Lesions distal to the origin may be treated by placing a stiff 0.014-in. guidewire. A stiff 0.014-in.-diameter wire is placed through the bifurcation and into the external carotid artery. Lesions at the very origin of the arch branches leave no place within the branch artery to put the sheath tip to make a stable system. The 0.014-in.-diameter guidewire is not as sturdy as 0.035-in.-diameter guidewire. Because of the location of the lesion at the origin of the artery, the only way to get a stable sheath position and to get the sheath close enough is to put the tip of the sheath up close to the lesion using a fairly heavy exchange guidewire. The lesion may be predilated or stented primarily. A premounted, balloon-expandable stent is advanced over the guidewire. The stent is advanced across the lesion. Small puffs of contrast may be performed to help position it. Just before placement of the stent, the sheath must be withdrawn slightly so that the lower end of the stent is able to clear the upper end of the sheath. When the sheath is withdrawn, it creates an inherently less stable situation, so care must be taken to maintain guidewire position without any withdrawal of the guidewire.

The advantage of the 0.035-in. system in this case is that this is a sturdier platform. The disadvantage is that the wire manipulation is quite limited and also that the stent delivery catheter fills the sheath and so quite a large sheath is required if the ability to inject contrast around the stent delivery catheter is going to be available. This ability is quite desirable since the placement of the stent can be challenging and it's good to be able to administer contrast in small puffs through the sheath to confirm the optimal placement of the stent prior to deploying it.

A lesion in the mid common carotid artery may also be encountered that is not at the common carotid artery origin. Because this is a relatively mobile artery, if the lesion does not involve the origin of the common carotid artery and there is a length of at least 1 cm of reasonably sized and nondiseased artery at the origin of the common carotid artery, the best option in this case is to use a self-expanding nitinol stent. Although the trailing end of the stent is difficult to place with a high degree of accuracy, if there is a centimeter of open space in the artery distal to its origin, this is usually adequate.

With respect to the innominate artery, sizing issues are often a problem. Because the artery is somewhat short, the placement of a self-expanding stent is not advisable in most cases. In addition, because the artery is larger in diameter than the other arch branches, if a balloon-expandable stent is to be employed, the balloon-expandable stents reach an adequate diameter of 10 mm or more are usually deliverable through a larger sheath and have a much larger crossing profile to get across the lesion in order to place the stent. Imaging during stent placement should be determined by whether the lesion is directly at the origin of the blood vessel or more distally close to the bifurcation because the origin is better seen in the LAO and the bifurcation of the innominate is better seen in the right anterior oblique (RAO) position of the image intensifier. The other thing about the innominate artery is that it's typically a very unstable place to have a sheath, especially when the origin of the innominate artery is being treated. Because this is an unstable system, consider using a stiff guidewire which extends out into the right subclavian and can be placed all the way down to the axillary artery if necessary to obtain more purchase. Another way to obtain more purchase and greater stability is to place two separate 0.014-in.-diameter guidewires, one into the common carotid artery and one into the subclavian artery and then to place a 0.035-in. compatible stent delivery catheter over the combination of the two wires. The combination of two different 0.014-in.-diameter guidewires is less than the diameter of a single 0.035-in.-diameter guidewire.

Most of these lesions can be treated using a transfemoral approach but sometimes the adjunctive addition of a transbrachial approach is quite help-ful. After stent placement whether it's balloon-expanding or self-expanding stent, a follow-up balloon angioplasty is performed. Care must be taken with placement of balloon-expandable stents to expand them adequately so that they are in a stable position but not to overexpand and cause injury to the artery and surrounding tissues. A completion study is then performed through the sheath and if this is satisfactory the guidewire and sheath are removed.

Transfemoral Approach to the Common Carotid Artery

If proceeding with a transfemoral approach, a guidewire and access sheath are inserted (Fig. 2). Heparin is administered intravenously, 75 to 100 U/kg. The tip of the guidewire is placed in the arch. A 6- or 7-Fr, 90-cm-long, straight sheath with a radiopaque tip is passed and the tip is advanced to within a few centimeters of the origin of the artery. The operator must decide whether to lead with the guidewire or to lead with the catheter. If the lesion is located at the very origin of the common carotid artery, either the catheter or the guidewire may be used to lead. Neither of these is optimal to lead because they will be protruding from the end of the sheath which is mobile within the arch and this is a relatively unstable position for the whole platform. If the lesion is distal to the origin of the vessel, lead with the catheter to cannulate the artery and then advance the guidewire. The appropriate selective cerebral catheter, 100 to 120 cm in length, is placed through the sheath. The head of the selective cerebral catheter extends beyond the end of the sheath. The cerebral catheter directs the guidewire into the origin of the common carotid artery.

The steerable guidewire is advanced carefully beyond the common carotid artery lesion and into the external carotid artery. The cerebral catheter may be advanced over the guidewire and into the external carotid artery. The steerable guidewire is exchanged for an Amplatz guidewire. After the stiff guidewire is in place in the external carotid artery, the cerebral catheter is removed. The dilator is replaced within the long sheath and the sheath is advanced carefully up to the artery origin. Avoid dottering the lesion with the dilator. It is usually best to advance the sheath directly over the dilator for the last few centimeters. After the tip of the sheath is in place, additional arteriography and heparin flushing may be performed through the sidearm of the sheath. The long sheath should be flushed regularly and care must be taken to avoid thrombus formation or microbubbles.

A carotid arteriogram is performed through the sheath with a small field of view. The usual diameters are 6 to 8 mm for the common carotid artery and 8 to 12 mm for the innominate artery. The most favorable lesions are focal and a 2-cm-long balloon is usually adequate. Usually, primary stent placement is performed. Orifice lesions are best treated with a balloon-expandable stent. Other lesions may be treated with either self-expanding or balloon-expandable stents, since these are relatively straight conduit arteries.

Self-expanding stent diameter should be 8 mm for a 5- to 7-mm common carotid artery or 10 mm for a 7- to 9-mm artery. The stent delivery catheters must be 120 cm. The length of the stent should be kept to a minimum. The stent delivery catheter is passed over the guidewire, through the sheath, and

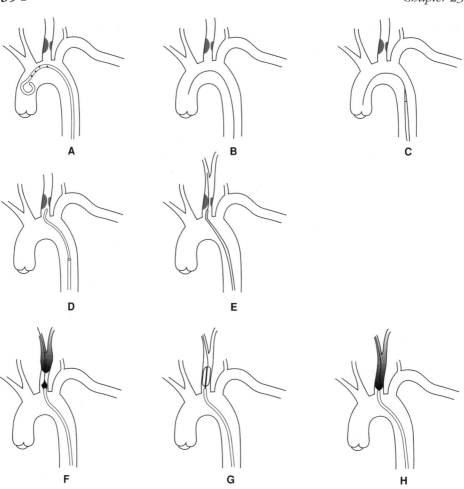

Fig. 2 Balloon angioplasty of the common carotid artery. (**A**) An arch aortogram is performed with a flush catheter. (**B**) The guidewire is replaced after the location of the common carotid artery origin and the lesion are identified. (**C**) A long sheath is placed in the proximal descending aorta. (**D**) A selective cerebral catheter is advanced through the sheath and used to cannulate the common carotid artery. The catheter must be at least 20 cm longer than the sheath. (**E**) The guidewire is directed into the external carotid artery. (**F**) The sheath is advanced into the proximal common carotid artery and an arteriogram is performed. (**G**) Balloon angioplasty is performed. If the lesion is in proximity to the bifurcation, the guidewire should be placed in the internal carotid artery. (**H**) Completion arteriography is performed through the sheath.

into position across the lesion (Fig. 3). The stent is deployed and postplacement dilatation is performed, followed by completion arteriography.

In each case, the sheath is close to the lesion and the sheath is withdrawn to uncover the stent and to deploy the stent. If landmarks require rechecking, contrast may be injected through the sheath prior to

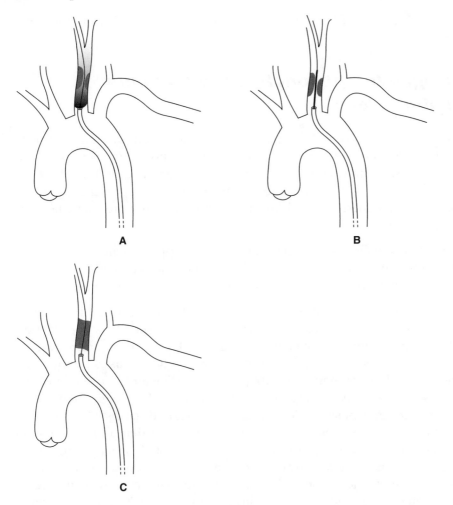

Fig. 3 Stent placement in the common carotid artery. (**A**) After guidewire and sheath placement, an arteriogram is performed. (**B**) A self-expanding or balloon-expandable stent is delivered to the site of the lesion or the angioplasty. (**C**) The stent is deployed while maintaining access to the common carotid artery with the sheath.

stent deployment. Afterward, completion arteriography may likewise be performed through the sheath.

Orifice lesions require a very high degree of placement accuracy since the proximal end of the stent should protrude into the arch enough to contain any arch plaque that has spilled over into the common carotid artery. Orifice lesions may also be challenging from a femoral approach because when the sheath is pulled back to expose the stent, the tip of the sheath loses its purchase on the origin of the common carotid artery. The sheath must be withdrawn carefully and the tip should be parked as close to the end of the balloon as possible without impinging upon it. After deploying the stent, postdilatation of both ends of the stent is performed using the same balloon.

Retrograde Approach to the Common Carotid Artery

Common carotid artery lesions may also be approached retrograde, usually through open exposure of the distal common carotid artery. This approach is usually best in the following circumstances: angulated arch anatomy or arch disease that is not favorable for an antegrade approach, an orifice lesion, or a combined carotid bifurcation lesion that requires simultaneous endarterectomy.

The two key factors for consideration in this approach are the very short working room between the access and the lesion and the need to clamp the carotid for a short period of time without options for a shunt.

The common carotid artery exposure is performed through a short incision and the artery is looped. Heparin is administered. It is usually best to place a transfemoral pigtail in the arch of the aorta for arteriography, even if the intervention is to be performed retrograde. This is because retrograde carotid arteriography is suboptimal at delineating the origin of the artery, especially in the setting of an orifice lesion. The image intensifier is placed in the LAO position. The artery is punctured as distally along the common carotid artery as possible but in a location that allows clamping and avoids any bifurcation disease. This helps to maximize working room. The guidewire is inserted through the needle, and fluoroscopy is initiated immediately since the lesion will be encountered within a few centimeters. After the guidewire is across the lesion, attempt to steer it into the descending aorta. This is frequently unsuccessful since the natural tendency is for the guidewire to direct itself into the ascending aorta. A short, bent-tip selective catheter, such as a Kumpe, is used to direct the guidewire into the descending aorta. A very short access sheath, preferably 8 cm or less, is placed in the retrograde position. A retrograde arteriogram is performed. If the image intensifier position has remained unchanged since the arch aortogram, this may be used for positioning. Otherwise, an arch aortogram may be repeated through the transfemoral pigtail catheter. The appropriate balloon and stent are selected and placed. The distal common carotid artery may be clamped during balloon angioplasty and stent placement. The artery is flushed and repaired after intervention.

The Subclavian and Axillary Arteries

Subclavian and axillary artery lesions can be approached antegrade (femoral artery access) or retrograde (brachial artery access). The best candidates for this procedure have symptomatic vertebrobasilar insufficiency or upper-extremity ischemia and a lesion that does not involve the origin of the vertebral artery. Whether planning an antegrade or a retrograde approach, arch aortography is performed through a femoral approach using a pigtail catheter. An image of the arch and the origins of its branches are used to guide catheter passage for lesions of the subclavian and proximal axillary arteries.

Transfemoral Approach to the Subclavian and Axillary Arteries

The lesion is usually identified during arch aortography. Heparin is administered, 75 to 100 U/kg. A 7-Fr, 90-cm-long, straight sheath with a radiopaque tip is passed and the tip is advanced to within a few centimeters of the orifice of the subclavian artery. The dilator is removed and the appropriate selective cerebral catheter (see chap. 6), 100 to 120 cm in length, is placed through the sheath. The tip of the selective catheter is placed beyond the end of the sheath. The steerable guidewire probes the orifice of the artery with support and direction provided by the selective catheter. The guidewire is advanced across the lesion and as far into the artery as possible to provide support for the catheter to be advanced (Fig. 4). The catheter is advanced into the subclavian artery. Selective arteriography may be performed if necessary. A stiffer guidewire, such as an Amplatz or a Rosen, is placed. The selective catheter is removed, the dilator is placed, and the sheath is advanced into the artery origin. Arteriography and heparin flush administration may be performed through the sidearm of the sheath.

The best lesions for angioplasty and stenting in this area are short and are located well proximal or distal to the vertebral artery. A lesion juxtaposed to the vertebral artery is better treated with open surgery. The balloon diameter is usually between 6 and 8 mm. The balloon catheter is placed across the lesion. The balloon is inflated and resolution of the atherosclerotic waist is observed using fluoroscopy (see chap. 16). Because the subclavian artery is soft and a rupture in this location has potentially disastrous consequences, it is important to avoid overdilatation. Completion arteriography is performed through the sheath. Selective stent placement is considered (see chap. 18). Subclavian artery orifice lesions are usually treated with balloon-expandable stents since these are often heavily calcified and spillover lesions from the aortic arch and the artery is relatively fixed in position at this site. Lesions in more distal locations are best treated with self-expanding stents, since the artery is more flexible and mobile in these areas and may be affected by external structures and forces. Stents should be avoided distal to the humeral head if possible since this is an area of very high flexibility.

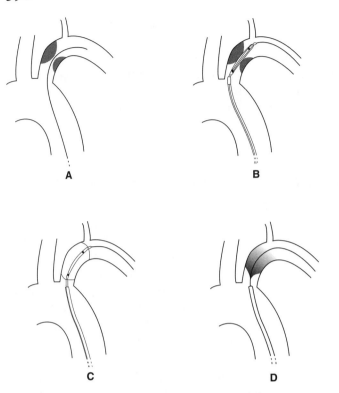

Fig. 4 Balloon angioplasty of the subclavian artery through a transfemoral approach. (**A**) A guidewire is placed in the subclavian artery and across the lesion. (**B**) A long sheath is placed with its tip in the subclavian artery. An angioplasty catheter is placed. (**C**) Balloon angioplasty of the subclavian artery lesion is performed. (**D**) Completion arteriography is performed through the sheath.

Stent placement considerations in the subclavian artery are similar to those for the common carotid artery. A premounted stent on the appropriately sized balloon with a 90- to 120-cm shaft length is used for orifice lesions (Fig. 5). The balloon and stent are passed through the sheath and across the lesion and the stent is deployed. Advancing the sheath across the lesion for stent delivery may not be necessary as long as the sheath tip has a secure purchase on the artery origin. Self-expanding stent diameter should be 8 or 10 mm and the delivery catheters are 120 cm. The delivery catheter is passed through the sheath and across the lesion, and the stent is deployed. Poststent balloon angioplasty is performed. Completion arteriography is performed through the sheath.

Lesions at the orifice of the subclavian artery pose similar challenges to those that occur at the common carotid artery origin. When the sheath is withdrawn to expose the stent, the tip of the sheath loses its purchase on the artery. When treating this type of lesion from a transfemoral approach, pull the sheath back slowly and place the tip of the sheath in the arch but

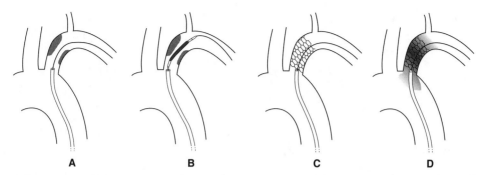

Fig. 5 Stent placement in the subclavian artery through a transfemoral approach. (**A**) A long sheath is placed in the proximal subclavian artery. (**B**) The stent is delivered to the site of the lesion. (**C**) Stent deployment is performed. Caution is exercised during stent deployment to avoid engaging the tip of the sheath with the stent and to avoid deployment in proximity to the origin of the vertebral artery. (**D**) Completion arteriography is performed through the sheath.

close to the origin of the artery. Another option is to place the stent through a retrograde, transbrachial approach, which is usually simpler.

If the lesion extends to the vertebral artery, care must be taken in deploying stents at this location as the origin of the vertebral artery is at risk for injury. This is also a location in the subclavian artery where there is some significant bending and tortuosity and curvature and therefore a self-expanding stent is useful when the lesion is up inside the artery and not directly at its origin. Avoid choosing a stent that's too long. To get the best view of the origin of the vertebral artery, sometimes it proceeds directly from the superior aspect of the subclavian artery but sometimes also it comes of the posterior aspect of the subclavian artery. A cranial–caudal angulation and a little bit of anterior oblique will help to bring out this area. After placement of a self-expanding stent, the balloon may be gradually upsized so that the artery is gently dilated and the risk of rupture is diminished. If the brachial approach is chosen, the catheter is advanced from the brachial side of the lesion and there's only really one place for this wire and catheter system to go and that is retrograde directly into the lesion.

Retrograde Approach to the Subclavian and Axillary Arteries

The transbrachial, retrograde approach to the subclavian and axillary arteries is direct and does not require selective catheterization from a remote entry site, as does the transfemoral approach (Fig. 6). The patient's ipsilateral arm is extended at the side. A working table is placed at the end of the arm board to accommodate the guidewires and catheters. The transbrachial

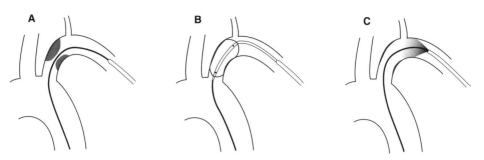

Fig. 6 Balloon angioplasty of the subclavian artery through a transbrachial approach. (**A**) A guidewire and sheath are placed through a brachial artery puncture or cutdown. (**B**) A balloon catheter is advanced through the sheath and into the lesion and balloon angioplasty is performed. (**C**) The balloon is withdrawn and completion arteriography is performed using a retrograde approach through the sheath.

approach may be performed through either an open exposure of the artery or a percutaneous puncture.

The guidewire is advanced retrograde using fluoroscopy. If stent placement is a likelihood, it is usually best to place a 7-Fr access sheath. Otherwise a 5- or 6-Fr sheath may be inserted. It is sometimes useful to place a longer sheath (20–40 cm), depending upon the location of the lesion, and perform retrograde arteriography through the sidearm of the sheath. Heparin is administered. The guidewire is advanced through the lesion. When the lesion of interest is at or near the origin of the subclavian artery, it is usually best to place a pigtail catheter through the femoral artery and perform an arch aortogram using a pressure injector. When a standard-length access sheath (12–15 cm) is used at the brachial artery entry site, retrograde arteriography through the sheath is usually not possible. After the guidewire is advanced across the lesion, a straight catheter with multiple side holes may be advanced over the guidewire until its tip is proximal to the lesion and this catheter may be used for arteriography.

If the lesion is proximal to the vertebral artery, the guidewire must be advanced into the descending aorta to maintain adequate control at the intervention site (see fig. 8 in chap. 9).The guidewire is directed into the descending thoracic aorta using a selective catheter with a bend at the tip. The balloon catheter with a 75-cm shaft is placed and the balloon is inflated. Completion arteriography is performed. Subclavian artery lesions often exhibit significant recoil after angioplasty and origin lesions contain spillover plaque from the aortic arch that can be recalcitrant to angioplasty. Either situation may necessitate stent placement.

Stenting of the orifice of the subclavian artery should be performed with a balloon-expandable stent. If the artery is too tortuous to safely pass a 7-Fr sheath through the lesion, the sheath is advanced as far as possible and then a premounted medium Palmaz stent is passed beyond the end of the sheath. Tortuous segments of the artery can be stented with self-expanding stents as with the transfemoral approach. The shaft length for self-expanding stents through the brachial approach is 80 cm. Stent placement across the origin of the vertebral artery is contraindicated. The long-term success of stents in the highly mobile segment of the subclavian–axillary artery as it crosses the first rib is not known but may be poor. If a lesion juxtaposed to the first rib requires stent placement, use a self-expanding stent. Consider first rib resection at a later time.

Selected Readings

Criado FJ, Wellons E, Ranadive RK, et al. Subclavian and vertebral arteries: Angioplasty and stents. In: Moore WS, Ahn SS, eds. Endovascular Surgery. Philadelphia, PA: W. B. Saunders, 2001:361–370.

Hobson RW. Innominate and common carotid arteries: Angioplasty and stents. In: Moore WS, Ahn SS, eds. Endovascular Surgery. Philadelphia, PA: 2001:371–374.

Hobson RW 2nd, Mackey WC, Ascher E, et al. Society for Vascular Surgery. Management of atherosclerotic carotid artery disease: clinical practice guidelines of the Society for Vascular Surgery. J Vasc Surg 2008; 48(2):480–486.

McKinsey JF. Symptomatic carotid stenosis: endarterectomy, stenting, or best medical management? Semin Vasc Surg 2008; 21(2):108–114.

Ricotta JJ 2nd, Malgor RD. A review of the trials comparing carotid endarterectomy and carotid angioplasty and stenting. Perspect Vasc Surg Endovasc Ther 2008; 20(3):299–308.

24

Visceral and Renal Arteries: Advice About Balloon Angioplasty and Stent Placement

The Celiac and Superior Mesenteric Arteries
Renal Angioplasty and Stenting
Selected Readings

403

The Celiac and Superior Mesenteric Arteries

A visceral artery occlusion identified on angiography usually appears longer than it actually is. Often, the occlusion starts at the origin of the artery and the precise location of the origin can sometimes be difficult to identify. Frequently, there are hints as to where the origin of the artery is located or if there is a beak of contrast or there is a significant amount of calcification in the area where the artery is located. Balloon-expandable stents are used to treat these lesions. This procedure may be approached from either a transfemoral route or a transbrachial route. The angles for cannulating a flush occlusion are fairly unfavorable from a transfemoral route. However, if the artery is still open or if there is a beak of entry contrast into the artery, then it may be possible to cannulate it in this way. It is usually a good idea to have a preprocedure study, which indicates the location and severity of visceral artery occlusive disease. In addition, a full array of premounted balloon-expandable stents should be available including low-profile systems.

Access is obtained through either the brachial or the femoral artery, which is determined to be the optimal approach from the preoperative studies. Systemic anticoagulation is administered. A sheath is placed that is usually 6 Fr in diameter and this sheath may have an angled hockey tip or a curved or renal double curved shape or it may be straight in shape. If a challenging angle is present during a transfemoral approach, consider using a curved sheath or guiding catheter such as a renal double curve or IMA shape. From the brachial route, a straight or hockey stick–shaped sheath tip is used. After sheath placement, the appropriately curved 4- or 5-Fr catheter is placed (Fig. 1).

The advantage of a more dramatically curved catheter is that it gives more angulation to the trajectory of the wire as you are attempting to cannulate an aortic side branch with an abrupt angle. The disadvantage of the more curved catheter is that as the guidewire enters the lesion, the catheter may buckle in an unfavorable way and create instability in the system. After the guidewire is in place, the catheter must be exchanged out and in this setting the curvature in the catheter may attempt to drag the guidewire out of the artery. The artery may be cannulated using either a 0.014- or 0.035-in. steerable guidewire. Choose the catheter with the least amount of curve needed to make the gap from the tip of the sheath to the origin of the diseased artery. Often times, it becomes apparent that it is useful to withdraw the sheath a little bit to allow the catheter to take its full shape and to have a full degree of mobility when attempting to cannulate the artery. If one finds that this position is not supportive enough, usually the sheath can be advanced directly over the catheter with the guidewire in it and protruding. The "no touch" technique is frequently employed when an artery origin lesion is expected. When the lesion is slightly farther from the origin of the artery so that there is a stump of relatively nondiseased vessel, cannulation is usually a little simpler. The opening of the artery is cannulated

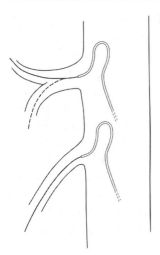

Fig. 1 Catheterization of the celiac and superior mesenteric arteries. A hook-shaped catheter is selected. The image intensifier is placed in the lateral or near-lateral position. The catheter tip is used to engage the orifice of the artery. A Glidewire is advanced. The celiac artery is usually short and the guidewire tip usually finds an early branch of the celiac and follows a curving path. Guidewire placement in the superior mesenteric artery usually follows a straighter, diagonal course.

with the catheter first and then the wire is placed through that location. Once the wire is in the lesion, care must be taken as you are crossing the lesion not to catch the wire on any undesirable locations or to create a subintimal channel. Keep in mind that the shape of the catheter will change as a longer distance of a guidewire and a stiffer portion of the guidewire is passed through the lesion and also through the catheter head. Once the guidewire is across the lesion, the same catheter can usually be used to exchange for a more favorable guidewire to perform the stent placement. As in the case of other aortic branch lesions, the celiac and superior mesenteric arteries can be treated using either a 0.035 system or a 0.014-in.-diameter system.

The advantage of the 0.014-in.-diameter system is that the sheath required is not quite as large and despite using a 6-Fr sheath or even a 5-Fr sheath, you can consistently get interim angiographic images by injecting contrast through the side arm of the sheath and around the treatment catheters. The other advantage of the small caliber system is that the balloons and the stents are much easier to make any sharp turns in the access sheath and pass across the lesion since they are so much lower profile. The 0.035 systems frequently require predilation in order to pass the stent into the lesion. The advantage of the 0.035 system is that it can be used with a larger and very stiff wire which can make the whole system, including the guiding sheath or guiding catheter, quite a bit more stable.

Once the wire is across the lesion, care must be taken to ensure that it's actually in the correct location. And even if it is in the correct artery, care must be taken to ensure that it hasn't gone into some small branch or collateral branch out of the main artery just distal to the lesion. With respect to the superior mesenteric artery, a left anterior oblique projection is often best since the superior mesenteric artery (SMA) tends to extend anteriorly and toward the right at its root. With respect to the celiac artery, a straight lateral is usually best but a substantial amount of image quality is lost in doing this since you are shooting X-rays through the wider part of the person from one side laterally to the other. Frequently, a steep oblique works well rather than a full lateral because of decreased image quality due to poor penetration. In addition, with a full lateral, it's usually best to put the arms above the patient's head and most patients can only tolerate this for a certain period of time before they become fatigued. The wire going into the superior mesenteric artery can extend for many centimeters distal to the lesion and into the distal SMA and this can provide a fairly good rail over which to work (Fig. 2).

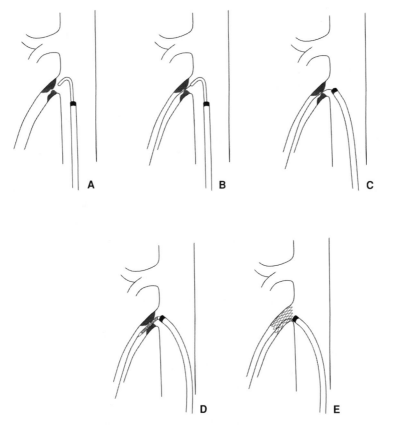

Fig. 2 Stenting of a superior mesenteric artery lesion. (**A**) The guiding sheath or catheter is advanced so that its tip is in proximity to the SMA. A hook-shaped angiographic catheter is placed. (**B**) A 0.014 in. guidewire is advanced. The angiographic catheter is used to support and direct the guidewire. (**C**) The catheter is removed. The guidewire is advanced into a stable position. (**D**) A pre-mounted, low profile, balloon expandable stent is advanced directly into the lesion. (**E**) The stent is placed at the orifice of the artery.

The celiac artery has some technical differences with the superior mesenteric artery. The artery begins to make turns immediately after its origin. It is not at all uncommon to place the wire within the celiac artery and have it only be within the artery for a few centimeters before it encounters resistance due to the tortuosity of the branches of the celiac artery. The artery is usually quite short and this requires great accuracy in placing stents. There is usually no available length of celiac artery in which the access sheath can be seeded. Try to choose the best celiac artery branch to provide stability. Once the guidewire is in place, the trick is to choose the right length and diameter of stent and to get it in the right spot so that the trailing end of the stent is flush with the aorta or it's protruding slightly into the aorta and so that the entire lesion may be treated. Because the celiac artery is often so short, the lesion may be the whole length of the celiac artery, with branches immediately distal to that. After stent placement, follow up with poststent angioplasty. If the artery is very short and the distal end of the lesion is very close to the branches, it is occasionally necessary to place a couple of guidewires into different celiac artery branches.

There are challenges in stent placement in the visceral segment. It is deep in a body cavity location and imaging is somewhat diminished. There is a continuous movement of vascular structures. Bowel gas often obscures the target site. This is an area where heavy calcifications may occur especially along the anterior wall at the origins of the visceral arteries and sometimes along the posterior wall where it is desirable to avoid embolization by disrupting this material. If there is a severe angle of exit from the aorta and especially if it's a superior mesenteric artery or if there is significant infrarenal pathology, then a transbrachial approach is more desirable.

In the case of a transbrachial approach, place a 4-Fr access in the left brachial artery using a micropuncture needle and a 4-Fr sheath. After placement of a 4-Fr sheath, administer systemic anticoagulation. A 90-cm omniflush catheter is passed along with a Glidewire. In the arch of the aorta, the omniflush catheter is turned posteriorly and is used to direct the guidewire into the descending aorta. The image intensifier is placed in the left anterior oblique position for this maneuver. A visceral aortogram is performed. The approximate distance to the lesion is estimated against the length of the catheter. A stiff guidewire is passed through the catheter and the catheter is removed. The 4-Fr sheath is removed from the arm and dilators are used and then a long 6-Fr sheath is placed so that the tip of the sheath is in the aorta just distal to the target lesion. Once the 6-Fr sheath is placed in the appropriate location, the oblique projections of the superior mesenteric and celiac arteries can be obtained and an angled tip long catheter, such as a 125-cm length 5-Fr vertebral catheter, is placed. After placement of the catheter, it becomes apparent where the tip of the sheath needs to be and the sheath is withdrawn slightly. It is not possible at this point to advance the sheath on its own without the dilator and the stiff guidewire and therefore, it is inserted beyond the point that it is required and then slightly withdrawn when the time comes. By pointing the angled tip catheter toward the origin of either the celiac or the superior mesenteric arteries, whichever requires treatment, the guidewire may then be advanced from the tip of the catheter. The shape of the aorta often causes a rotational bias in the sheath, and when this happens it may point toward the lesion intended for treatment or it may point away.

The same steps are followed as described above for the transfemoral route. The major difference in the transfemoral route is that the access site management is a little simpler but the actual access to the visceral artery for stenting is often more complex. This has to do with the extreme angles of origin of some visceral arteries. After the sheath is placed and the lesion is crossed, the sheath and the guidewire may try to pop out during the case.

Renal Angioplasty and Stenting

The technique of renal angioplasty and stenting has been greatly simplified by the introduction of the 0.014-in.-diameter systems in renal revascularization. The renal arteries are usually approached retrograde, but an antegrade approach through a brachial puncture site can be used when the angle of the renal artery takeoff from the aorta is narrow or when severe aortoiliac disease prohibits catheterization of this segment. Renal revascularization may also be performed using IMA-shaped guiding catheter with the use of a manifold device and also with the possibility of a distal protection device. Chapter 9 contains a detailed discussion of renal artery catheterization. Chapter 10 provides information about aortorenal and selective renal arteriography. Supplies required for renal artery intervention are listed in Table 1.

In deciding whether to treat a renal artery from the transfemoral route or the transbrachial route, there are a few considerations. Most of the time it's fairly simple to treat a renal artery stenosis from a transfemoral route. The distance is shorter, the imaging is simpler, and the procedure is overall safe and reliable. But, it can also be among the most challenging of endovascular cases. One disadvantage of the transfemoral route is that there may be some associated infrarenal aortic pathology such as an abdominal aortic aneurysm, mural thrombus, and other lesion, which may substantially influence the safety of the case. If there is substantial iliac tortuosity, frequently this will bias the catheter or sheath toward one side or the other and create extra challenge. This may work within your favor if this is the side you are treating; however, it may work aggressively against you and serve to turn the catheter and/or sheath to the side opposite that you desire throughout the procedure. The third situation in which it is helpful to abandon the transfemoral route and go with the transbrachial route is when there is a severe and acute angle of takeoff of the renal artery so that it is significantly downsloping similar to a superior mesenteric artery. Although this is usually possible to do through a transfemoral route, having a critical or even preocclusive lesion near the origin of the renal artery is sometimes

Table 1 Supplies for Renal Artery Intervention

Guidewire	Starting guidewire	Bentson	145-cm length	0.035 in. in diameter
	Selective guidewire	Magic torque	180 cm	0.035 in. (marker tip)
		Glidewire	180 cm	0.035 in. (angled tip)
Catheter	Exchange guidewire	Rosen	180 cm	0.035 in. (J tip)
	Flush catheter	Omniflush	65-cm length	5 Fr
	Selective catheter	Cobra C1, C2	65, 65, 80	5 Fr
		Renal double curve	65, 80	5 Fr
		Renal curve 1, 2	65, 80	5 Fr
		SOS omni 2	80	5 Fr
Sheath	Selective guide sheath	Ansel 1, 2, 3	45-cm length	6 Fr, 7 Fr
		RDC	55 cm	
Balloon	Balloon angioplasty catheter	Balloon diameter	4, 5, 6, 7 mm	5 Fr
		Balloon length	2, 4 cm	
		Catheter shaft	75 cm length	
Stent[a]	Balloon-expandable stent	(Premounted) Stent diameter	5, 6, 7 mm	
		Stent length	12–29 mm	
		Shaft length	80 cm	

[a] No stents are approved by the FDA for routine usage in this vascular bed.

extremely difficult to cannulate when coming from a transfemoral route. After the guidewire is across the lesion, the more angulated the approach, due to the curvature imposed by the turn from the aorta into the renal artery, the less stable the system and the less pushability and trackability the operator has.

After retrograde femoral puncture, the guidewire is passed to the level above the upper abdominal aorta. A 4- or 5-Fr flush catheter is placed and the guidewire is removed. The catheter head is placed at the junction of the first and second lumbar vertebral bodies. It is best to perform a complete aortoiliac arteriogram if renal function permits. This allows accessory renal arteries and other variations to be identified, as well as disease that is present along the approach to the renal arteries. The operator then knows where other disease is located that may potentially cause complications during intervention. After this is performed, a magnified view of the aorta and renal artery origins should be obtained. The image intensifier usually has an obliqued orientation slightly toward the side of probable intervention. After the image intensifier is optimally located, it is usually best to leave it in that position until after the artery is cannulated.

The renal arteries are unique in terms of their mobility with breathing. The origins of the renal arteries are relatively fixed in place by the diaphragmatic crus. The renal parenchyma and surrounding tissues within

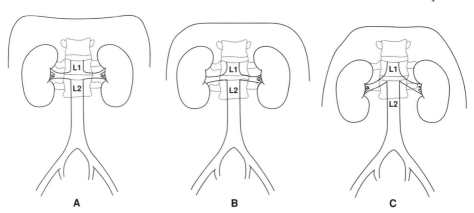

Fig. 3 Renal artery position is (dependent upon diaphragmatic motion. (**A**) At full exhalation, the kidney position is high in the retroperitoneum and the angle at the renal artery origin is affected accordingly. (**B**) During midinhalation, the angle of takeoff at the renal artery origin becomes more acute. (**C**) At full inspiration, the renal artery origin is at an even more acute angle.

Gerota's fascia are mobile with diaphragmatic excursion. The result of this anatomic arrangement is that the angle of takeoff of the renal arteries from the aorta varies with the ventilatory cycle. The anatomic picture portrayed with arteriography varies depending upon how the diaphragm was held during arteriography. A fully held breath tends to accentuate the acute angle at the origin of the renal artery by pushing the kidney caudad (Fig. 3). Because the kidneys move up and down continuously with the breathing cycle, it is frequently helpful to have the patient hold their breath prior to angiogram but also prior to stent placement itself so that accuracy of stent placement can be achieved. Frequently, a deep breath causes too much displacement and it will help to force the kidneys inferiorly and accentuate the angle of origin of the renal arteries. Often it is helpful to have the patient exhale and hold the breath while in exhalation so the kidneys are elevated and this tends to deaccentuate the angle of takeoff of the renal artery.

The renal arteries tend to egress from the aorta in a posterolateral direction so it's frequently valuable to use an ipsilateral anterior oblique of anywhere from 5 to 15 degrees in order to see the renal artery origin. If the preoperative study obtained is either a CAT scan or an MRA, this can be used to assess the best angle for visualizing the renal artery origin. Even though many arteries will be seen in their best projection by a slight anterior oblique, some arteries don't follow that rule. If the aorta is a little rotated, one artery may even originate a little bit anteriorly.

Systemic heparin is administered. A 6-Fr sheath or 8-Fr guide catheter is advanced over the guidewire (Fig. 4). The guiding sheath or guiding catheter is selected that best fits the angle and curvature of the renal artery origin. There are numerous shapes, specially designed for renal artery intervention,

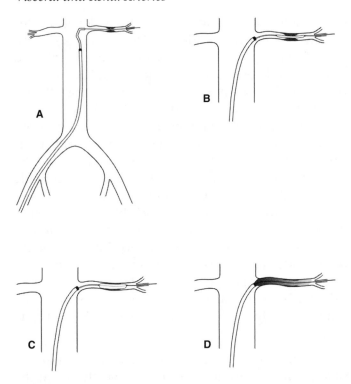

Fig. 4 Balloon angioplasty of the renal artery. (A) The left renal artery is cannulated with a cobra catheter and the guidewire is advanced across the stenosis. (B) An angioplasty balloon is advanced over the guidewire and across the lesion. (C) Balloon angioplasty of the left renal artery is performed. (D) Completion arteriography is performed by removing the guidewire and withdrawing the balloon enough to administer contrast through the balloon catheter. This is a simple maneuver but if there is a problem at the angioplasty site, it must be recrossed. (E) Another option for completion arteriography is to place another catheter through an alternate site, which ensures guidewire control of the lesion. (F) Angioplasty can also be performed through a guiding catheter advanced into the renal artery orifice. (G) A completion renal arteriogran is obtained by injecting contrast through the guiding catheter.

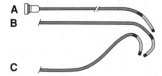

Fig. 5 Access for renal artery intervention. The Ansel (Cook, Inc.) renal guiding sheath tips are shown here. These sheaths have a hemostatic valve, a sidearm, and a dilator. The Ansel 1 (A), Ansel 2 (B), and Ansel 3 (C) sheaths are used for progressively more acutely angled renal arteries.

which are available through different companies. The Ansel guiding sheaths are produced by Cook, Inc. Bloomington, Indiana, U.S.A. There are three different curves to choose from (Fig. 5). The tip of the sheath is soft and radiopaque. The transition from dilator to sheath is smooth, and the distance that the dilator extends beyond the sheath is very short. This permits the tip of the sheath to be placed within the renal artery without a long segment of leading dilator tip advancing into the distal renal artery. A guiding sheath with a 6- or 7-Fr shaft and a 45-cm length is adequate. If a guide catheter is selected, it may have an IMA shape or some other curve. The tip is curved but it is somewhat flexible. A guidewire is advanced through the IMA guide catheter. When the tip of the catheter falls into the orifice of the renal artery, the guidewire is advanced (Fig. 6). If this is an unfavorable angle, another option is to place a C2 Cobra catheter or other appropriate curved tip catheter and use one of these catheters to cannulate the renal artery. The renal artery is cannulated, the 0.014-in. guidewire is advanced across the lesion and into the distal renal artery, and the guide catheter tip is placed close to the lesion. The guidewire choice should be one that has a relatively stiff body across the location of the lesion and also has a floppy wire tip so that injury to the renal parenchyma may be avoided.

A critical orifice lesion may make it difficult to enter the renal artery. In this case, the steerable guidewire tip must be used to gently probe the origin of the artery. After the guidewire traverses the lesion, it is advanced into a secondary branch. This is done to maintain as much purchase on the artery as possible. However, the guidewire should not be forced or advanced against resistance because it can perforate the parenchyma. Another option is to use the "no touch" technique. The sheath is advanced into the aorta in the proximity of the renal artery (Fig. 7). A stabilizing guidewire is placed which protrudes into the aorta and lays against the wall of the aorta to hold the tip of the sheath in a steady position. Through the tip of the sheath, the renal artery lesion is probed with a directional guidewire and crossed with the least amount of trauma.

A selective catheter is passed over the guidewire into the renal artery if selective arteriography or pressure measurements are required or if a different guidewire is desired over which to perform stenting. Nitroglycerine may be administered through the catheter to help prevent renal artery spasm. Attempting to assess the hemodynamic significance of the renal lesion by measuring pressure across it can be challenging. It is not well understood if a pressure drop across the lesion is significant and how much of a drop there has to be to represent a physiologically significant change. In addition, measuring the pressure using a 4- or a 5-Fr catheter there may be some decrease in pressure because of occupation of the residual lumen of the renal artery by the pressure-measuring device. In order to accurately measure pressure, it means potentially crossing the lesion more than once by placing the pressure measuring catheter across the lesion and then withdrawing it. As the

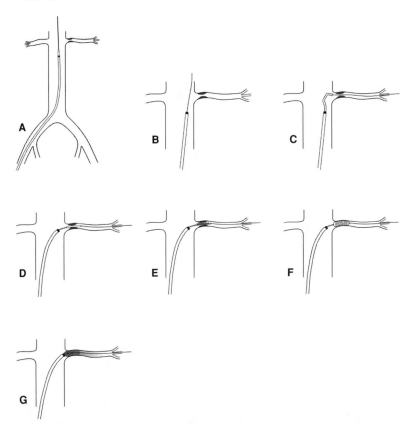

Fig. 6 Balloon angioplasty and stent placement through a guiding sheath. (**A**) A guidewire and guiding sheath are placed in the aorta. (**B**) The dilator is removed. (**C**) A selective catheter, such as a C2 cobra, is placed through the sheath and into the renal artery. Guidewire access across the lesion is obtained. (**D**) The balloon catheter is advanced through the guiding sheath and over the guidewire. The tip of the guiding sheath is maintained in proximity to the renal artery origin. (**E**) A premounted, balloon expandable stent is placed at the location of the lesion. (**F**) The stent is placed with balloon inflation. (**G**) Post-stent angiography is performed through the sheath while maintaining guidewire access.

kidney loses its ability to vasodilate distal to the stenosis, it may become more resistive. This will tend to equalize the pressures proximal and distal to the lesion and this may be the explanation for why sometimes an apparently significant appearing lesion has a less than significant pressure drop across it. Likewise, with vasodilatiing agents, if the kidney is physically unable to vasodilate any further than it already is, this will lead to a less dramatic hemodynamic response than one would anticipate based on the severity of the lesion.

After these maneuvers, a guidewire is inserted into the catheter and across the lesion for treatment. Keeping the guidewire in the correct place is

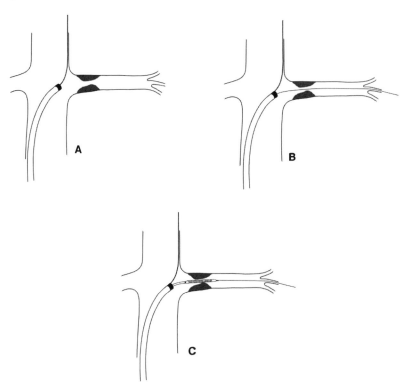

Fig. 7 No touch technique. (**A**) The guiding sheath or guiding catheter is stabilized by passage of a guidewire that leans on the side wall of the aorta. (**B**) The tip of the sheath is stable and avoids direct encounter with juxtarenal aortic disease. A 0.014 in guidewire is passed through the same access and into the renal artery. (**C**) The pre-mounted stent delivery catheter is advanced into position.

a challenge throughout the remainder of the case. Every maneuver tends to move the guidewire and tension builds up around the sharp turn form the aorta into the renal artery. The end organ is so close that only a short length of relatively soft (atraumatic) guidewire can be maintained within the artery.

The guiding sheath or catheter may be advanced close to but not into the lesion over the selective catheter and the guidewire. Prior to stent placement, predilatation may be performed using a 2 to 4 mm balloon to create a tract for stent delivery. The angioplasty balloon is usually 2 cm in length and has low-profile features with a monorail system. Atherosclerotic renal artery origin lesions usually require stents to achieve a substantial improvement from endovascular intervention, and most operators perform stent placement in this situation. After balloon angioplasty, the guiding sheath or guiding catheter may be gently advanced using the angioplasty catheter for support. The balloon catheter is removed. After the stent is placed on the wire, it is advanced into position. It is quite common to have a challenge getting the stent across the lesion and forceful advancement when the stent is not going easily may force the guidewire and/or the guide catheter to back up in an undesirable way. This is where system stability is important to permit the operator to push when needed and get acceptable results. Contrast is puffed from the sheath to assess landmarks again for correct placement. Because the premounted stent and its catheter may fill the lesion l, there may not be any filling of contrast into the artery past the stent until the stent is deployed. However, the contrast should puff around the origin of the artery and give an identification of the location of the stent at the origin of the renal artery. When the stent is appropriately positioned, it is rapidly deployed and after deployment the balloon is deflated. The same balloon is used to expand and flare both the proximal and distal ends of the stent. Occasionally, a slightly larger balloon is used to flare the proximal end of the stent in the aorta.

The stents used for the renal arteries range in length from 10 to 30 mm and in diameter from 4 to 7 mm. The tendency by eye is to overestimate the length of the stent required. These stent delivery catheters are 0.014-in. compatible, monorail system devices. The very low profile helps in getting the stent to make the turn in the guiding sheath into the renal artery and in crossing a lesion that may have a very narrow residual lumen. The low-profile nature of these stents also permits the administration of contrast around the stent delivery catheter while in the sheath and just prior to deployment. In general, the shortest length stent that will cover the lesion should be deployed. If the renal artery has substantial tortuosity, the stent will straighten a segment of the artery, leaving all the curvature over a shorter segment of remaining nonstented vessel. This can inadvertently create an undesired kink in the artery. Efforts should be made to avoid this situation.

A final diameter of 5 or 6 mm is usually adequate. The balloon and mounted stent are advanced through the sheath and across the lesion. The guiding sheath is gently withdrawn to uncover the back end of the stent. The stent is placed so that the aortic end is deployed to treat the aortic plaque as it spills over into the renal artery, usually about a mm in the aortic flow stream. Aortic wall calcium deposits often provide a good landmark for this deployment. Inflation is observed using fluoroscopy and may cause flank pain. Completion arteriography is performed through the sheath. After balloon inflation of a balloon-expandable stent, the balloon occasionally becomes stuck. If this occurs, do not yank the catheter. Deflate the balloon very well, then advance the catheter a bit to dislodge it from the deployed stent. If the balloon is difficult to withdraw from the stent, advance the tip of the sheath to about the edge of the stent so that the position of the stent is not loosened by catheter withdrawal.

The smaller caliber guidewire systems have the advantages of crossing critical lesions with lower-profile guidewires, permitting balloon angio-plasty with a very low-profile balloon, and allowing complex intervention through smaller caliber sheaths. The disadvantages are that the smaller caliber guidewire is not as radiopaque and it provides less support than a 0.035 in, system.

At some point, it may be appropriate to perform renal stenting with distal protection devices in order to limit distal embolization. There are disadvantages of the existing distal protection devices as applied to renal stenting. None of the currently available protection devices have a short enough landing zone to be adequate for most renal arteries. Most of the existing devices are based on guidewires that are not stiff enough to be stable in the setting of the acute turn from the aorta into the renal artery as is required.

Recurrent renal artery stenosis is notoriously difficult to assess on plane angiography. The best way to evaluate the degree of stenosis in this situation is with intravascular ultrasound. Treatment options for recurrent renal artery stenosis are standard balloon angioplasty, repeat stenting, cutting balloon angioplasty, or cryoplasty.

Selected Readings

Burkett MW, Cooper CJ, Kennedy DJ, et al. Renal artery angioplasty and stent placement. Am Heart J 2000; 139:64–71.

Corriere MA, Pearce JD, Edwards MS, et al. Endovascular management of atherosclerotic renovascular disease: Early results following primary intervention. J Vasc Surg 2008; 48(3):580–587.

Dubel GJ, Murphy TP. The role of percutaneous revascularization for renal artery stenosis. Vasc Med 2008; 13(2):141–156.

Hood DB, Hodgson KJ. Renovascular disease. In: Moore WS, Ahn SS, eds. Endovascular Surgery. Philadelphia, PA: W. B. Saunders, 2001:341–354.

Jaff M, Mathiak L. Four-year follow-up of palmaz-schatz stent revascularization as treatment for atherosclerotic renal artery stenosis. Circulation 1998; 98:642–647.

Lee RW, Bakken AM, Palchik E, et al. Long-term outcomes of endoluminal therapy for chronic atherosclerotic occlusive mesenteric disease. Ann Vasc Surg 2008; 22(4):541–546.

Rosenfield K, Fishman RF. The techniques of performing endovascular renal artery stenting. In: Jaff MR, ed. Endovascular Therapy for Atherosclerotic Renal Artery Stenosis. Armonk, NY: Futura, 2001:55–81.

Sarac TP, Altinel O, Kashyap V, et al. Endovascular treatment of stenotic and occluded visceral arteries for chronic mesenteric ischemia. J Vasc Surg 2008; 47(3):485–491.

van den Yen PJG, Kaatee R, Beutler JJ. Arterial stenting and balloon angioplasty in ostial atherosclerotic renovascular disease: A randomized trial. Lancet 1999; 353:282–286.

25

Complex Lower-Extremity Revascularization

Recanalizing Iliac Artery Occlusions

There are many treatments now available for iliac artery occlusive disease. The previous gold standard of aortobifemoral bypass is rarely performed at the present time. Other options include a variety of extra-anatomic bypasses, such as axillofemoral and femoral–femoral bypass. A combination of extra-anatomic bypass and some endovascular inflow may also be performed. Previous treatment for unilateral iliac artery occlusion was frequently a femoral–femoral bypass. At the present time, it is possible to recanalize most iliac artery occlusions. Unilateral iliac artery occlusion is most common and there is often stenosis of the contralateral side. Bilateral iliac artery occlusions may also be treated using a bilateral endovascular approach. If one of the iliac arteries can be reopened and the other one cannot, stenting on one side can be performed followed by a femoral–femoral bypass.

Figure 1 shows a variety of occlusions involving the aortoiliac segment. Aortic occlusions that begin distally and extend into the iliac arteries can often be opened. Aortic occlusions that are flush with the renal arteries are more dangerous due to the risk of expressing compacted thrombus into the renal arteries. The patients in whom iliac artery recanalization is ill advised are those in whom disease extends in a severe manner into the common femoral artery. In this case, either the procedure should be changed or the iliac artery recanalization can be combined with a femoral endarterectomy.

By way of assessment of iliac artery occlusions, it does make a difference as to whether these lesions are located in the common iliac artery alone or the external iliac alone or whether it involves both the common and external iliac artery. With respect to common or external iliac arteries, if the proximal end of the artery at the lesion has a beak of patent artery either just above it, this will enhance getting into the occlusion in the best location (Fig. 2). The beak or stub can be used to enter the occlusion, either by coming in proximally from the brachial artery or by coming in over the aortic bifurcation from the contralateral side. Getting the guidewire in the correct place with respect to the proximal end of a common iliac artery occlusion is often challenging when coming from below (Fig. 3). The guidewire often will pass into the subadventitial space posterior to the aortic bifurcation. The distal aorta and proximal iliac arteries are often fused together in one big cast of calcium. So when the subadventitial guidewire comes in from below, sometimes it will resist breaking through this calcium in order to pass back into the true lumen. It is preferred to approach a common iliac artery occlusion from the proximal end, especially if there is a stump or beak of open artery that shows the way into the lesion (Fig. 4). In recanalizing common iliac artery occlusions, it may be necessary to approach the occlusion from both ends. The distal end of the external iliac artery lesions are also challenging to manage because they must reconstitute at the common femoral artery and a smooth junction between the external iliac artery and common

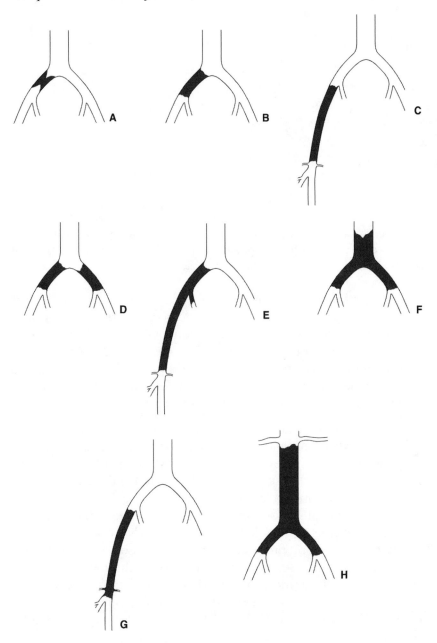

Fig. 1 Patterns of aortoiliac occlusive disease. These lesions are arranged in order of those which are simplest to treat with endovascular intervention to those which are the most complex. (**A**) Iliac stenosis is the most favorable situation for use of endovascular techniques. (**B**) Common iliac artery occlusion. (**C**) External iliac artery occlusion. (**D**) Bilateral common iliac artery occlusion. (**E**) Combined common and external iliac artery occlusion. (**F**) Combination of infrarenal aortic occlusion and bilateral common iliac artery occlusion. (**G**) Iliac occlusion combined with common femoral artery occlusion. (**H**) Iliac artery occlusion combined with extensive infrarenal aortic occlusion that extends from the level of the renal arteries.

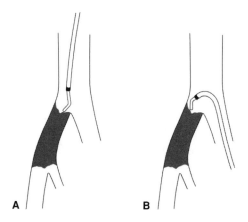

Fig. 2 Approach to a common iliac artery occlusion. (**A**) A common iliac artery occlusion may be recanalized from a proximal approach, through a transbrachial access. (**B**) Another option is a contralateral approach.

femoral artery must be created. This requires true lumen reentry precisely at the junction of the external iliac and common femoral arteries. There is also a limitation to the use of stents at the reentry zone, because it is undesirable to place stents that extend into the common femoral artery. An external iliac artery occlusion is difficult to approach from the common femoral artery side because of the inadequate working distance between any common femoral artery puncture site and the beginning of the external iliac artery.

Assess the aortoiliac segment based on preoperative imaging so that plans can be made ahead of time. These procedures may be time consuming and may involve different devices. If stent–graft relining of the occlusion is anticipated, it will affect the size of the sheath selected. If there is the possibility of a combined open and endovascular approach (e.g., adding a femoral endarterectomy or femoral–femoral bypass), it will influence the choice of anesthesia and the sterile preparation. An aortogram or an MR angiogram or a CTA may be used for preprocedure evaluation. Assess whether there's any hidden aneurysmal disease, which may have led to thrombosis of either a common or internal iliac artery or any significant tortuosity. Usually, a preoperative study can assess whether the common femoral artery is going to be adequate. The length and caliber of the occluded artery can also be estimated.

Needle access is usually obtained into the contralateral groin, assuming a unilateral occlusion. If there is bilateral occlusion, needle access is usually obtained at the brachial artery. If the common iliac artery is occluded but the external iliac and common femoral arteries are patent, needle access may be gained on the ipsilateral side. A guidewire is advanced under fluoroscopic guidance and a 6-Fr sheath is placed. Frequently, there is iliac artery occlusive disease, either stenosis or occlusion, that's contralateral to the iliac artery which requires treatment and frequently guidewire passage will require some effort or extra steps. Once the guidewire is in the infrarenal aorta, a flush

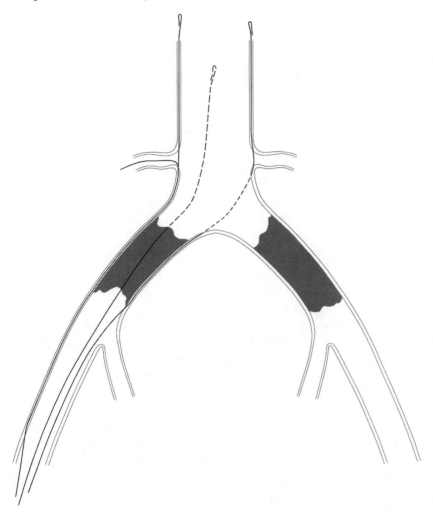

Fig. 3 Passing a guidewire retrograde through a common iliac artery occlusion. It is usual for the guidewire to enter and progress through the lesion from a retrograde approach. However, after the guidewire enters the subintimal plane, it may be challenging to re-enter the true lumen proximally. This is especially the case when there is a substantial atherosclerotic disease burden of the aortic bifurcation or severe calcification of the infrarenal aorta.

catheter is placed over the guidewire. The patient is given systemic anticoagulation with heparin. In the setting of extensive occlusive disease, flow in the aortoiliac segment may be slow and this observation should prompt more aggressive systemic anticoagulation during the procedure.

An aortoiliac arteriogram is performed with delayed filming so that reconstitution on the side of the occlusion can be imaged. Recanalizing an occlusion requires setting up an adequate treatment platform which includes placement of a sheath. If the lesion is an external iliac artery occlusion or a common iliac artery occlusion which has a decent beak of artery at its origin, place a longer sheath, 30 to 45 cm, 6 Fr into the iliac artery. Be sure

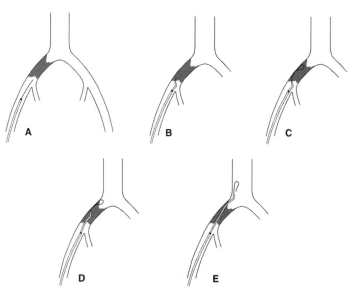

Fig. 4 Iliac artery recanalization. (**A**) A sheath is placed to provide a platform. (**B**) A braided, angled tip catheter is placed and a Glidewire is advanced through it to probe the lesion. (**C**) Using the catheter and the sheath for support, the guidewire is pushed into the most promising location and the guidewire buckles. (**D**) The guidewire loop progresses through the subintimal space and re-enters the true lumen. (**E**) The catheter is advanced over the guidewire to gain access to the true lumen.

the sheath tip has a radiopaque marker. In the case of a common iliac artery occlusion, a hook-shaped or U-shaped catheter is placed through the sheath over the aortic bifurcation the same way you would to go over the aortic bifurcation for routine contralateral catheterization (Fig. 4). The closer the occlusion initiates to the bifurcation, the more a stiff, hook-shaped catheter is needed. Catheters to consider for this include an inferior mesenteric artery catheter, a Sos omni, a Motarjeme catheter, or any variety of hook-shaped visceral catheter. Once the catheter tip is engaged in the beak of patent artery, a Glidewire is advanced into the occluded artery. Sometimes this is a relatively short distance and the guidewire tip will remain straight and resist going into the occlusion and will attempt to push the catheter out of the bifurcation every time forward pressure is placed on the guidewire. Sometimes it forms a loop as it goes into the subintimal space. If the loop won't form in the subintimal space or it tries to push the catheter out with each application of forward pressure, you have other options. One is to use a catheter with a stiffer tip to support the wire better. Another option is to approach the occlusion from the brachial artery and push straight into the occlusion. Yet another option is to puncture the common femoral artery ipsilateral to the occlusion and pass the guidewire and catheter retrograde.

After the loop forms and there are several to many centimeters of guidewire and catheter on the contralateral side, frequently the 6-Fr sheath can be advanced over the aortic bifurcation directly over the guidewire and catheter combination. This step helps to provide additional support for pushability in the direction of the occlusion. The loop of Glidewire is advanced and often will pop back into the true lumen distal to the occlusion. Another option, other than a looped subintimal hydrophilic guidewire, is to use a low profile 0.018- or 0.014-in. compatible, stiff tip exchange catheter (Quick cross catheter, Spectranetics). This is a microcatheter with a stiff tip that can be passed directly through a 5-Fr angiographic catheter and that combined with a stiff, low-profile guidewire, frequently is enough to push across an occlusion.

Reentry catheters are discussed in more detail later in the discussion on femoral–popliteal occlusive disease. It is possible to use reentry catheters in this situation but it may be challenging. The reason is because the Outback catheter (Cordis) and the Pioneer catheter (Medtronic), which are the available reentry catheters, are both relatively stiff. Yet, they are designed to pass over a 0.014-in. guidewire. They are also large in caliber and fill a 6-Fr guiding sheath quite snugly. If one is progressing up and over the aortic bifurcation, the system may not have the structural support to permit passage of the reentry catheter. To be effective, it must be passed all the way to the end of the position of furthest most guidewire progress. Because a long length of guidewire past the bifurcation is not possible and because these are relatively stiff 6-Fr catheters, it's usually not possible to pass these up and over even using a heavy 0.014-in. wire. A reentry catheter is usually easier to use when it is passed retrograde from the ipsilateral common femoral artery and into a common iliac artery occlusion. This will aid in reentry into the true lumen in the distal aorta. There are no significant turns to be made and the puncturing needle is directed into the location closest to where the common iliac artery origin is located.

In treating a common iliac artery occlusion, it is frequently of value to perform an ipsilateral retrograde approach, especially if there is no success coming from the proximal end or some reason why this approach should be avoided. Just remember that when an artery access site is created distal to an occlusion, if the reconstruction is not successful and pressure at the access site remains low, the opportunity for puncture site thrombosis to occur is increased. Ipsilateral retrograde access can be performed using a micropuncture needle. The micropuncture needle can be entered into the artery in several ways. Sometimes with a common iliac artery occlusion, there is still a palpable pulse as pulsatile blood flows through internal iliac artery collaterals. Also, injecting contrast into the aorta from some other route will reconstitute femoral artery and this can be road mapped. The road mapped image can be used to puncture with the micropuncture needle. Ultrasound guided puncture is also helpful, although the artery may be quite small in diameter due to hypoperfusion.

In the case of a common iliac artery occlusion with a patent external iliac artery, there is frequently enough artery so that an acceptable length of guidewire can be passed retrograde so that a sheath can be placed from the groin area. If an acceptable length of guidewire is not possible then sometimes an angled catheter can be advanced either 4 or 5 Fr directly over the initial guidewire and that can be used to cannulate the internal iliac artery and advance into the internal iliac artery so that a short stiffer wire can be used. This will allow placement of a short 6-Fr sheath. I recommend using a 6-Fr sheath with a radiopaque tip so that the tip of the sheath can be advanced directly up to just below the occlusion. Through a 6-Fr sheath, most reconstructive options are available. From this position, a couple of different angles are obtained to help see where the best place is to approach the lesion. There are various options for approaching the lesion and these include passage of a Glidewire and possibly forming a loop and a subintimal angioplasty as described earlier. Another option is to use a Quick Cross catheter directly from below. This type of catheter is used with a stiff guidewire. The catheter and guidewire are advanced in a step-by-step manner: one and then the other until the occlusion is crossed. If this is not successful, a reentry catheter may be advanced over the guidewire through the 6-Fr sheath and a reentry needle can be placed just proximal to the origin of the occlusion.

If the occlusion is near the origin of the common iliac artery or flush at the origin with the bifurcation of the aorta being somewhat obscured, then a kissing stent should be placed on the contralateral side so that any debris or compacted thrombus which is located at the bifurcation may be caged at this point and not forced into the patent contralateral side (Fig. 5). A common iliac artery occlusion that originates within 1 cm of the bifurcation will require bilateral access and will probably also require kissing stents to reconstruct. If the occlusion involves the infrarenal aorta to some degree and the iliac arteries, then an aortic stent can be placed first followed by kissing bilateral iliac stents.

External iliac artery occlusions have some nuances that make them somewhat different from common iliac artery occlusions. They are almost always approached in an up and over manner because of the challenge of getting working room when you puncture the ipsilateral side, as mentioned earlier. The challenge with an external iliac artery occlusion is getting back in at the appointed location at the junction between the external iliac and common femoral arteries. The patient is fully anticoagulated. The guidewire and catheter system is advanced into the internal iliac artery. A 6-Fr sheath is passed over the aortic bifurcation on a stiff guidewire and the 6-Fr sheath tip can even be advanced all the way into the internal iliac artery to get as close to the origin of the occlusion as possible. The stiff guidewire is removed and an angled tip catheter is placed into the 6-Fr sheath. The sheath is then withdrawn just a little bit and readjusted until you see a clunk or a slight movement at the tip of the sheath which indicates that it has popped from the internal and back into the distal common iliac artery. A couple of different angiographic angles are obtained by injecting contrast through

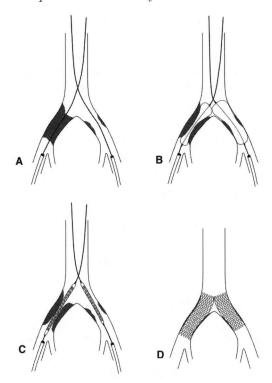

Fig. 5 Kissing stents of the aortic bifurcation. (**A**) Bilateral guidewires and balloon catheters are placed. Because the right side has a significant lesion and because it is also very near the bifurcation, both arteries are accessed. (**B**) Kissing balloon angioplasty is performed. The balloon in the left iliac artery is used to 'protect' the artery. (**C**) There is a substantial residual stenosis on the right side and the intended stent will be required to raise the bifurcation to treat the lesion. (**D**) Kissing stents are placed to raise the aortic bifurcation.

either the catheter or the sheath, with the catheter pointing directly down the barrel of the external iliac artery. At this point, one has a choice of either using a Glidewire and forming a loop and going subintimal through the external iliac artery or using a combination of a Quick Cross catheter and a 0.014-in. diameter guidewire. Whatever is chosen to cross the occlusion, it often breaks back into the true lumen on its own. If there is challenge in reentering, this is a good position for placement of a reentry catheter and using the needle on the reentry catheter enter the true lumen. The location of the sheath is also perfect because injecting through the sidearm of the sheath will allow reconstitution of contrast into the location where reentry is desired.

After the occlusion has traversed either common iliac or external iliac artery, the operator has the choice of how to reconstruct the lesion. Ample evidence shows primary angioplasty without stenting to be inadequate for iliac artery occlusions. Most experts advise stenting the lesion or placing stent–grafts. In the external iliac artery, stent the entire occluded segment using self-expanding stents. Accurate stent placement is required on the distal end of the occlusion because stent placement into the common femoral artery should be avoided. This is facilitated by the over the bifurcation approach because the self-expanding stents are deployed from the tip end to the hub end. In the common iliac artery, one has a broader choice of self-expanding or balloon expanding stents. If the aortic bifurcation is heavily calcified and/or there is a lot of distal aortic disease, balloon expandable stents are used. They have superior radial strength. They have some limitation in length and to cover he whole common iliac artery may require more than one stent on each side. Self-expanding stents are a reasonable choice for longer occlusions, or in arteries that are somewhat tortuous, especially if there is less aortic disease. If they extend into the aorta, they must be placed carefully so that they are equal on the bilateral sides. If there is a lot of disease in the distal aorta and/or the aortic bifurcation must be raised quite a bit, self-expanding stents do not work as well.

The biggest challenges with iliac artery recanalization are these. One is the situation where you've got through an external iliac artery occlusion but are unable to enter at the appropriate location at the external iliac common femoral artery junction. Another is when disease extends from an occluded external iliac artery directly into a heavy calcified and possibly even occlusive common femoral artery. These are difficult to treat from an endovascular standpoint if not impossible. Another scenario is when there is a combined occlusion of both common iliac and external iliac artery. These are challenging to cross and often require some innovative steps to do it. Another scenario is in recanalizing a common iliac artery but then having the distal aorta be so calcified that it's impossible to break through to get back into the true lumen. Once the iliac artery is recanalized the worst possible thing that can happen other than rupture which is rare, is distal embolization. This is the reason why I like to avoid predilatation and also like to cover the whole occlusion if at all possible.

Some operators like to use covered stents or stent–grafts to cover the occlusion. It is not necessary to achieve reasonable long-term patency. If a stent–graft is selected, some of the features which must be considered are the following. A larger sheath may be required depending on the finished desired diameter of the stent–graft. It is likely that there will be some predilatation required because the stent–graft no matter how tightly packed on its delivery catheter is somewhat high profile and has some rough edges which may catch on the lesion and may not want to pass. Therefore, predilatation is usually required. Lastly, perfect placement is usually required because one would not want to cover the collaterals at the medial and lateral iliac circumflex or cover the internal iliac artery or extend one end of the stent–graft up into the aortic bifurcation unless it was met on the contralateral side with an opposing structure such as a contralateral kissing stent–graft.

Femoral–Popliteal Occlusive Disease: When to Use Each Method of Revascularization?

There is no dominating option for reconstruction of femoral–popliteal occlusive disease that is more successful than all the others. There is a significant overlap in 6-, 12-, and 24-month patencies between many of the different methods of revascularization. One of the notable features of endovascular approaches to the lower extremity is that as we have become better at getting across challenging lesions, but not necessarily better at keeping these open. Lesion length is clearly important in determining long-term success. With respect to recanalizing occlusions, other important factors in success is whether it crossed a joint space and also whether the entry and exit segments into the subintimal space were well treated at the time of the reconstruction. There are multiple adjunctive tools for getting across lesions and also multiple tools for reconstructing arteries, many of which are discussed in chapter 22. It probably doesn't matter how one crosses the lesion.

For the femoral and popliteal arteries, there are several different methods of reconstruction after crossing a stenotic or occluded lesion. These are demonstrated in Figure 6. The method of reconstruction with the longest track record is standard balloon angioplasty. This is still a reasonable option and has reasonable long-term outlook. The problem with standard balloon angioplasty is that the patencies are only very satisfactory for focal lesions. The longer and more complex the lesion becomes, the less satisfactory the long-term patency. A second option is balloon angioplasty with selective stenting. This is an option which is practiced very widely. In this situation, balloon angioplasty alone is performed of a superficial femoral artery or popliteal artery lesion and if after balloon angioplasty there is an evidence of significant residual stenosis or a significant dissection, then stent placement is performed. Stent placement has improved significantly over the past several years as there are multiple choices of different kinds of stents, multiple different types of designs, and many options for stent placement. Because stents are relatively low in profile none require more than a 6-Fr sheath. They don't add much morbidity or time and the added risk of stent replacement is quite low at least during the immediate timeframe or first 30 days. The longer-term issue around stent placement has to do with the fact that recurrent stenosis occurs often and has not treatment. When recurrent stenosis develops, it often involves the whole length of the stent. Stents also develop fractures which are related to external compressive forces. Because of the combined issues around recurrent stenosis and stent fracture, there is enthusiasm for the idea that stent placement should be as limited as possible. Another option is to proceed with primary stenting. There is some evidence that at one year primary stenting produces better results than balloon angioplasty and selective stenting. In addition to having no treatment for recurrent stenosis and stent fractures, stents which are placed at specific locations may

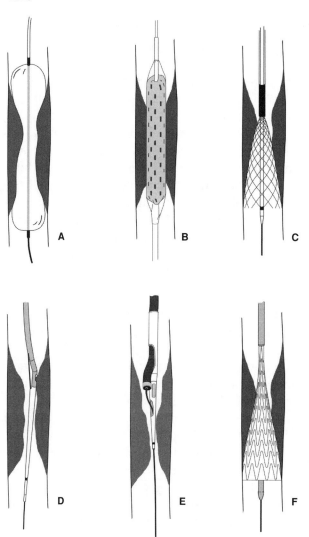

Fig. 6 Multiple methods of reconstruction are available for superficial femoral and popliteal artery lesions. (**A**) Plain old balloon angioplasty (POBA). (**B**) Cryoplasty. (**C**) Self-expanding stents. (**D**) Atherectomy. (**E**) Laser atherectomy. (**F**) Stent-graft.

cause other problems. Between the adductor canal and the popliteal artery the artery must be flexible with bending at the knee. Stents in this location are avoided if possible.

Other options include cryoplasty, atherectomy, stent–grafts, and cutting balloon angioplasty. These are described in a following section.

Most of the new devices and techniques are based on the 0.014-in. platform. One of the best ways to gain experience with 0.014–in. diameter systems is to use them routinely for infrainguinal interventions. Experience may be gained with a variety of different types of wires from the softest, floppiest, and least traumatic to hydrophilic coated to stiffer wires which can be used as exchange guidewires. There are numerous balloon catheters both monorail and coaxial that are compatible with 0.014-in. diameter systems. There are also numerous stents that are available on 0.014 systems. When the desired stent is only available on a 0.035 system, it can still be placed over a 014 guidewire. The 014 guidewire has the added advantage of being compatible with multiple other devices including aspiration catheters, atherectomy devices, and reentry devices.

When initiating a case, use a standard Glidewire and diagnostic catheter to pass over the aortic bifurcation and then once the aortic bifurcation has been crossed to place a stiff exchange guidewire through the catheter and then remove the catheter. A series of dilators are used at the femoral access site and then the access sheath is placed over the exchange wire. The tip of the exchange wire is placed into the largest branch or collateral near the lesion if possible to get the tip of the sheath as close to the lesion as possible. A decision must be made in infrainguinal work whether the tip of the sheath will enter the superficial femoral artery or whether it will be placed in the common femoral artery in order to treat a superficial femoral artery lesion. This decision is made based on the location of the lesion. If a popliteal or even tibial artery lesion is being treated and the superficial femoral artery is relatively free of occlusive disease, the sheath is advanced well into the superficial femoral artery.

Subsequently, the stiff exchange wire and the dilator for the sheath are removed and the 0.014-in. diameter guidewire is placed. A curve is created at the tip of the wire and the wire is advanced into the sheath. After the wire reaches the tip of the sheath contrast is administered though the side arm of the sheath and the lesion and the area that must be crossed is road mapped. The 014 wire has a steerable component with a torque device and this is placed on the guidewire and using the roadmap and the steerable wire the lesion is crossed. After this is performed, 0.014-in. compatible repair devices or reconstruction devices are used. This might include angioplasty balloon, stents, or other devices. During this process, the manipulation and handling of 0.014-in. diameter guidewire is performed on a regular basis. Practice in keeping the tip of the wire stable and also in passing these low-profile devices can be obtained. The operator learns how to get the tip of the sheath close to the target lesion and how to save contrast and manipulate the imaging so that the most direct information can be obtained. The likelihood that a 0.014-in. diameter guidewire or the low-profile catheters would occlude flow is low and this also helps with visualization.

Femoral–Popliteal Occlusive Disease: Subintimal Angioplasty

Subintimal angioplasty is a generalized description of use of the subintimal plane in order to pass the guidewire beyond the lesion. The general nomenclature of subintimal angioplasty tends to include all types of reconstructions which are placed in the subintimal space. There are differences between transluminal and subintimal passage. For example, with transluminal passage of the guidewire, one leads with the tip. In the subintimal space, one leads with the loop of the guidewire. In complex lesions, especially if short occlusions are present, sometimes the operator does not know if the guidewire is subintimal or transluminal. The endovascular treatment of long occlusions, anything more than a few centimeters, depends on passage in the subintimal plane. This technique, more than any other single maneuver, has significantly decreased the need for femoral–popliteal bypass. Use of the subintimal space for reconstruction is all about passing the guidewire out of the true lumen and into the subintimal segment and then along the subintimal passageway and then reentering into the true lumen. These specific steps are described herein.

Set yourself up for success by placing an adequately sized sheath and placing the tip of it close to the lesion. Also, get good runoff pictures so you know where the reconstitution is located and know hat this si not an isolated segment and know that by opening the lesion, it will have the desired affect from a hemodynamic standpoint. Anticoagulate the patient well, even before entering the occlusion because thrombus formation is enhanced in these low flow circuits. Subintimal angioplasty is described in general in chapter 22.

The key to entering the subintimal space is locating the correct origin of the occlusion (Fig. 7). If there is a stump of open superficial femoral artery, an angled-tip catheter is placed in it with the end of the catheter pointed at the plaque/artery wall interface. It is usually best to point the catheter opposite to the side with the largest collateral. Put the tip of the catheter right into the plaque and push a Glidewire. The tip of the Glidewire catches and a loop forms right behind it that travels along the subintimal plane. If there is no stump of proximal superficial femoral artery, the location of the artery can often be identified by the presence of calcification or the presence of engorged vasa vasorum the line the wall of the occluded artery. Point the catheter tip away from the profunda femoral and toward the side of the superficial femoral artery and push the guidewire. A selective catheter with a relatively stiff tip and a hockey stick shape works best for this.

After the guidewire is in the subintimal space, advance the catheter behind it (Fig. 8). Leave the loop intact, but advance the catheter to support it and enhance the pushability. The loop works best if it is not too wide. This tends to occur if the guidewire gets too much ahead of the catheter. The best part of the guidewire to lead the loop, is the segment right behind the more flexible couple cm of tip. If the loop becomes too wide, it tends to spiral around the artery more and is also less successful at forcing its way into the true lumen at the distal reconstruction site.

Reentry into the true lumen is usually accomplished with the loop itself (Fig. 9). The tip of the sheath proximally should be at a location where

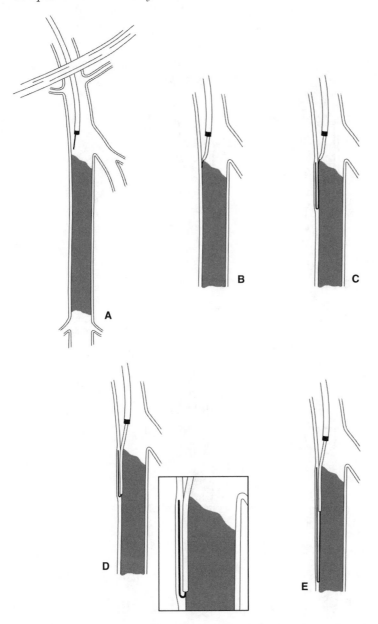

Fig. 7 Entering the subintimal space. (**A**) A sheath is placed in proximity to the occlusion. In this case, since the occlusion begins in the proximal superficial femoral artery, a sheath is placed over the aortic bifurcation, using the profunda femoris artery to anchor an exchange guidewire during sheath insertion. (**B**) An angled tip catheter is used to direct the guidewire tip away from the profunda femoris or any large branches. Take advantage of any available stump that provides entry to the occlusion. (**C**) The tip of the Glidewire buckles and advances into the subintimal space. (**D**) The catheter is advanced over the guidewire. (**E**) The loop is carefully maintained.

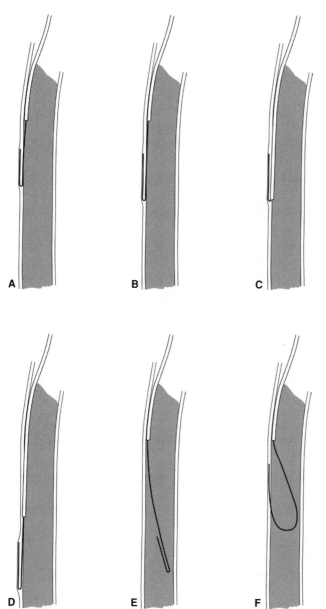

Fig. 8 Passing along the subintimal space. (**A**) The guidewire loop must be well managed. The best way to do this is to advance the catheter incrementally to support the guidewire. (**B**) The guidewire is advanced as long as the loop itself passes easily and the loop remains narrow. (**C**) After several cm of guidewire have passed out of the catheter, the catheter is advanced. If the loop has hit an area of increased resistance in the occlusion, the catheter may be advanced up to the base of the loop. (**D**) The guidewire may then be advanced again ahead of the catheter. (**E**) If the guidewire is advanced too far ahead of the catheter, the guidewire may begin to follow a spiral or diagonal pattern. (**F**) Avoid permitting the loop to get too big. It will follow less predictable patterns and will not be effective as a re-entry tool.

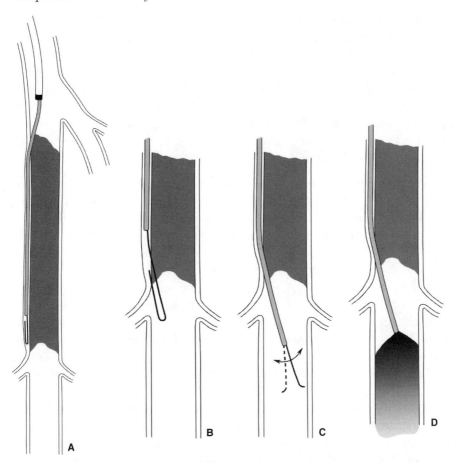

Fig. 9 Re-entry into the true lumen. (**A**) The patent distal segment is visualized by administering contrast through the sheath and having it travel through profunda collaterals. The loop of Glidewire and supporting catheter are advanced. (**B**) The loop of guidewire inself usually re-enters the true lumen. (**C**) The loop is withdrawn and the guidewire is rotated to show that it is free and not trapped in the subintimal space. (**D**) Contrast is administered to confirm the presence of the catheter in the distal reconstituted true lumen.

contrast administration will illuminate the distal reconstituting segment by flow through collaterals. The advancing loop is supported by the catheter right behind the loop. The ability of the loop to enter the true lumen depends on a differential in wall stiffness between the occluded segment and the patent, reconstituted segment. At some point, the path of least resistance for the loop is to enter the true lumen rather than the more resistive space of the subintimal space in a softer and patent artery. Keeping the loop small in diameter seems to facilitate this. When the loop breaks into the true lumen, it changes in appearance as the wire enters a free space. After this occurs, advance the catheter into the true lumen and pull the guidewire out to make sure there is backbleeding. If so, administer contrast to see the runoff.

Occasionally, the catheter will be in a collateral. If the distal reentry site is heavily calcified, the loop may bounce off of it and fail to reenter. There are some tricks that can be used but none of them work very well. One is remove the loop and push the stiff catheter tip up to the reconstituted segment and push with the guidewire, directed and with maximum support. Another option is to place an angioplasty balloon over the subintimal wire and perform angioplasty to fracture the plaque and create a space to reenter. Yet another is to inflate the angioplasty balloon to use this as support and push the guidewire through it.

The best option if the loop does not reenter is go straight to a reentry catheter (Fig. 10). The reasons are several. One is that you can spend a lot of valuable time attempting maneuvers with only a low likelihood of success. Another is that the subintimal space at the level of the reconstituted segment may become beaten up and patulous with all these maneuvers. This makes the reentry catheters less effective. These catheters rely on the ability to be passed into a tight subintimal space and to use that for leverage to support needle passage into the true lumen. Reentry catheters are useful when no other maneuver will do the job. A 6-Fr sheath is required. The subintimal space may be gently dilated over the length of the occlusion with a 3- or 4-mm balloon if the device will not advance in the subintimal space. Support for the device is limited by the fact that a 0.014-in. guidewire is used and also that the device must be passed right to the end of the guidewire. This does not provide much of a rail over which to work. Pass the reentry catheter along the subintimal space so that the location from which the needle protrudes (which is not at the very tip) is opposite the segment desired for reentry. Even if the guidewire has slipped too far down the artery on previous attempts, the catheter can be directed toward the best place to reenter. This often means, however, that the actual tip of the device will be nestled in a tight spot more distally to the location where the needle will be placed. The device is oriented using either intravascular ultrasound (Pioneer catheter) or an external marker (Outback catheter). The needle is placed in the true lumen and the 0.014-in. guidewire is advanced. The needle is retracted. The guidewire is carefully maintained in place as the reentry catheter is withdrawn. Be careful to use a long guidewire initially, usually 300 cm, to accommodate the long reentry catheter and also the distance inside the patient.

Atherectomy, Stent–Grafts, Cryoplasty, and Cutting Balloons to Treat Infrainguinal Disease

These tools are discussed in brief in chapter 22. They play some role in infrainguinal revascularization. This is probably because no one option is dominant in terms of clinical and technical success, affordability, or ease of

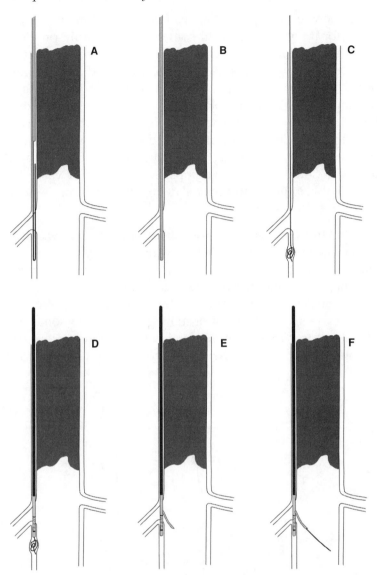

Fig. 10 Using a re-entry catheter. (**A**) The guidewire and catheter have been advanced along the subintimal space but were unable to re-enter. (**B**) The guidewire and catheter are advanced in the subintimal space past the lesion. (**C**) A stiff 0.014 in. guidewire is buried in the subintimal space along a segment of artery that is even with the true lumen. (**D**) A re-entry catheter is advanced, in this case the Outback catheter (Cordis), and oriented toward the true lumen. (**E**) The needle on the tip of the catheter is deployed. (**F**) The 0.014 guidewire is advanced into the true lumen. The needle is withdrawn and the re-entry catheter is removed, leaving the guidewire in place.

use. Whether the guidewire passage was transluminal or subintimal, there are multiple options for reconstruction of the artery. Atherectomy provides the potential to debulk the lesion. Stent–grafts offer the most complete type of reconstruction considering the lesion is completely covered and the new pathway is relined. Cryoplasty offers an upgrade on standard balloon angioplasty without leaving an implant. Cryoplasty has the potential that it may diminish long-term likelihood of restenosis. There is also the empirical observation that it tends to cause less postangioplasty dissection. Nevertheless, many dissections and residual stenoses are present after cryoplasty and these must still be managed. Cutting balloon angioplasty is mostly of value for stenoses in infrainguinal vein grafts and may also be used for focal de novo lesions, especially in the tibial arteries.

Directional atherectomy catheters are available from Fox Hollow. Additional atherectomy catheters will be available within the next two years. The directional atherectomy catheter has a cutting chamber that is advanced along the artery, cutting and removing plaque as it progresses. Atherectomy may be used as a mainstay of treatment for the superficial femoral and popliteal arteries but it is somewhat time consuming and there is some risk of embolization. Atherectomy may be performed with the concomitant use of a distal protection device (Fig. 11). Most operators use atherectomy for

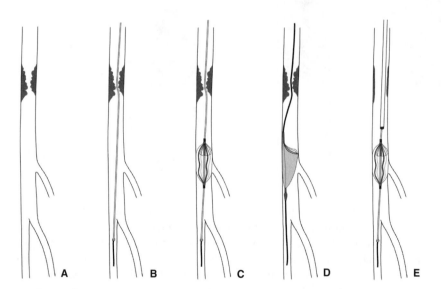

Fig. 11 Using a distal embolic protection device. (**A**) An embolizing femoral-popliteal artery lesion is identified by arteriography. (**B**) A free-wire system is used. The designated guidewire is passed beyond the lesion and into the tibial runoff. (**C**) An Emboshield filter (AbbottVascular) is passed beyond the lesion and deployed proximal to the trifurcation. The guidewire is permitted to float distally in the tibial artery. (**D**) Another free-wire filter choice is the Spider filter (EV3). (**E**) After treatment of the lesion, a filter capturing catheter is placed to retrieve the filter.

reconstruction in areas where stent placement is not desirable. These include the common femoral artery, profunda femoris artery origin, the proximal superficial femoral artery, and also the no-stent zone of the knee (from the adductor canal to the popliteal artery).

The atherectomy catheters pass over a 0.014-in. guidewire. The tip of the sheath is placed close to the lesion. The atherectomy catheter is advanced over the guidewire in its nonengaged state to be sure it will go through the lesion. The catheter is withdrawn and is oriented so that the cutting chamber faces the plaque. Upon engaging the cutting motor, the angle created in the catheter fully exposes the cutting chamber. The device is advanced very slowly down the artery. Despite attempts to remain steady, there are segments of plaque where the device skips a bit. This is not surprising since a very homogeneous substance is being cut. It is best to start cutting just mm proximal to the lesion and to conclude cutting just mms distal to the lesion. After cutting in one orientation, the cutting chamber is closed, the catheter is withdrawn, and reoriented in another direction, and another cut is performed. Usually after a few cuts, depending on how long it is, the chamber becomes full and is cleaned. After several cuts, angiography is performed. To the extent possible, the atherectomy device is used as a sole method of reconstruction, but sometimes it requires stent placement to treat loose flaps.

Another debulking option is excimer laser assisted angioplasty. The excimer laser is useful for recanalizing occlusions and burring holes through occlusions that will assist in guidewire placement using a step-by-step approach with the guidewire. The excimer laser is also useful in debulking superficial femoral, popliteal and tibial arteries lesions. One big advantage of the excimer laser over the atherectomy device is that the excimer laser is a little bit faster and it can also be used to dissolve some emboli if they should occur during the process of debulking. The laser may be passed more than once at progressively higher power levels, but it achieves a proscribed diameter of the artery, based on the size of the catheter and whether a turbo booster was used.

Another method of reconstruction is to place one or more stent–grafts. The stent–grafts produced by Gore, the Viabahn, have a superficial femoral artery indication and is the most widely used in practice. One major advantage of the Viabahn is that the luminal flow surface is completely relined and the damaged or diseased flow surface is excluded. In-stent restenosis is limited because it is not possible for intimal hyperplastic tissue to grow through the graft itself. Restenosis may occur at the end of the graft. The Viabahn requires a slightly larger sheath so this must be planned during sheath placement. The Viabahn grafts may be placed in a manner that cover the collaterals. This should be avoided. If the graft fails at a later time, it might go into a fast fail mode where the outflow thromboses when the graft goes down. Viabahn stent grafts may be used as an alternative to stenting in the superficial femoral artery and popliteal artery. Deployment accuracy is only fair since the stent–grafts deploy with a rip cord pull. If the stent–graft is oversized too much, there is a potential for wrinkling and bunching of the material. After placement, balloon angioplasty is performed, not with an oversized balloon but with one that is sized to the graft. Balloon angioplasty is restricted to the length of the graft itself, to avoid dissection along adjoining segments of artery. If more than one stent–graft is required, major overlaps in the devices will leave a lot of excess material in the lumen. Stent–grafts may be placed across the knee joint in the treatment of popliteal aneurysms but this maneuver is not as clearly acceptable for occlusive disease.

Cryoplasty is an option to be considered in areas where it is desirable to avoid placing a stent such as the common femoral artery, origin of the profunda or superficial femoral artery and also the tibial trifurcation, tibial arteries and the flexion point around the knee. A larger sheath is required than with standard balloon angioplasty. The balloon catheters are coaxial in design. Anecdotal experience suggests that there is less dissection with cryoplasty. This may be because of the cooling effect but it may also be because of the fact that the balloon inflation is a slow and highly coordinated process to a specific pressure level and a gentle inflation that may help limit the random nature of the dissection that occurs during inflation.

Cutting balloon angioplasty works well for infrainguinal vein graft stenosis (Fig. 12). This tends to be composed of intimal hyperplastic tissue which is focal in the graft. The tip of the sheath is placed close to the graft origin and the patient is anticoagulated. A 0.0140-in. guidewire is passed into the graft and across the lesion. Balloon inflation is performed slowly and with an undersized balloon. A standard angioplasty balloon of the size desired for the finished diameter is placed to further enlarge the graft. Focal tibial artery lesions and focal but heavily calcified lesions of the superficial femoral and popliteal arteries may also be treated with cutting balloon angioplasty.

Tibial Artery Occlusive Disease: Angioplasty and Stenting

Focal tibial artery lesions that cause limb-threatening ischemia are unusual but these can be treated readily with angioplasty in an attempt to achieve at temporary limb salvage. More recently, success has been achieved in recanalizing tibial artery occlusions. This is a far more common presentation in patients with limb threat due to infrageniculate occlusive disease. Tibial revascularization is a rapidly growing part of endovascular practice. Many of the principles, techniques, and devices required to make this happen have been adopted from other vascular beds. The best factors suggesting success

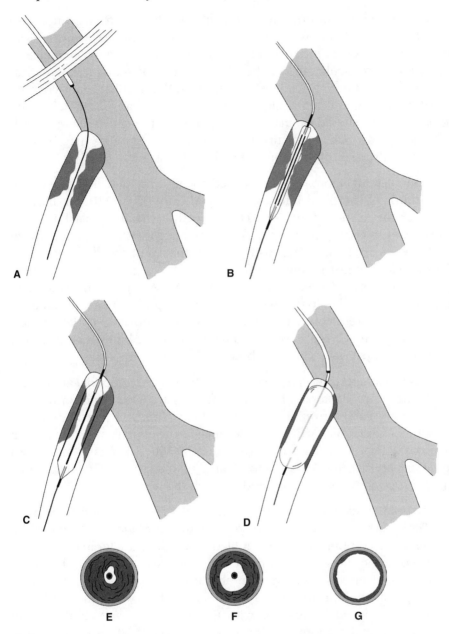

Fig. 12 Use of the cutting balloon to treat infrainguinal bypass graft stenosis. (**A**) A sheath is placed in the artery proximal to the anastomosis. An 0.014 in. guidewire is passed into the bypass graft. (**B**) An undersized cutting balloon is placed in the stenosis. (**C**) The cutting balloon is inflated to cut the intimal hyperplastic lesion. (**D**) A standard angioplasty balloon that is sized to the desired diameter of the graft is placed and inflated. (**E**) The cutting balloon is placed in the lesion. (**F**) The cutting balloon is undersized in comparison to the graft diameter to avoid rupture. When the undersized balloon is inflated, the leisn is cut in several places. (**G**) After standard balloon angioplasty, the lumen assumes a much larger configuration.

are in cases where the foot damage is minimal an also where the runoff into the foot is intact. Patients with major foot damage or the exposure of vita structures or with severe intrapedal occlusive disease have a poor chance of salvage with endovascular approaches. Because endovascular revascularization rarely provides the robust level of perfusion that results from bypass to the tibial arteries, it is often desirable to open more than one tibial artery. After that, the foot should be managed aggressively to achieve wound healing. The long-term patency of tibial angioplasty and stenting may be only fair but limb salvage is often achieved without bypass.

A contralateral approach is preferred for lesions involving the proximal two-thirds of the tibial arteries. A long sheath, 90 or 110 cm, may be placed over the aortic bifurcation. The tip of the sheath is placed in the popliteal or even the tibial artery. Inflow lesions of the iliac and superficial femoral arteries are treated aggressively. With the tip of the sheath close to the lesion, less contrast is required for interval arteriography and less time and fuss is necessary for exchanges of catheters. An ipsilateral antegrade approach is direct and helps to maintain control of guidewires and catheters (Fig. 13). This is preferable when treating the distal tibial or pedal arteries. An antegrade approach is also preferred when the aortic bifurcation is hostile but is difficult in patients who are obese.

Selective catheterization is described in chapter 9. Tibiopedal arteriography is discussed in chapter 10. Longer guidewires are used to perform selective tibial artery catheterization, usually 300 cm. This will provide enough length so that exchanges can be made outside the vascular system with a 140 cm coaxial catheter if needed. Heparin (75–100 U/kg) is administered prior to tibial artery catheterization for treatment. If spasm occurs in the tibial arteries, nitroglycerine is administered through the access catheter.

A 0.014-in. guidewire is placed in the tibial artery. A 4- or 5-Fr catheter with a Tuohy-Borst adaptor is used along with the guidewire to enter the tibial artery. The combination of the angled tip on the catheter and the steerable, angled tip on the guidewire make it possible to reach artery branches with all kinds of angles. The angiographic catheter also provides support for the long guidewire. If the lesion is a stenosis, the low-profile guidewire can usually be placed by leading with the tip of the wire. If the lesion is an occlusion, make an extra effort to obtain good images of the runoff arteries distal to the occlusion. Place a low-profile exchange catheter with a stiff tip, such as the Quick Cross catheter (Spectranetics). The catheter tip is advanced into the occlusion. When the catheter tip meets resistance, do not push any further and definitely do not buckle the catheter. Place a relatively stiff, low-profile guidewire (CTO guidewire) and advance the guidewire tip beyond the tip of the catheter. The guidewire may pass easily for a cm or more or may only gain a few mm. When the guidewire meets resistance, stop pushing. Advance the exchange catheter and often this will

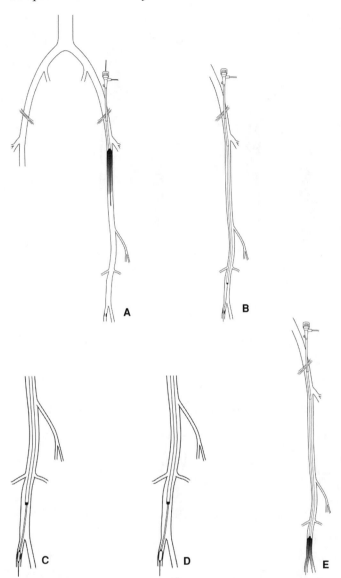

Fig. 13 Balloon angioplasty of the tibial artery. (**A**) Femoral arteriography is performed. (**B**) The guidewire is advanced through a posterior tibial artery stenosis. (**C**) The angioplasty catheter is positioned across the lesion. (**D**) Balloon dilatation of the posterior tibial artery is performed. (**E**) The balloon is removed and completion arteriography is performed.

pass well beyond the end of the guidewire. Continue this alternate push or "hopscotch" maneuver until the guidewire breaks into the true lumen on the distal end. This maneuver is usually successful in recanalizing tibial artery occlusions. If the guidewire passes outside the adventitia, it is only rarely of any clinical significance. Pull the catheter back a bit and see if the catheter tip can be advanced into a slightly different pathway. If this is unsuccessful

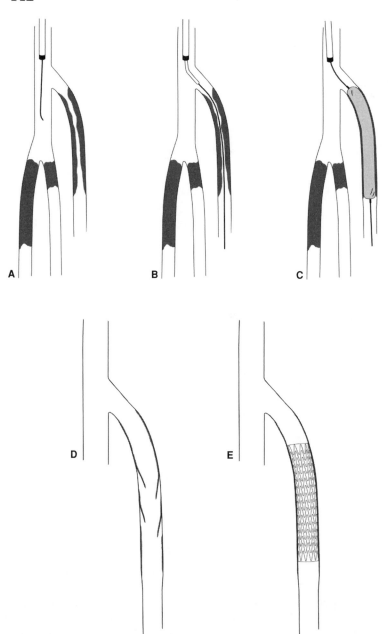

Fig. 14 Tibial artery balloon angioplasty and stenting. (**A**) A sheath is placed just proximal to the lesion. (**B**) A directional catheter is used to help direct the guidewire into the appropriate tibial artery. (**C**) A low profile angioplasty balloon that covers the length of the lesion is placed and inflated. (**D**) A significant post-angioplasty dissection is present. (**E**) A self-expanding nitinol stent is placed to treat the dissection.

and there is access to a laser, consider using a 0.9-mm probe to create a new channel.

Balloons range from 1.5 to 4 mm in diameter. Longer balloons are now available for the tibial arteries, up to 15 cm. The best way to treat the lesion is to place a low-profile balloon angioplasty catheter, 0.014-in. compatible platform, with a balloon that is long enough to cover the whole lesion with a single inflation (Fig. 14). The balloon is inflated slowly until it reaches its full profile and inflation is maintained for a few minutes. Completion arteriography is performed through the sidearm of the sheath. If significant dissection or residual stenosis is present, repeat balloon inflation is performed. Stents are used sparingly. If a stent is required in the proximal segment, near the tibial artery origin, a balloon-expandable stents is placed. This permits the greatest accuracy of placement. This is a location in the limb, between the tibia and fibula, that is relatively protected from external forces. If stent placement is required in the remainder of the artery, a self-expanding stent is used to accommodate the more flexible and mobile artery segments. There are no stents which are designed to work well at the ankle and foot.

Selected Readings

Antusevas A, Aleksynas N, Kaupas RS, et al. Comparison of results of subintimal angioplasty and percutaneous transluminal angioplasty in superficial femoral artery occlusions. Eur J Vasc Endovasc Surg 2008; 36(1):101–106.

Bargellini I, Petruzzi P, Scatena A, et al. Primary infrainguinal subintimal angioplasty in diabetic patients. Cardiovasc Intervent Radiol 2008; 31(4):713–722.

Ramjas G, Thurley P, Habib S. The use of a re-entry catheter in recanalization of chronic inflow occlusions of the common iliac artery. Cardiovasc Intervent Radiol 2008; 31(3):650–654.

26

Coiling of Peripheral Aneurysms

445

Coils

These devices are designed to occlude blood vessels in various situations (Fig. 1). There are many different scenarios in which coils and/or occlusion devices may be of value. Coiling is sometimes undertaken of a hypervascular tumor prior to removal. Coiling and/or occlusion of the internal iliac artery may be performed on one or both sides prior to abdominal aortic stent graft placement to avoid a type I or major type II endoleak. The internal iliac artery may itself be aneurysmal and require occlusion. Coiling and occlusion devices may be required in all sorts of arrangements in which aneurysm disease is being treated. Coiling is also required whenever there is flow in undesired side branches. When there is an iatrogenic or traumatic event, which creates an unwanted leak or communication between artery and vein, coiling is considered. Available coils are delivered using standard catheters. Larger coils fit through either a standard 4- or 5-Fr angiographic catheter and are 0.035 in. in diameter, the same as a guidewire that would be used for that catheter. The smaller caliber coils for peripheral use fit through a microcatheter of approximately 2.5 Fr and the coils are 0.018 in. in diameter.

The key to coil embolization is to provide excellent positioning and platform support. One of the challenges associated with coiling is getting adequate position of the delivery catheter and keeping it stable during the coiling process. Even when the catheter is perfectly positioned for coil delivery, the act of passing the coil and the pusher through the catheter may change the catheter position. The best way to set up a coiling case is to do it in a telescoping manner. An example of this would be to use a 6-Fr sheath and to advance the tip of the sheath as close to the target lesion as possible. And then to extend from beyond the tip of the sheath, a 5-Fr catheter which could be used to enter the lesion and deliver the coils. Additional levels of telescoping can also be performed by using a sheath within a sheath and then a catheter and then the coils delivered to that. Another maneuver that is not often required is to place the microcatheter (2.5 Fr) through the 5-Fr angiographic catheter to approach the lesion. This is performed whenever the larger caliber diagnostic catheter cannot be advanced into the lesion as desired.

It is usually best to place the catheter into the area of treatment a little farther than you think it needs to be. Everything that happens after that tends to put force on the catheter that makes it back out. If by stiffening the catheter slightly by advancing the coil the catheter retracts or buckles backward a slight amount, it will still be in adequate position. It is usually best to advance the coil all the way to the end of the catheter and recheck the position. If the catheter is in too far at that point, withdraw the catheter somewhat and then go ahead and push the coil through. As soon as the

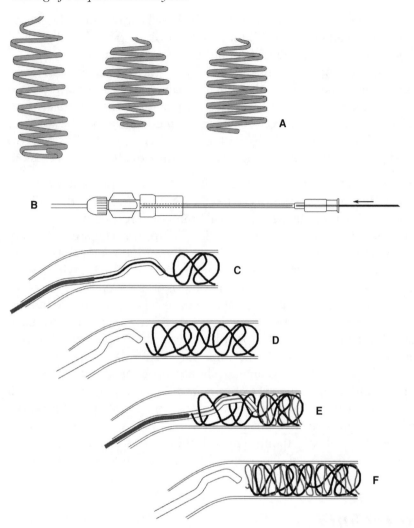

Fig. 1 Coils in the peripheral arteries and coil placement. (**A**) Multiple different configurations of coils are available. The diameter of the coil should be oversized to the artery that is being treated with the coil to help prevent the coils from migrating after placement. (**B**) Coils are pre-packaged in a metal tube. The tube has an adapter that is connected to the angiographic catheter that has been placed at the site intended for coil placement. A guidewire tip is used to advance the coil through the catheter. (**C**) The guidewire is used to push the coli out of the catheter. Immediately upon exiting the catheter, the coil begins to assume its shape. (**D**) The coil is permitted to wander along a short segment of artery. (**E**) The catheter is re-advanced and additional coils are placed. (**F**) The coils are interwoven with each other. The tip of the catheter can be used to tamp the coils and compress them into a plug.

leading end of the coil extends beyond the end of the catheter, it begins to take its shape. The catheter can still be pushed a bit or pulled back a bit if more preside placement is needed. When the first coil is placed it should be placed in the deepest position anticipated. When placing subsequent coils, the catheter tip may be pushed though the coils that are already placed but this is not a reliable plan and it is best to place them sequentially and deliberately if possible. As the coils are being placed, the tip of the catheter may be used to tamp down or to bunch up or compact the coils. This helps to create a good plug to serve as a nidus for thrombus formation and occlusion.

Several different companies make coils. The coil is straight while it's within the catheter, but as soon as it reaches an environment that allows it to expand to a larger diameter, it will immediately begin to coil. Be sure to match the appropriate-sized coils with the appropriate-sized delivery catheter. If a 0.018-in. coil is placed inadvertently into a standard 4- or 5-Fr catheter, it will begin to coil within the catheter and the catheter will have to be removed and replaced because it won't be possible to remove the coil or to push it out. The patient is anticoagulated during coiling. There are numerous different shapes of coils but there is no clinically apparent advantage of one shape over another for the peripheral indications. The final resting diameter intended for each coil is the important factor. Whether the coil is tapered or a tube shaped, the diameter should be oversized by at least a couple of millimeters to the artery to be treated. If the coil is undersized, it will be free floating when placed in the artery. Some coils have thrombogenic attachments on them that are designed to generate thrombus around the coil. When the coils are tightly packed, they act as a plug, which will induce thrombus formation and cause occlusion of the intended artery.

Coiling Technique

A stiff wire is placed near the target. The patient is heparinized. A sheath is advanced, usually 5 Fr or 6 Fr. If an occlusion device other than standard coils will be required, a larger sheath will be needed and this must be check ahead of time. If the target is too delicate to have an exchange guidewire go through it, like in the case of a splenic artery aneurysm, don't overdo it by attempting to get the sheath tip too close. Place the sheath as far as it will comfortably go. Place a 5-Fr angiographic catheter over the stiff guidewire and through the sheath. If the sheath position is inadequate, it can usually be advanced a bit further toward the target by pushing it over the combination of the angiographic catheter and the stiff guidewire. The 5-Fr angiographic catheter, usually with a simple curve angled tip, often a Glidecath, is advanced to the end of the exchange guidewire. The exchange guidewire is removed and a Glidewire is placed. The anatomy is road mapped, usually by administering contrast through the sheath. The Glidewire is advanced beyond the site where the coils will be placed and the Glidecath is passed over it. When the catheter is in the appropriate position, the Glidewire is removed.

The coils with the intended diameter are prepared one by one since they are packaged separately. The metal tube housing the coil is locked onto the catheter. The stiffer end or back end of a Bentson guidewire is used to push the coil out of its canister and for several centimeters into the catheter. Once that is accomplished the guidewire is turned around and the soft end of the guidewire is passed into the catheter and is used to deliver the coil. Although the stiff end of the guidewire could be used to deliver the coil, this may present a problem at the treatment end by inappropriately stiffening the catheter and the entire system may begin to move in an unwanted direction. Therefore, a relatively floppy guidewire tip is used to advance the coil into position. The guidewire used to push the coil must be of the same diameter as the coil itself (use 0.035-in. guidewire for 0.035-in. coil). The coil is pushed quickly along the long distance of the catheter, but as it nears the treatment site, it is best to slow down so that the catheter does not whip around. The coil is radiopaque and can be visualized well using fluoroscopy. The coil begins to twist as soon as it exits the catheter and can be observed as it begins to twist. The coil and the guidewire that is used to push it have about the same radiographic consistency. This means that it is not always simple to know when the coil has been fully deployed from the catheter. Watch the coil carefully so that it can be observed separating from the catheter. The key thing is not to let the catheter tip withdraw or retract and allow the following end of the coil to end up in an unwanted position. During coil delivery, sometimes it is necessary to administer forward pressure on the catheter. In between placing coils the catheter itself may be advanced all by itself and the blunt edge of the catheter used to reposition or to clump the coils together.

When a very remote target requires embolization or the vessels along the pathway to the target are small in caliber, even more telescoping is required. Embolization of a type II endoleak in an aortic aneurysm sac through the collaterals of the superior mesenteric artery is an example of this type of situation. A 6-Fr sheath is placed well into the superior mesenteric artery. A long 5-Fr angiographic catheter is used to select the best superior mesenteric artery branch to use as a pathway and the catheter is placed as far into that branch as possible. A microcatheter, usually 2.5 Fr and 150~cm in length, is advanced through the 5-Fr catheter is advanced to the target. The coils are placed through the microcatheter. Because of the small diameter of the microcatheter, it is not easily aspirated of blood and the system is usually quite circuitous. It also may be challenging to push the coil with a guidewire all the way through the microcatheter. If this is the case, a 1- or a 3-cc syringe filled with saline may be used to flush the coil out of the microcatheter by injecting into the microcatheter forcefully. The coil will shoot out the other end. This is a very fast way to deliver the coil but is somewhat less accurate and care should be taken to position the catheter carefully prior to injecting with saline.

It is quite common in the fully heparinized state for the patient to still have some flow of blood through the area which has been coiled. This makes it extra challenging to decide if additional coils are required. In general, it's best to make a plug of coils but it is also best to try to be precise in the placement so that additional areas are not occluded. In addition, at some point in creating a plug, there will be insufficient room to place additional coils and the trailing end of the most recently placed coil may drag into another blood vessel and this should be carefully monitored to avoid.

Coiling the Internal Iliac Artery

A very common maneuver that is used as an adjunct to stent–graft treatment of aortic aneurysms is coiling of the internal iliac artery. This may be required to actually treat an internal iliac artery aneurysm. It may also be required that a relatively normal internal iliac artery be coiled to prevent backbleeding from it after it is covered by a stent–graft limb (Fig. 2).

When coiling an internal iliac artery as an adjunct to stent–graft exclusion of an aortic aneurysm, it may be performed prior to aneurysm treatment or at the same time. A 6-Fr sheath may be placed from either the contralateral or ipsilateral femoral access, depending on the angulation revealed by aortography. Patients with nonaneurysmal disease usually have an angle of origin of the internal iliac artery that is acute and is not simple to cannulate when coming from the ipsilateral femoral artery. Internal iliac artery cannulation is simpler in this case from the contralateral side coming over the aortic bifurcation. The tortuosity of the aortoiliac segment in patients with aneurysm disease may completely change these relationships and make ipsilateral access a reasonable choice. In addition, there may be occasions when it is not desirable to pass the sheath through a particularly friable or diseased segment of contralateral iliac artery.

If the origin of the internal iliac artery is all that requires coiling, the tip of the sheath is placed in the origin of the internal iliac artery. The 5-Fr catheter is advanced over a guidewire and into the internal iliac artery. The area of the neck of the internal iliac artery is investigated, often with several different views. The usual goal is to place a plug of coils in the origin of the artery without occluding more branches than necessary. Sometimes the plug will migrate a bit further into the artery as the coils are being placed. After the best view is identified, the position of the image intensifier is maintained. The coil is selected, placed into the catheter with the stiff back end of the Bentson guidewire, and then advanced the rest of the way to the target

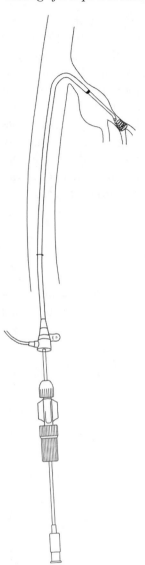

Fig. 2 Coiling of an internal iliac artery aneurysm. A telescoping system is constructed. A 6 Fr sheath is placed in the internal iliac artery. A 5 Fr catheter is placed through the sheath and used to direct the placement of the coils. The coils are placed through the 5 Fr coil.

area by advancing the soft end of the guidewire. Before the coil comes out of the catheter, the tip is readjusted, usually withdrawn slightly. The coil is deployed. After several coils are deployed, the coil mass is shaped a bit using the head of the catheter to tamp them into a plug. After coil placement is complete, a completion arteriogram is performed and the sheath is removed.

In the case of an internal iliac artery aneurysm, the outlet branches to the internal iliac artery must be occluded as well as the internal iliac artery itself. Finding all the branches leading out of the aneurysm can be a challenge. In this case it helps to place the tip of the sheath all the way into the aneurysm and then to use the angiographic catheter to select out the branches and coil them one at a time. The aneurysm itself is also filled with coils. If the aneurysmal dilatation is larger, more than a couple of centimeters in diameter, it can be filled with many coils or can be filled with a few longer pieces of guidewire. This can be done by taking a removable core guidewire, taking out the core, cutting it into longer pieces that may be many centimeters in length, and placing these as one would place a coil. Then the sheath is withdrawn so that its tip is in the internal iliac artery proximal to the aneurysmal dilatation and coils are placed to occlude the inflow.

Selected Readings

Bharwani N, Raja J, Choke E, et al. Is internal iliac artery embolization essential prior to endovascular repair of aortoiliac aneurysms? Cardiovasc Intervent Radiol 2008; 31(3):504–508.

27

Making a Clean Getaway: Puncture Site Management

Obtaining Hemostasis
Holding Pressure
Timing the Sheath Removal
Closure Devices
Managing Puncture Site Complications

Obtaining Hemostasis

In a manner similar to the performance of open surgery, wound complications present a low-level but constant problem. Access related complications are still the most common complication of endovascular procedures. These complications are not usually threatening but they may add substantially to the morbidity of the procedure and may necessitate additional procedures. Obtaining hemostasis after a percutaneous intervention has the same importance as surgical wound closure. Percutaneous closure devices are not covered in depth in this text. However, these devices are here to stay and each has its own learning curve.

Obtaining hemostasis is made safer and simpler when the arteriotomy site is selected well and the puncture site is managed properly during the procedure. Puncturing the artery with satisfactory technique, holding pressure during exchanges, using dilators to prepare the tract and the arteriotomy, and upsizing the sheath only when necessary all help to maintain the arteriotomy. If the initial puncture site is poorly placed and the patient requires a larger access for intervention, it is safer to get access in another location than to risk bleeding or thrombosis at the puncture site. A damaged sheath tip may injure the artery at the access site. During sheath placement, if the tip of the sheath is damaged, crinkled, or accordioned by a poorly prepared tract, a fresh sheath should be placed after the arteriotomy is better prepared. During the procedure, avoid inflating a balloon in the end of the sheath. Fully deflate an angioplasty balloon before withdrawing it into the sheath.

Ensure that the patient is comfortable prior to pulling the sheath. Drain the bladder if needed. Avoid agitation and discomfort due to bladder distension after the diuresis caused by contrast administration. Some patients are uncomfortable after lying on the angio table because of back or limb pain. These patients may need a short break or additional sedation. If blood pressure is elevated, it can make hemostasis more difficult to achieve. Consider antihypertensive medication. If any significant amount of heparin was administered, measure the activated clotting time and wait to remove the sheath until it is 180 seconds or less. Administer additional local anesthetic at the access site if the procedure has gone on for more than an hour.

Holding Pressure

When the plan is to hold pressure, the hemostatic access sheath is removed in the recovery room rather than in the operating room. The patient is placed in the supine position. If there is a large pannus, an assistant retracts the skin fold to achieve a horizontal working surface. Pressure is applied before the catheter or sheath is removed. The fewest number of gauze pads possible are used, usually just one is best, to hold pressure so that the pulse is readily

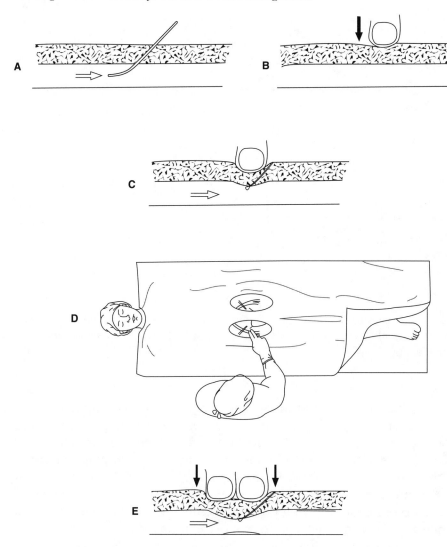

Fig. 1 Puncture site management. (**A**) A percutaneous catheter is placed. (**B**) Pressure is held at the arteriotomy site after the catheter is removed. (**C**) Digital pressure does not occlude flow. Platelets deposit at the arteriotomy site as digital pressure prevents leakage of blood from the artery. (**D**) The ipsilateral foot is exposed during pressure application to continuously evaluate the color of the foot. (**E**) Even if greater pressure is required for hemostasis, flow is not occluded.

palpable while holding pressure. If pressure is applied in the correct location, there should be minimal bleeding.

Following a retrograde femoral artery puncture, digital pressure is held at the location of the arteriotomy that is proximal to the skin puncture site (Fig. 1). In the case of a retrograde femoral artery puncture, the tract leading from the skin to the arteriotomy is also compressed. But, no amount of tract

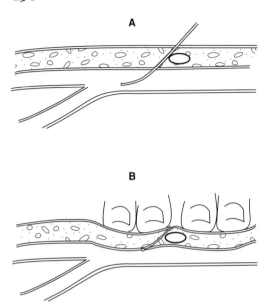

Fig. 2 Hemostasis after antegrade puncture. (**A**) An antegrade catheter is placed. (**B**) After the catheter is removed, pressure is applied both above and below the inguinal ligament.

compression is of value if the arteriotomy is not adequately compressed. The ipsilateral foot is exposed while pressure is held so that the color of the foot can be continuously assessed. The goal is to prevent bleeding from the artery while maintaining flow through it and permitting a platelet plug to form on the flow surface. Too much pressure applied occludes the artery while too little pressure applied in the wrong place allows continued hemorrhage or may even promote it. Applying pressure to the artery distal to the puncture site increases resistance, which forces more extravasation.

Antegrade femoral artery puncture requires a two-handed technique. One hand is placed proximal to the inguinal ligament to apply pressure over the distal external iliac artery to decrease the head of pressure flowing through the punctured segment and to diminish any oozing into the retroperitoneal space (Fig. 2). The goal is not to occlude arterial flow, even temporarily. The other hand places point pressure over the area of arterial puncture just distal to the inguinal ligament and over the arteriotomy. The distal hand can also assess the pulse and ensure that the pressure exerted by the proximal hand is not significant enough to stop flow. Pressure is usually held for a minimum of 15 minutes. Patients who are on antiplatelet agents or hypertensive or who have larger arteriotomy sizes (>7 Fr) probably need to be compressed for longer. Managing the puncture site is a routine task, but doing it improperly guarantees a complication. Therefore, stay actively involved and do not delegate it completely to someone else.

Timing the Sheath Removal

The sheath is usually removed at the completion of the study unless heparin was administered. An activated clotting time may be useful to help time sheath removal. If the sheath is to remain in place for more than an hour, consider a low-dose heparin drip through the sidearm of the sheath. If the access site is to be handled with a closure device, this is done on the table at the conclusion of the procedure regardless of whether the patient is anticoagulated.

Closure Devices

Many practices have evolved to a point where the preferred method for all patients is to use closure devices. The advantages of closure devices are significant. They allow for early ambulation and discharge of the patient. The patient also avoids the experience of having someone pressing on the groin. Many patients have back or joint problems that are exacerbated by a prolonged period in the supine position. The closure devices are better at achieving hemostasis for larger sheaths (>7 Fr). Closure devices can be used while the patient is ill anticoagulated, without waiting to a later time to manage the sheath. So why not use a closure device on all patients? Problems with closure devices include cost, a small rate of failure, the hole must be enlarged to 7 or 8 Fr (which seems a little silly if the arteriotomy is only 4 or 5 Fr), and the rare but devastating complication like limb loss or distal embolization. Closure devices are only approved for retrograde femoral punctures.

The main reason not to use a closure device is some technical or anatomical issue that precludes its use. A severely diseased, calcified, or stenotic femoral artery is most common. If the puncture site is low, at the femoral bifurcation, or in the profunda femoris or superficial femoral artery, it is better off being held by hand. When a treatment site, such as an external iliac artery stent, is close to the puncture site, there is a risk that the device will catch on the stent.

There are two kinds of closure devices: those that place a stitch (e.g., Pro-glide) or rivet (e.g., Pro-star) and those that place a collagen plug (e.g., Angio-seal). There are more examples of each of these types of closure devices that are not mentioned here. Both types have been widely adopted and have acceptably low complication rates. Each type of device has its nuances and tricks and each is being continually refined.

Managing Puncture Site Complications

Several factors contribute to percutaneous femoral artery puncture site hemorrhage: anticoagulation or bleeding disorders; presence of severe common femoral artery calcification; high puncture, involving the distal external iliac artery; low puncture, involving the crotch of the femoral bifurcation or proximal deep femoral artery; a puncture site that lacerates the side of the artery; or a large-caliber arteriotomy (especially 10 Fr or larger). Puncture site management is often relegated to a member of the team with the least experience or understanding of the procedure performed. However, managing a complication after it has occurred requires more energy and expertise than is needed when the puncture site is managed well to begin with.

28

Endovascular Complications Can Be Avoided

Selecting the Appropriate Patient
Selecting the Appropriate Technique
Selecting the Appropriate Approach
Knowing When to Quit

Selecting the Appropriate Patient

The best candidates for endovascular intervention have either lesser forms of disease or strong indications for intervention with prohibitive operative risk. Endovascular surgery provides valuable therapeutic options in these two groups of patients. The challenge is that as the techniques and equipment improve, the forms of vascular disease that can be treated continue to expand. This creates a dynamic process that must be constantly realigned. The temptation is never ending to apply endovascular intervention to all patients; however, there are many in whom the benefits are not so clear-cut.

Endovascular skills and the interventions derived from them are most effective in serving patients in need when they are used in a fashion that is complementary to, rather than exclusive of, other treatment options. Physicians must be dedicated to the treatment of patients with vascular problems, not to one type of procedure or another. One of the significant judgment challenges in endovascular interventions is that the natural history of some vascular processes may be the same as or better than the outcomes possible with intervention.

Selecting the Appropriate Technique

After endovascular intervention has been selected as the best among available options, there are many techniques from which to choose. In general, the simplest intervention that gives the longest-term solution to the clinical problem is best. It is easy to become sidetracked with the latest and greatest, only to realize afterward that its clinical value was marginal, or worse, that the patient suffered because of it. The clinical applicability of each new technique must be carefully evaluated.

Most patients who undergo endovascular procedures can also be treated with standard surgery. The reason that standard surgery is not performed, even though it is generally more durable, is because an endovascular procedure holds the promise of lower complication rates. If an endovascular procedure has a high risk of complications, it should not be performed, or at least this should be included in the risk–benefit analysis. Many new techniques do not have well-established complication rates and each has a learning curve.

Selecting the Appropriate Approach

After selecting the appropriate patient and technique, choosing the right approach ensures a smooth entry and exit. The best approach is almost always the simplest, shortest, and most direct route to the target. The more understanding the operator has about the presentation, physical findings, and noninvasive physiologic data, the more likely he or she is to choose the simplest approach with the fewest surprises.

The entry artery, not just the pulse, should be palpated prior to cannulation. A severely calcified artery can lead to puncture site complications. The operator should work on the forehand side as much as possible. A double-wall puncture creates extra holes and is almost never required. An alternative approach is occasionally required and is always better than forcing a complication. When converting an arteriographic procedure to a therapeutic one, a second well-placed puncture site that provides direct access to the target is often simpler.

If pressure is not held adequately and precisely at the puncture site after the procedure, a complication is virtually guaranteed. This mundane task must be well performed to avoid trouble. Pressure must be sufficient to occlude the arteriotomy without stopping flow.

Knowing When to Quit

Not every patient should undergo a procedure and not every lesion should be treated with endovascular techniques. When the risk of an endovascular procedure is too high or the potential for success is low, other alternatives should be considered. Sometimes this point in the decision tree arises during an endovascular procedure! This is a major reason why the techniques of endovascular intervention should be performed by those who regularly manage vascular patients.

The quest for the perfect cosmetic result of a reconstruction is seductive, but it does not guarantee long-term patency and may cause a short-term disaster. The temptation to become a lesion-oriented physician, rather than a patient-oriented physician, is counterproductive. Clinical orientation is crucial because the best results come from doing only what is indicated by the clinical condition of the patient.

Index

1
2
3
4
5
6
7
8
9
10
11
12
13
14
15
16
17
18
19
20
21
22
23
24
25
26
27
28
29
30
31
32
33
34
35
36
37
38
39
40
41
42
43
44
45